Turn Up the Heat

Turn **Up the Heat**

Unlock the Fat-Burning Power
of Your Metabolism

Philip L. Goglia

Viking

VIKING
Published by the Penguin Group
Penguin Putnam Inc., 375 Hudson Street,
New York, New York 10014, U.S.A.
Penguin Books Ltd, 80 Strand,
London WC2R ORL, England
Penguin Books Australia Ltd, 250 Camberwell Road, Camberwell,
Victoria 3124, Australia
Penguin Books Canada Ltd, 10 Alcorn Avenue,
Toronto, Ontario, Canada M4V 3B2
Penguin Books India (P) Ltd, 11 Community Centre, Panchsheel Park,
New Delhi - 110 017, India
Penguin Books (N.Z.) Ltd, Cnr Rosedale and Airborne Roads, Albany,
Auckland, New Zealand
Penguin Books (South Africa) (Pty) Ltd, 24 Sturdee Avenue,
Rosebank, Johannesburg 2196, South Africa

Penguin Books Ltd, Registered Offices:
Harmondsworth, Middlesex, England

First published in 2002 by Viking Penguin,
a member of Penguin Putnam Inc.

1 3 5 7 9 10 8 6 4 2

Every effort has been made to ensure that the information contained in this book is
complete and accurate. However, neither the publisher nor the author is engaged in
rendering professional advice or services to the individual reader. The ideas,
procedures, and suggestions contained in this book are not intended as a substitute
for consulting with your physician. All matters regarding your health require
medical supervision. Neither the author nor the publisher shall be liable or
responsible for any loss, injury, or damage allegedly arising from any information
or suggestion in this book.

LIBRARY OF CONGRESS CATALOGING IN PUBLICATION DATA
Goglia, Philip L.
Turn up the heat : unlock the fat-burning power of your metabolism / Philip L. Goglia.
p. cm.
ISBN 0-670-03085-6
1. Reducing diets. 2. Energy metabolism. I. Title.
RM222 2.G568 2002
613.2'5—dc21   2001057914

This book is printed on acid-free paper. ∞

Printed in the United States of America
Set in Sabon
Designed by Jaye Zimet

To all of my clients with whom I have partnered so many health victories:
My wish to improve the quality of your lives now and in the future
is the essence of this book, my gift to you.

Preface

Frank Sinatra used to sing, "When I was twenty-one, it was a very good year . . ." By the end of the song Frank is past thirty-five. "I'm in the autumn of my years," he croons. As a young man, I used to shake my head: autumn after thirty-five? My father would nod. He warned me about the midlife crisis I could expect to face. It was inevitable.

My boss hammered the point home: "After forty it's all maintenance and repair." The message was clear: I was heading downhill. I would never feel as healthy as I did when I was twenty-one. By the time I turned forty I'd be past my prime.

Three years ago, I saw a poster of Brendan Fraser in *George of the Jungle*. Swinging on a vine in his loincloth, Mr. Fraser had a body to envy. And I stood there envying it. After all, I had been working out since I was sixteen years old and I still couldn't get rid of the love handles, still couldn't find enough discipline to avoid those late night visits to Pepperidge Farm. Although it was easy to conclude I'd never look good swinging on a vine, that I was a victim of unlucky genetics, a friend set me wise. The guy who turned Brendan Fraser into George of the Jungle was Phil Goglia.

I did some checking and discovered Phil was a nutritionist with a degree from Duke. He was an ex-body builder. He had a wall full of glamorous celebrity portraits in his office full of praise I didn't quite trust. After all, I've tried too many diets. Read too many books. Channel-surfed through too many infomercials. But since the consultation was free . . .

It didn't take long to discover that Phil is the Ernest Hemingway of nutritionists. He is the master of the unminced word. With a minimum of adjectives and a maximum of verbs he will strip away long-cherished beliefs and superstitions about your body. He will reveal the lies about weight loss that most people continue to believe. That the only way to lose weight is to eat less. Wrong. That if something tastes good it's bad for you. Wrong. That self-denial and suffering are the only way to look good and feel your best. Wrong. That cheating isn't permitted. Wrong, wrong, wrong.

You will not believe Phil's method works. And then, if you stick with it, you will not believe what you see in the mirror.

Take a look at the photograph of Phil on the back cover. You'd never guess that, as an overweight little boy, Phil was plagued by health problems that changed his life and the course it would take. Phil determined to learn as much as he could about how his body worked. He discovered amazing things. And now, for the first time, he's sharing those discoveries in this book.

This year I will be forty-six. I've never been in better shape. My body fat is down to 4 percent. My energy is through the roof. I work out six days a week. I would lick my twenty-one-year-old self any day. In short, I'm in my prime. And the reason is Phil Goglia. I urge you to read this book, so that you, too, will have a very good year.

—Glen Berenbeim
Executive Producer,
Touched by an Angel

Acknowledgments

I would like to acknowledge the following people for the support they have given me in my life and the contributions they have made toward helping this book become an advancement in the technology of health and nutrition.

To my parents, Charles and Patricia Goglia, for the wings they have given me along with the courage to use them.

To my sister, Catherine, who showed me what it takes to be a hero in this world as she battled and beat breast cancer.

To Carol, who has gifted me with the essence of unconditional love.

To my son, Gibson, who, through his birth, has shown me the wonder of the human spirit and its power.

To Matt, my business partner, who has given me vision and the strength to act upon it.

To Scott, my other business partner, who has provided me with a stable platform to globally share my nutritional knowledge.

To Joy Parker, my collaborator and client, who with infinite patience and the greatest degree of integrity captured not only my voice and wisdom but the true science of nutrition in a concise, very special, and almost magical way. It is because of her talent that each word in this book speaks, that each sentence can be heard in a way that will cause a new paradigm in the future of nutritional science and the coaching of health.

To Bonnie Solow, my literary agent and client, who believed in me from the very beginning. She knew that, without a doubt, the contents of this book would change the face of nutrition forever. I am in awe of her ability to expertly balance the business, the science, and the human spirit of this book.

To Karen Murphy, my editor, for so enthusiastically supporting me and helping this book to become a clear source of information that distinctly answers the question, How do I lose weight and keep it off? She expertly edited my book with an insight into the world of health and nutrition that was pure and true.

To Clare Ferraro, my publisher, and everyone at Penguin Putnam, who so powerfully took a stand in the need to compile and distribute the special information contained within this book and to give it a global voice that could, in turn, change the health of a nation.

To Erin Pasternack, who was able to condense my nutritional protocols into easy-to-use formats and still maintain her sense of humor.

And, finally, to my high school wrestling coach, Eric Suby, who taught me about possibilities through a single phrase so simple yet more powerful to me than anyone will ever know. When I was a young wrestler standing on the edge of the mat, waiting for my match to be announced, terrified of the possible, perhaps painful, outcome, Coach Suby would walk up beside me, put his arm around me, and say, "Just go out there and have fun. What's the worst thing that could happen?" And he was right. To take on the possibility of succeeding is always a better choice in life.

Contents

Introduction
If We Are All on a Diet, Then Why Aren't We Thin?

My twenty years of experience in nutritional counseling has shown me that none of the popular diet programs on the market have worked in the long run for any of my clients, making them feel "broken" and inadequate. Truly, it is not we who are inadequate, but the information we are currently being taught about nutrition, weight management, and exercise. As a nation, we have been misled by faulty premises reported as weight-loss "science" in the media, by misinformation about what kinds of foods are "good" for us and what kinds are "bad," and by diet gurus who have been telling us that one-size-fits-all food plans are the answer to our *individual* nutritional needs.

The truth is: *Each one of us is metabolically unique.* That is why most popular diets fail—their one-size-fits-all approach ignores the fact that *everyone does not utilize fats, proteins, and carbohydrates with the same amount of efficiency.* Only when people eat and exercise for their *own* metabolisms will they see remarkable and *permanent* results in the areas of weight loss, energy levels, and overall health.

Through extensive medical research and nutritional evaluations of thousands of different clients, I have identified three basic metabolic types. They are:

The fat-and-protein-efficient metabolism (74 percent of the population). This metabolism can more efficiently utilize fats and proteins than carbohydrates, creating a physique that is naturally strong.

The carbohydrate-efficient metabolism (23 percent of the population). This group easily digests and utilizes carbohydrates, creating a physique that has a tremendous endurance capacity.

The dual metabolism (3 percent of the population). This third type has the very special ability to utilize all three nutrients—fat, protein, and carbohydrate—with equal ease, creating a physique that equally combines both strength and endurance.

This book teaches you how to identify your specific metabolic type and to dynamically fuel it for weight loss, greater health, increased performance levels, and healthful longevity.

■ The Problem with "Diets"

All of the most popular diet books on the market today take a one-size-fits-all approach to weight loss, and most are based upon the faulty premise that one has to reduce caloric intake to lose weight. Ironically, the opposite is true: One becomes fat because of eating inconsistently and, ultimately, too little. Caloric deprivation will cause you to lose weight in the short term, but in the long run you will experience a rebound effect that will leave you heavier and less healthy than when you started. Eventually, your metabolism will cool to a point at which you stop utilizing calories efficiently. The cooler your metabolism becomes, the less efficiently it can utilize nutrients, causing you to hoard body fat as a protective survival mechanism. The result is unwanted weight gain.

Another problem with popular diet programs is that they are nutritionally static. They do not change as body composition (fat to lean muscle ratio) and metabolic efficiency change. My nutritional program, on the other hand, is designed to be dynamic, changing from week to week to promote continued weight loss as your changing body composition demands different fueling patterns. I offer an easy-to-follow twelve-week program designed so that your weekly menus vary just enough to keep you from reaching a weight-loss plateau. On this program, your body composition will continue to change (losing fat and gaining lean muscle). And you can continue to cycle through these twelve weeks until you have reached your weight loss and physique goals.

Metabolically appropriate food programming will also *make you healthier from the inside out.* If you are following a diet that is inappropriate for your metabolic type, it will undermine your health—perhaps even kill you in the long run. Through accurate metabolic typing and metabolically compatible food protocols, all of my clients consistently lower their total cholesterol, triglyceride, and body fat levels. The result is always a healthier and more fit physique, and an active and youthful lifestyle.

This book provides you with a system to determine your metabolic type and compatible food programs that you can follow for the rest of your life. Because the menus are specifically tailored for your unique metabolic type, you will experience consistent weight loss while always feeling nutritionally satisfied, energized, and vitalized. In the pages that follow, I will coach you through simple steps that will help you to discover your individual metabolic type and efficiency. I will teach you about how to gradually increase the caloric and nutritional content of your meals until they correctly support your specific metabolic needs. Because you will be eating three main meals and three to five snacks daily, you will never feel the pangs of hunger or the anxiety associated with caloric restriction.

If you are facing a weight-loss emergency, such as an upcoming wedding, a family gathering, or a class reunion, this book also offers you a Quickstart Program that will help you to maximize your weight loss and energy levels immediately. On Quickstart you will be able to lose as much as 2.5 percent body fat and 5 pounds per week.

Most important, as you experience the benefits of this program, you will begin to develop a more positive image of your body. And I'm not just talking about a "mental attitude" here. There is no one alive who does not have a dream of the "ideal" body they would love to have. The nutritional plans and exercise protocols in this book will help you make that dream come true. The exercise chapter offers three basic workouts, each specifically designed to capitalize on the strengths of your metabolic type.

Until you try this program, you can't even imagine the incredible transformations that metabolically appropriate food programming can make in your life. The power of food—to build health, stamina, and high performance—is almost unimaginable. I know firsthand how hard—emotionally and physically—diets are on the body. And I understand and empathize with the anxiety, frustrations, and fear associated with trying to lose weight, because as a child, I was 140 pounds overweight and suffered from very poor health. That was the genesis of my quest to uncover the secrets of weight loss and good nutrition. That journey eventually inspired me to earn a master's degree in nutrition, become a world-class champion bodybuilder, and found my own clinic so that I could dedicate my life to sharing with thousands of others the health, vitality, and self-esteem I have discovered through metabolic food programming.

This book is my legacy to you. It is my hope that these pages will be the final stop on your journey to nutritional health, elevated performance levels, and weight control. It will teach you how metabolism truly functions and how appropriately fueling yourself can transform your life and give you a youthful future. This book is designed to be an instructional and educational tool that provides you not only with scientific nutritional enlightenment but also with behavioral coaching that will help you understand how you got where you are in the first place. If you simply allow yourself to be coachable enough to follow this program, it will change you in ways you've never dreamed possible.

Part I

The **Program**

I. Why America Can't Stay Thin

Exposing the Myths Behind Dieting and Uncovering the Mystery
Behind How Our Bodies Work

As we enter the twenty-first century, the United States has become one of the most overweight nations on earth. Currently, 59.4 percent of the adult population, approximately 97 million people, are overweight or obese. In other words, more than one out of every two people—every other person that you see—has a weight problem. This figure has increased by 8 percent in the last ten years—and is continuing to rise with no end in sight. Of that number, 12.5 million are severely overweight and 2 million are morbidly obese, meaning that they are severely at risk for life-threatening health conditions such as heart disease, cancers, stroke, diabetes, and atherosclerosis. And these figures represent only adults over the age of 20. During the last couple of decades, childhood obesity has also been on the rise. At present, 27.1 percent of children ages 6 to 11 are obese, as are 21.9 percent of adolescents between the ages of 12 and 18.

Back in 1900, only 5 percent of Americans were obese. This figure is amazing when one considers that never before have people spent so much time, money, and energy trying to find out what causes them to be overweight and how to take off unwanted fat. We have more diet books, food programs, and health and exercise books to choose from than ever before. At any given time, 40 percent of all women and 25 percent of all men are dieting, and about one in three of these people are trying to maintain their weight. But according to the American College of Sports Medicine, people who diet gain back 67 percent of their lost weight within a year, and the remainder within a five-year period. These individuals spend approximately $30 billion per year on commercial weight-loss programs and about $6 billion on weight-loss products. If you add to this the money spent on medical treatments and work days lost due to obesity-related illnesses, the total cost to society surpasses $100 billion per year.

In spite of the huge sums of money invested in weight loss and health care for the obese, each year Americans, as a whole, continue to become *more* overweight and unhealthier, not less so. While ten years ago only a quarter of the population was obese, now that figure has risen to a third. In fact, since 1943, the Metropolitan Life Insurance Company has had to change their height-and-weight tables three times to accommodate the changing state of American weight. More than 250,000 deaths a year are due to obesity-related health problems, making this the second-greatest *preventable* cause of death in the United States.

These figures prove that there are widespread misconceptions about how we become overweight in the first place, what constitutes proper nutrition, and the relationship between exercise and body composition. All of us start out on an even playing field as infants, instinctively knowing that we have to eat regularly to fuel our metabolisms. When a baby is hungry, it cries until that need is satisfied. But as we get older, we become inculturated with the idea that hunger is a *positive* thing; we begin to associate the pain of wanting food as something that is *good* for us because it will keep or make us thin. Therefore, we eat less and develop inconsistent caloric patterns. But one day we wake up and see an overweight man or woman staring out at us from the mirror, and we don't have a clue about how we *really* got that way in the first place. We do not realize that the cultural effects of how we have been fueling ourselves have had an adverse metabolic impact on our bodies. We wound up getting fat because we did not provide our bodies with the right nutritional management system.

The bottom line is that the diet and food-management programs currently available to us are *not working*. If they were, the people who follow these food programs would become fit, lean, and healthy—and they would stay that way. But they aren't and they don't. The saddest part of all is that every one of us who has been on a diet and gained back the weight—and who hasn't?—feels that he or she has failed. It is not uncommon for my clients to tell me that they have tried four or five different diets in their attempt to lose weight and to get healthier.

A very successful 38-year-old man named Paul told me at our first meeting that he had been on numerous diets over the last few years. Paul is 5 feet 11 inches tall and weighed 275 pounds. He had tried almost every popular diet program, including the Zone, the Atkins Diet, the Grapefruit Diet, and ultra-low-calorie programs, such as Optifast and Medifast. While he had lost many pounds in the short term, the extreme caloric deprivation coupled with the emotional and physical stresses of all these diet programs caused him not only to gain back the lost weight, but to gain even more. By the time he came to me for nutritional counseling, he was completely confused about the proper nutritional choices for his performance level, weight loss, and future health.

There is only one way to experience permanent weight loss, greater energy, vibrant health, and improved quality of life: *Adopt a food program based on one's metabolic type and unique nutritional requirements, and couple it with the appropriate exercise program.* Proper nutrition is not something a person can figure out by looking at the current diet fads and marketing strategies that are being used as a ploy to get us to buy low-fat, low-sugar, and low-calorie products. We must be taught about foods and how they affect our bodies. We must learn how to chose reliable teachers and how to become "coach-able" regarding food management and proper exercise. We need to get onto the playing field of nutrition and see how certain concepts can dramatically improve our daily performance.

■ Myths and Misconceptions About Why We Can't Keep Off the Weight

As I have worked with thousands of clients over the last eighteen years, from professional actors and athletes to housewives and attorneys, counseling them on the varying principles of normal, therapeutic, and sports nutrition, I have noticed that there are certain specific misconceptions about food that many people hold as fact. Your body is a magnificent chemical factory governed by rules of cause and effect: what you put into it is what you get out of it metabolically. It has been evolving and interacting with its environment for hundreds of thousands of years, and many of the ways it responds to food— such as hoarding fat—have developed as survival strategies during times of food scarcity and physical trauma. But your average person has no idea how all these finely tuned processes work together to create health and fitness. To really understand why we have become so fat, it is necessary to look closely at some of the myths and misconceptions about how foods affect the body.

Myth 1: All Metabolisms Are Created Equal

Even though the great majority of diet books on the market operate as if this axiom were true, all metabolisms are *not* created equal. We all do not utilize fats, proteins, and carbohydrates in the same manner. There are three basic and very different metabolic types, each with its own unique nutritional requirements. The first, the **fat-and-protein-efficient type,** makes up about 74 percent of the population. People in this group can most easily metabolize and utilize fats and proteins, but are the most carbohydrate sensitive of the three types. Ideally, they should eat 50 percent protein, 25 percent fat, and 25 percent carbohydrate. The second, the **carbohydrate-efficient type,** which comprises approximately 23 percent of the population, metabolizes carbohydrates with great ease and, therefore, has a strong, stable insulin response. These individuals should ideally ingest 20 percent protein, 12 percent fat, and 68 percent carbohydrate. The third metabolic type is the **dual metabolism,** about 3 percent of the population. People in this group metabolize fats, proteins, and carbohydrates with equal efficiency, so their ideal daily diet should consist of 33.3 percent of each of these food groups.

Identifying your metabolic type and eating accordingly will decrease unwanted scale weight, improve your fat-to-lean-muscle ratio, increase your energy level, and improve your health and well-being. Understanding your metabolism is truly the cornerstone to a successful weight-management program and unlocking the mystery of how to spearhead the development of a youthful future.

Myth 2: All Calories Are Created Equal

Since the use you get from calories depends upon your ability to metabolize them, it is important to look at not only *how many* calories you are ingesting, but at *what kinds of calories* make up your daily food plan. For example, if you have a fat-and-protein-efficient metabolism but eat mostly carbohydrate-rich foods, the type of calories you are ingesting will not efficiently repair and fuel your body.

At present, Americans are obsessed with the idea of low-fat/no-fat. They have confused excess body fat with the fats found naturally in foods. The fats in foods are much needed nutrients that provide us with energy, strengthen cell membranes, and support nerve and hormone function in the body. The issue is not to avoid fats, but to eat them in the proper dietary proportions in support of one's individual metabolic type.

A certain amount of body fat is necessary for survival. While there is a healthy and unhealthy percentage of body fat for each individual, based upon frame size, in general, men should have between 15 percent and 17 percent body fat and women should have between 18 percent and 22 percent.

People do not realize that when fats are removed from processed foods, sugars are added in their place—otherwise, there would be no flavor. Since three out of four people are fat-and-protein-efficient, and, therefore, cannot efficiently utilize large amounts of sugars, eating tremendous amounts of low-fat foods will actually cause the body to store sugar as unwanted body fat while elevating triglycerides. Many people also avoid eating a lot of protein because they are afraid of fat. Again, three out of four people are cutting themselves off from the food source that they can metabolize most efficiently, the nutrients they most need to repair and fuel their bodies. Since adequate protein intake is the foundation of a strong immune system, they are also lowering their resistance to disease and potentially causing a severe decay in their future health.

Myth 3: Carbohydrates Are Better for You Because They Are Easier to Digest Than Fats

One reason that many diets and nutritional programs are low in fats is because, in general, people tend to believe that fats are harder to digest than carbohydrates and, therefore, get stored more easily as excess weight. How you utilize fats and carbohydrates has little to do with which one digests quicker. If you are a carbohydrate-efficient individual, you will always be able to utilize foods from that group more efficiently than fats. If you are a fat-and-protein-efficient individual, you will metabolize fats and proteins with more effectiveness than carbohydrates. If you have a dual metabolism, you will be able to utilize fats, proteins, and carbohydrates with equal ease. Digestion is not the issue; the issue is what happens *after* digestion.

Myth 4: You Must Reduce Your Caloric Intake in Order to Lose Weight

Along with the misconceptions about low-fat and sugar-free foods, people also believe that foods labeled "low calorie" are generally healthier choices than ordinary foods. The danger in this case is that low-cal also means "empty calories"—a lot of food volume with limited food value. While eating reduced-calorie foods may temporarily satisfy your appetite, in many cases they do not adequately support your body's nutritional needs. To understand why this is so, it's important to take a look at the definition of a calorie.

A calorie is a heat-energy unit that the body uses either as an energy source or to repair tissue. Each person has a particular daily caloric requirement, based upon the minimum amount of calories that his or her body needs to function properly. When you do not ingest enough calories to efficiently fuel your metabolism, you will lose some superficial weight over the short term. But eventually your metabolism—as a result of reduced caloric heat—will cool down to the point at which it will stop utilizing calories efficiently and your weight loss will stop. If your body does not have enough calories to adequately fuel and repair itself, it will be forced to cannibalize its own muscle tissue for energy, gradually increasing your fat-to-lean-muscle ratio. In fact, I have found that most of the people who come to me with weight and health problems are usually *already* ingesting *far fewer calories* than they should in order to efficiently fuel their bodies. Therefore, their metabolism, the body's calorie-burning furnace, is already running 25 percent to 60 percent below its ideal metabolic-efficiency level. In turn, the body is storing much of the limited amounts of food these individuals eat as fat and wasting muscle tissue as an adaptive mechanism to create an alternative energy source.

Most people have an adversarial relationship to food. They see calories as the enemy that has created their unwanted body fat. Fat has become the thing they fear—it has reduced their self-esteem and made them feel self-conscious and undesirable. The idea of *increasing* caloric intake to lose weight not only goes against what they have been told, it is also downright frightening to them. Recently, a client named Eric, who weighed 285 pounds, came to my office for nutritional counseling. Eric was eating only 1,200 calories a day—two meals and three pieces of fruit. Yet he was unable to lose any weight. When I started him on Stage One of his food program, a 2,800-calorie nutritional plan designed for his metabolic type, he was scared to death. "I can't eat all this food," he told me. "Food is what made me fat in the first place. If I eat all this, I will gain weight, not lose it."

I told Eric what I tell all of my clients: that he needed to simply have the goodwill to give the program a try. "You've already been on several other diets," I said. "What would it be worth to you for this to be the last food program you were ever on? What would you give to know that you didn't have to feel hungry every day to be lean, healthy, and strong? Relax. Be coach-able."

Eric agreed to try the program. This was a huge step of trust on his part because years of evening news, television talk shows, magazines, and books had sent a message that he was fat because he was eating too much. In seven days, Eric lost five pounds. His metabolism was being stimulated for the first time in decades. When he got off the scale, he was ecstatic.

Since then Eric has continued to lose scale weight. Over a ten-month period, he has gone from 285 pounds to 253. Most important, he has lost considerable body fat and gained several pounds of lean muscle. He started off with 38 percent body fat and dropped to 23.5 percent, a loss of 14.5 percent.

If I break this dramatic physique change down according to weight, it looks like this: Eric began his food program with 108.4 pounds of body fat and 176.6 pounds of lean muscle on his frame. He ended up with 59.5 pounds of total body fat and 193.5 of lean muscle. This means that he lost 48.8 pounds of fat and gained 16.8 pounds of lean muscle. While his scale weight change was only 32 pounds, he experienced a total body conversion of 65.6 pounds!

Even though it goes against what we have been taught, the bottom line is this: No one can lose fat and keep it off without giving the body the appropriate caloric support needed to create an efficient metabolism. The key to losing inches and improving body composition is to eat enough of the *right kinds of foods* for your metabolic type, and to eat enough so that your metabolism is at peak efficiency, burning red hot. Proper food programming is not about caloric restriction, but about consistent, healthy *caloric management.*

Myth 5: Americans Have Become Fat Because We Are Overeating and Underexercising

It is simply not true that everyone who is overweight or obese is a couch potato. In my experience, people are exercising more than they ever have. There have never been more gym enrollments; more clubs for running, walking, or mall walking; more people participating in things like yoga or Pilates; more classes for spinning, aerobics, or stair stepping. Two years ago, the number one product sold on an infomercial was Billy Blank's Tae-Bo video, breaking sales records worldwide.

But exercise is not the key to weight management. If it were, then those of us who are consistently exercising would not be overweight. And it is not the amount of exercise that a person does that changes his or her physique—a physical workout merely breaks down muscle tissue, creating the *potential* for physique change. *The key to changing the physique is proper nutrition—the foods a person eats to repair that broken-down muscle tissue.* You can't change your weight and body composition for the better unless you add appropriate nutrition to your exercise program. In the long run, exercise without proper nutritional support for your metabolic type often does more harm than good, creating a wasting effect on the body. I often ask new clients to stop exercising for a week or so to give their food program time to repair the long-term damage to their tissues.

As I mentioned previously, most clients who come to my office for nutritional counseling are eating far fewer calories than they need in order to maintain an efficient metabolic temperature for their physiological structure. I have also observed that many of them are exercising a great deal. In fact, a national survey of methods people employ for weight loss found that 84 percent of women were eating fewer calories and 60 to 63 percent were increasing the level of their physical activity. The same is true for men: 76 to 78 percent were eating fewer calories and 60 to 62 percent were increasing their physical activity. Yet obesity is still on the rise.

Sarah, a fat-and-protein-efficient woman, noticed that she was becoming very sturdy and muscular when she exercised. Because she wanted to be slender and willowy, she decided to severely drop her caloric intake, to cut most of the protein from her diet, and to increase her exercise regimen to two and a half to three hours per day. Instead of getting firmer and leaner, however, she started becoming soft and "mushy." Reducing her caloric intake and the types of nutrients she needed made it metabolically impossible for her body to adequately repair her muscle tissue. When she came to me for nutritional counseling, I increased her protein intake to a point that would properly nourish her but would not add an excessive amount of muscle to her frame, and I reduced her exercise regimen to about an hour per day. I explained to her that she simply could not exercise for three hours a day unless she wanted to eat like a bodybuilder—and look like one.

Even though Ted weighed only 148 pounds, he decided that he wanted to get rid of the fat around his waist. To accomplish this, he severely decreased his caloric intake and increased his exercise levels. He, too, began exercising about two hours a day, taking spinning, aerobic, and yoga classes, and lifting weights. But instead of getting rid of his fat, Ted found that his body began wasting muscle tissue and hoarding fat. After assessing his nutritional needs, I increased his daily caloric intake and decreased his exercise level. As a result of eating a metabolically appropriate food program, Ted's body fat dropped and his lean muscle increased.

One of the first steps to losing unwanted weight and improving health and quality of life is to learn to separate nutritional fact from fiction.

■ "Science" That Has Led Us Astray

Where do these myths come from? Why do people believe in them so faithfully in spite of the obvious evidence that these dietary strategies do not help them to achieve any long-term weight loss or greater health benefits? Part of the problem is our steadfast belief in the power of science to always provide us with the correct answers. Most of the clients who come to me have been searching for years for answers to their questions about weight loss and health, and they have taken much of what they have read or heard in the media as scientific fact. The inherent problem is that much of this information does not work for them, or only works if they have a particular metabolic type that randomly matches the nutritional findings of the study. For example, there is a lot of information out there about high-carbohydrate diets, yet 74 percent of people in America are fat-and-protein-efficient and require 25 percent fat, 50 percent protein, and 25 percent carbohydrate in their daily diet in order to adequately fuel their bodies metabolically. With diabetes on the rise (a 33 percent increase over the last decade alone), it is clear that people are not receiving accurate information about *how to manage carbohydrates* in their food plan.

In the scientific research I have read over the last couple of decades, I have found many inconsistencies and half-truths in what is presented to the general public as "science." All too often the results of nutritional research are based upon original faulty premises or test groups that are too small or limited in range. Here are some of the most common studies and theories, as well as their inherent inconsistencies and flaws.

Genetic Studies

A great deal of research has been done on how an individual's genetic heritage affects their nutritional patterns for weight gain and weight loss. First, you must realize that inherited characteristics do not give us the whole picture. Environmental factors have fully as much to do with how our bodies utilize nutrients, store fats, and lose weight as does our genetic heritage. While it is true that metabolic types do have strong genetic associations, no one should ever believe that just because Mom, Dad, and Sis are overweight, he or she, too, is doomed to a life of obesity. Your lifestyle patterns of weight gain and loss have fully as much to do with whether or not you are ingesting the proper nutrients for your metabolic type, whether you are eating enough calories to efficiently fuel your individual metabolism, whether you are correctly exercising for your metabolic type, whether you are ingesting enough water, what your stress levels and sleep patterns are, and hormonal changes over the course of a lifetime—for both men and women.

One recent study in the *American Journal of Clinical Nutrition* involved a group of women ages 38 to 60 who were fed a diet composed of 40 to 45 percent fat. The study found that over a six-year period, some of the women gained from 7.7 to 11.4 pounds. Others did not gain so much weight. What this study claimed to have discovered was that some women have a *genetic predisposition* to become overweight or obese. In other words, if you have the "fat gene," you're out of luck—it will be very hard for you to avoid becoming fat.

While this study is correct in stating that not all metabolisms are created equal, it did not take into consideration that there are three distinct metabolic types and three different ways of fueling those types. If a woman has a dual metabolism, or is fat-and-protein-efficient, of course she will be able to better handle eating a diet of 40 percent fats than a woman who is carbohydrate-efficient and should *never* consume more than 12 percent of her diet as fats. If you feed a person whose metabolism does not efficiently utilize fats more than three times the amount of fats that she requires for optimum metabolic efficiency, *of course she is going to gain weight*. There is no issue of genetic superiority, inferiority, or digestive efficiency involved here.

Studies also do not take into account all-important lifestyle issues, such as activity levels or current eating patterns. What kinds of foods were they eating to begin with—and how much? If some were already ingesting inappropriate nutrients for their metabolic types, then their metabolisms would be inefficient from the start. If others just happened to be eating the proper proportions of nutrients, then their metabolisms would have started with a higher level of efficiency.

The Fat Cell Theory

To understand this theory, it is necessary to see how fat cells develop within the body. We are all born with a certain number of fat cells. The number of cells we have multiplies during the growing years and levels off as we approach adulthood. An older version of this theory claimed that we do not develop any additional fat cells when we become adults, but that the ones we have simply continue to fill with fat. More recent research states that when a person gains 60 percent above his or her ideal weight and the body's fat cells expand in size eight- to tenfold, they may reach the limit of their storage capacity and divide to form new cells (this is known as *hyperplasia*). Statistically, a nonobese person has about 25 billion to 30 billion fat cells; a moderately obese person has approximately 60 billion to 100 billion; and a seriously obese person has close to 200 billion fat cells.

The main point of the contemporary version of this study is that even when an obese person loses weight, he or she will have more difficulty maintaining their weight than a person with fewer fat cells. Even though the large cells in the obese individual shrink with weight loss, they are supposedly more "eager" to fill up with fat than the fat cells in a "normal" person.

This study implies that even when an obese person loses weight, he or she is doomed to gain it all back. My experiences working over the long term with hundreds of obese clients simply do not bear out this theory. Whether or not my clients have been able to keep off the lost weight has everything to do with environmental factors and lifestyle choices, such as how closely they stick to the food and exercise programs tailored to their metabolic types. It is somewhat ridiculous to assume that how well we can maintain our weight is simply based upon how many fat cells we have and their "eagerness" to store fat. There are many, many other processes in the body connected to weight gain. These include the efficiency of the adrenal system, thyroid function, hormonal patterns, the endocrine system, and sensitivity to insulin. I myself was 140 pounds overweight as a child and an adolescent—the years when my fat cells were most rapidly developing. But for more than three decades I have eaten and worked out according to my metabolic type, and I have no trouble at all maintaining my weight—albeit as a bodybuilder, I weigh more than the average man my height. In spite of that, my ratio of fat to lean muscle is 10 percent and has been for years.

The Body's Use of Insulin

There has been much discussion recently in popular diet books about the role of insulin in maintaining body weight. It is generally believed that many individuals become "insulin resistant" when they gain weight; that is, they lose their ability to efficiently release insulin.

This, in turn, leaves a person with a surplus of glucose in the body, much more than it needs for its immediate metabolic needs. When this occurs, the pancreas cannot produce the proper amount of insulin to meet the needs of efficient glucose utilization. The result is often adult-onset diabetes (Type 2) and unwanted weight gain.

In my experience, insulin-resistance and blood-sugar diseases such as diabetes occur when a fat-and-protein-efficient individual eats excessive amounts of carbohydrates and not enough fats and proteins over an extended period of time. I have never seen a carbohydrate-efficient individual, and have rarely seen a dual metabolism, with any form of blood sugar problem because both these metabolic types efficiently utilize carbohydrates. Given the large amount of carbohydrates in the American diet, and the hidden sugars found in all of the low-fat foods we ingest because of our fear of fats, it is no wonder that the 74 percent of us who are fat-and-protein efficient are experiencing difficulties with insulin levels, body fat, and energy levels.

The 33 percent increase in diabetes over the last ten years is certainly proof that we do not all process carbohydrates equally well. With the proliferation of fast food, junk food, low-fat foods, and vegetarian diets that derive much of their protein from dairy (more hidden sugars), the amount of carbohydrates in the American diet has risen drastically. Because we live in a society that has been taught that all metabolisms are created equal and that we should all be eating the same amounts of fat, protein, and carbohydrate, even when we do try to "eat healthy" only some of us succeed. Many nutritional aids such as the U.S. Department of Agriculture's Dietary Guidelines for Americans recommend that everyone eat the same, somewhere in the neighborhood of 30 percent fat, 12 percent protein, and 58 percent carbohydrate. Seventy-four percent of the population, roughly three out of every four individuals, simply cannot metabolically utilize a diet of more than 25 percent total carbohydrate. It is no surprise that diabetes is on the rise. Clearly, one can see that this is a result of eating too much of the *wrong* types of foods—not too much food.

The Setpoint Theory

The setpoint theory states that each of us has an ideal weight range that is determined by genetic factors. Therefore, if you diet and lose weight, the body will feel hungry again, and you will eat until you re-gain the weight you have lost. The idea that a "setpoint" weight ex-ists for each person is controversial, but some researchers suggest that a person's setpoint can be reset to a lower point by a combina-tion of exercise and diet.

The idea of a setpoint comes up each time I work with my clients. One of the main questions they ask me is, "How much should I ide-ally weigh?" I explain to them that instead of focusing on some sort of ideal weight or image of physical slimness, it is better to concen-trate on becoming internally lean and healthy. When I see a client's body fat percentage, cholesterol, and triglycerides drop; their perfor-mance level increase; and their energy levels soar, that is every bit as important to me—and them—as are the inches and scale pounds they are losing. Weight management is as much about quality of life as it is about how much one weighs and how thin one looks.

So, do I feel that everyone has an ideal weight, a setpoint their body should settle into once they are properly nutritionally fueled? In a sense, yes, but clinically that weight should be based more on body composition, height, and frame than on genetic factors. Each person requires a certain minimum amount of muscle in order to maintain proper posture. When I see a person with unusually poor posture, I can guarantee that when I measure their ratio of body fat to lean muscle, their fat percentage will be much higher than it should be. They will also have significantly fewer pounds of lean muscle on their frame than they should have because of muscle lost due to years of poor nutritional habits. If you are eating for your metabolic type, your body will find and maintain an appropriate and healthy setpoint.

Weight Cycling

This concept, also called the "yo-yo effect," states that each time a person returns to a higher weight after dieting, his body fat percent-age rises, making it more difficult to lose weight on the next diet. Eventually, a person reaches a point of diminishing returns where it not only takes longer to lose the weight each time he diets, but his body fat keeps rising every time he gains back the weight. The theory behind this is that the body becomes more and more adept at protecting itself against what it interprets as a food shortage and, there-fore, learns how to more quickly lower its metabolic temperature to avoid starving. The fact that most contemporary diets are low in calories contributes to this cycle because people lose muscle mass and gain body fat on such stringent food programs.

I have found that it is not only the *frequency* of dieting that causes people to experience a cooling of their metabolisms and an in-crease in body fat, but also their metabolic type and how well their chosen diet meets their nutritional needs. The amount of lean muscle lost on any low-calorie program is greatly influenced by whether or not the foods allowed on that diet match your nutritional require-ments. For example, a fat-and-protein-efficient individual is likely to lose a great deal of muscle mass on a high-carbohydrate diet that pro-vides a limited-protein intake.

The individuals whose bodies suffer the most from dieting are those who not only diet frequently, but who try a wide variety of ap-proaches. The woman who does a fasting diet one month, a grape-fruit diet six months later, a high-fat diet the next time, then a low-fat, high-carbohydrate diet the next time is a lot worse off than someone who just goes to Weight Watchers whenever she wants to drop 10 pounds. Some diets will do more harm to your body than others, depending upon the needs of your metabolic type.

One of the problems with the concept of weight cycling is that it causes people to just give up after a while. Since most of the clients who come to me for nutritional counseling have already been on four or five diets, I know from experience that it is still possible to lose weight and build up your lean muscle, no matter how many food programs you have tried. It might take some people a bit longer than others—depending upon factors such as age and how much abuse their bodies have had to endure. But I have found that every one of my clients is able to restore metabolic efficiency and a proper ratio of fat to lean muscle by eating and exercising according to their meta-bolic type. The reason for this is that I give them a new definition of the word "diet." Yo-yo dieting is a completely different concept than food programming or food management for one's metabolic type. When a person eats correctly with the best proportions for his me-tabolism, the body will no longer have to hoard fat to adapt to strange diet regimens.

The truth of this statement can be seen in what I call the "10-pound syndrome." Everyone who goes on a diet will tell you that the last 10 pounds are the hardest to lose. That is because those last 10 pounds are the fat that your body is hoarding to protect itself against what it perceives as nutritional inconsistency and trauma. Hanging on to that last 10 pounds is your body's way of adapting to an inappropriate diet—caloric deprivation—and food percentages and combinations not suited to your metabolic type. If you eat appropriately for your metabolic type, losing the last 10 pounds should be no harder than losing the first.

The Myth That Diets Do Not Work Without Exercise

This theory implies that it is a waste of time to bother eating correctly if you don't exercise, and that exercise should always come first. But if a person who believes this chooses a low-calorie food program and starts to exercise, he will only waste muscle tissue, hoard fat, and will ultimately injure himself. Exercise only utilizes calories as energy and creates the potential for greater muscularity by breaking down muscle tissue. Since proper nutrition is needed to repair that muscle tissue, exercising like crazy on a food program that is inadequate for your nutritional needs will do more harm than good. One of my clients told me about the drop-out rate in her gym. Since she's been on my program for the past seven months, she's watched a number of obese individuals join her gym, exercise like crazy for a few weeks, then suddenly disappear. "I know that they aren't getting the food they need to fuel their workout," she said. "I can see that their bodies aren't changing. Eventually, they get so discouraged you never see them again."

Nutrition is so important for successful weight loss and management that a person should not attempt strenuous exercise if he cannot commit to the proper evaluation of his current nutrition program, and a plan to improve it. Nutrition is of critical importance because it stabilizes proper caloric intake, preserves and builds muscle mass, increases metabolic rate, and controls appetite. An increased metabolic rate (or *metabolic temperature*) is determined by the amount of muscle tissue you repair and develop. And that, in turn, controls your body's daily caloric request.

■ Why Most Modern Diets Work over the Short Term and Not over the Long Term

Let me begin by saying that there is no question that many people *do* lose weight on current diet programs. The main reason for this is that most of us have such inconsistent eating patterns that almost *any* program, followed carefully, will give the body enough nutritional consistency and stability that it will drop a few superficial pounds of body weight. The crux of the matter, as we have seen, is that people usually *do not keep off the weight* they lose on such programs because they are not designed for either their metabolic type or for long-term maintenance. Because these programs are defined as a "diet," the results are only a temporary fix.

The average man and woman judges the value of weight-loss programs according to how much weight they or their friends have lost on that regimen. If you are obese or overweight, losing pounds is a good thing. But my question to you is, what else have you lost? Have you also lost muscle mass? While you were on this diet for months, did you lose your emotional balance? Were you irritable and short-tempered? Did your relationships at home and in the workplace suffer? Has the diet you've been on promoted an extraordinary life, or did it ultimately cause your life to decay?

In my experience, the criteria by which you should choose a weight loss or weight-management program must be broader than just how much weight you will lose. To increase your chances of success over the long run, you should ask yourself the following questions.

■ Will this diet effectively increase your internal health and promote a youthful future?

Since there are three metabolic types with very different nutritional needs and nutrient-metabolizing abilities, you should never pick a dietary program that does not address your innate capacities. For example, if you are a carbo-hydrate-efficient person, your body will have difficulty efficiently utilizing nutrients from a diet that is high in fats and protein. You will feel tired, lethargic, and on edge because you are not ingesting enough of your primary energy source, carbohydrates. Even though you may appear externally thinner at the end of a few months, you will be less healthy than when you started. As cholesterol levels elevate, you will become fatter on the inside. And you will be emotionally erratic. As your health decays, your performance levels will deteriorate as well.

■ What *kind* of weight will you lose on this diet?

Will you lose pounds of body fat while you build lean muscle, or will you lose a percentage of what lean muscle you have, which in most cases is already lower than it should be? Most of the clients who come to me have a much higher percentage of body fat than is healthy for their gender, age, and frame size, regardless of their weight. I have one 47-year-old female client who is 5 feet 8 inches tall and, when she first came to see me, weighed 158 pounds. Her body fat percentage was 34.25 percent. Even though her scale weight indicated that she was merely overweight, her body fat made her technically obese. It was a full 10.25 percent over the 20 to 24 percent recommended for women. Because of her small frame size, she should even perhaps aim for the lower end of that recommended spectrum. Just because a person is skinny does not mean that he or she is healthy, or even lean. She can be thin and overfat simultaneously. Many fat-and-protein-efficient vegetarians who do not ingest a metabolically appropriate balance of nutrients in their diet are technically obese because they carry such a large percentage of body fat in comparison to lean muscle.

On ultra-low-calorie diets—less than 1,000 calories per day—40 to 45 percent of weight loss comes from the body cannibalizing its own muscle tissue in order to produce enough glucose to operate its basic life-supporting functions. A person may look slimmer but could end up carrying at least 30 percent body fat, making him or her technically obese, though not overweight. You do not have to look fat to be fat.

■ What sort of maintenance does your choice of diet offer you?

Can a particular diet *keep* you lean, healthy, and energized for the rest of your life? For example, if a food program is calorically restrictive, it is unlikely that you will be able to stay on it for more than a few months. The stress your body experiences when undernourished is extreme. People are unaware that the body experiences hunger as *trauma*. To protect itself, it will respond by cooling your metabolism and hoarding fat. The body has numerous ways of adapting to inadequate caloric intake. Eventually weight loss will end as your metabolism becomes more adept at making do with less. When you do not ingest the correct caloric amounts and the proper proportions of the appropriate nutrients that your body needs to repair and nourish itself—according to your metabolic type—you will feel exhausted, anxious, and irritable. This is not a healthy physical, mental, and emotional state to be in for weeks or months on end. Somehow you have been taught to attach value to these symptoms, seeing them as positive indications that the diet is successful.

■ **Is your food program static? Or is it dynamic, changing as your body composition changes and as your metabolism becomes more and more efficient?**

The problem with most current food programs is that they are static, not changing as your body changes. Their caloric patterns do not shift from week to week as you incur weight loss and changes in body composition (fat-to-lean-muscle ratio). Eventually on these diets you will reach a weight-loss plateau because the caloric pattern you are following now supports and matches your new body weight. Static food programs do not allow for continued weight loss.

■ **Is your diet program a one-size-fits-all program, or does it recognize the unique nutritional needs of your metabolic type?**

The problem with most current foods plans is that they are one-size-fits-all regimens. That's why two of your friends may have lost fifteen pounds each on a high-protein diet, but you and your sister bottom out at a loss of eight pounds, no matter how long you stay on the program. If your friends are fat-and-protein-efficient, which means that their metabolisms are well fueled on a food plan high in those nutrients, of course they will lose weight. But if you and your sister are carbohydrate-efficient, you will not have enough carbohydrates to efficiently fuel your tissues and maintain stable energy levels on such a regime. Since you can't possibly utilize all of those fats and proteins, you will begin storing some of them as fat, which will eventually raise your body fat percentage and cholesterol levels. The result is disappointing, ineffective weight loss, and a decay in health that you might not even be aware of.

■ **Does your diet plan require you to drink adequate water?**

There is a lot of confusion about how much water is enough for our daily metabolic needs. Most traditional medical doctors recommend eight 8-ounce glasses a day, regardless of whether you are a 125-pound woman or a 300-pound man. This is absurd considering that 70 percent of our body is fluid based. Another widely held rule of thumb is that you should drink half of your scale weight in ounces. In other words, if you weigh 180 pounds, you should drink 90 ounces of water. My research, and my experience working with thousands of clients over the last sixteen years, has shown that because of water's vital role in maintaining the core metabolic temperature of your body, **the**

correct daily amount of water intake is approximately one ounce of water per pound of scale weight. So, under my program, that 158-pound woman I mentioned would drink 158 ounces of water per day, which translates to twenty 8-ounce glasses, or about three of those 1.58 quart bottles of water found in any store. (I discuss the role of water in the body in greater detail later, on page 50.)

Keeping these basic principles in mind, as you read through this book you will see that one of the main differences between metabolic food programming and most diets is that this program will teach readers the *trade* of weight management, the science behind it. Other programs rely on the *tricks,* gimmicks that will help you to lose superficial weight, but for how long—and at what cost to your health, immune system, energy levels, longevity, and general well-being?

As you read my book and learn more about how to create a food program that is dynamic, not static, based upon your metabolic type and caloric needs, you will begin to see the advantage of leaving behind one-size-fits-all, cookie-cutter diets and nutritional theories. You will discover how much healthier you will be if you eat according to your own unique metabolic requirements. In a very short time, you will begin to watch yourself lose weight, gain lean muscle, develop tremendous energy, and experience more health, well-being, joy, and self-confidence in your daily life. You will start repairing the damage that dieting has caused in your body over the years and begin creating a vitally rich and healthful future for yourself.

■ The New Weight-Loss Paradigm

We have taken a look at some of the most common misconceptions about food. If I am asking you to leave behind your old ideas about nutrition and dieting, what, then, are the new guidelines? They can be summed up in five statements:

1. All metabolisms are not created equal. There are three different unique metabolisms.
2. Because of this, all calories are not equal. There are distinctly different ways to efficiently utilize the calories found in fats, proteins, and carbohydrates.

3. Since calories are heat-energy units, metabolism is a function of caloric heat. For this reason, a person's caloric intake must be managed daily in order to create enough consistent caloric heat to release fat as an energy source. It has been historically proven again and again that calorically restricted dieting does not work.

4. Your caloric pattern changes as your body composition changes. Your nutritional regimen must be dynamic, not static.

5. Once you are satisfied with your particular body composition, you can stabilize your food pattern, maintain your weight with healthy nutritional choices, and free yourself from excessive food concerns.

Some of the ideas in this chapter might seem new and unfamiliar to you. But keep in mind that the old dieting rules that we have loyally followed have consistently let us down. It's time to re-evaluate much of what you thought you knew about food and embrace a paradigm shift in food programming. All I ask of you as you read this book is that you allow yourself to be "coach-able" enough to faithfully follow the nutritional plan based on your metabolic type and to make exercise a part of your lifestyle. It may seem unrealistic at first to believe that eating *more* food than you already eat daily—but the right kinds of food—can actually create a leaner and more fit you. You may ask yourself, "Is it *really* necessary to eat three meals and three or four snacks per day to create an appropriate amount of metabolic heat? Or to drink all that water?" But if you are willing to have the goodwill to follow this food program, you will watch your body, your energy levels, your health, your relationships, and your life change in ways you never dreamed possible. This book will be the tool through which you design a youthful future and live your dream of fitness and health.

This book will teach you how to energize your every waking hour and develop vibrant and long-lasting health. It will show you how to use nutrition to avoid and prevent illnesses such as diabetes (which has increased 33 percent in the last decade), heart disease, and atherosclerosis. It will explain the importance of proper hydration and how drinking enough water daily helps to keep your metabolic thermostat at the right "temperature" so that your body will not hoard fat. It will show you how to exercise safely and effectively, according to the needs of your specific metabolism. Once you have learned how to eat and exercise according to your metabolic type, you will never again have to live hungry, controlled by calorically re-stricted food regimens. As you discover how to satisfy your nutri-tional needs, you will experience the freedom of not being ruled by food cravings and the need to binge. You will learn the science of making food work for you as an ally, not as an adversary, supplying your body with the fuel it needs to perform at its highest level. Most important, you will discover how to own your food choices and ex-perience life at your personal best.

2. Turning Up the Heat

Discovering Your Metabolic Type and Making It Work for You

Most of the people who come to my office for a consultation have been trying to take off extra pounds for years. Typically, a client will say to me, "I've been eating all these healthy foods and exercising so hard, so why am I still gaining weight?" The problem is not with his or her intentions. People really want to be leaner and healthier, and invest much precious time, energy, and money toward reaching that goal. As we have seen, one of the major problems is in the accuracy of the information presented in the media—the false claims about food and exercise. Every time a person picks up a magazine, goes to the bookstore, or turns on the television, he or she is inundated with confusing, contradictory, and incomplete information. To begin this program, we first need serious re-education about how food really works as fuel in the body.

Albert Einstein once said that insanity is expecting different results from doing the same thing over and over again. When I explain to clients the basic science behind weight loss, I always see those light bulbs click on in their heads. Their eyes light up because they realize that they have finally found a food-and-exercise plan that makes sense to them.

The bottom line is, if people want to lose fat and gain lean muscle, they have to eat enough of the foods appropriate *for their metabolic type* to create sufficient caloric heat to make their me-

tabolisms efficient. Just because something is considered a healthy food doesn't make it a healthy choice for everyone.

For example, I see clients every week who have Type 2 diabetes (adult onset), or some kind of blood sugar problem in their family. They know they feel physically sick every time they overindulge in sugars, so they try to control their carbohydrate intake, which makes logical sense. But they've also been told by the media and by diet books to stay away from foods that are high in fats. For this reason, it has never occurred to them that fats, inherently found in protein, could be an effective source of energy for them. In fact, when I ask them if there is any coronary disease in their family, they almost always say no, which is one of the factors that indicates a genetic predisposition to efficiently utilize fats.

I see other clients who are trying to eat an organic, mostly vegetarian diet who have no idea how to get enough protein into their bodies. Someone told them that animal protein was not healthy for them. So instead they try to supply their bodies with protein from non-animal foods, such as soy, dairy, legumes, white or brown rice, and whole wheat, which do not perfectly match the animo acid profile that humans require to repair muscle tissue. While these foods do contain some protein, they are primarily carbohydrate and, therefore, will be reduced to glucose as they are metabolized. The body uses these foods first as carbohydrate and only secondarily as a protein.

If a person is efficient at utilizing carbohydrates, and they want to eat soy, dairy, grains, and vegetables, they've made some good food choices. But people who are best at utilizing fats and proteins (three out of four) are at a disadvantage on a vegetarian or vegan diet, and will have difficulty appropriately fueling and repairing their bodies. For this reason, it is very easy for vegetarians to inadvertently waste muscle tissue. They may have the appearance of being thin, which our culture equates with being "healthy," but will most certainly have an unhealthy percentage of body fat versus lean muscle. Thin does not automatically mean "lean" or healthy.

I also explain to my clients, many of whom excessively exercise in the gym, that they must remember this: **Exercise itself does not change one's physique; it merely creates the opportunity, or potential, for physique change.** Exercise does not rebuild muscle tissue. The foods that people eat before and after exercise repair muscle tissue. People cannot change their weight and body composition for the better unless they supplement their exercise program with appropriate nutritional support. In fact, in the long run, exercise without the proper nutrition often does more harm than good.

There is a third concern associated with this undereating-overexercising syndrome: *How long can a person sustain a low-calorie diet and an intense workout schedule?* It is only a matter of time before exhaustion and eventual injury intervene—with health decay as the final result. What happens when the exercise and diet fads fail to deliver on their promises to help us achieve a superior quality of life and level of health? Instead of achieving lasting results on the diet programs we so arduously follow, we usually end up weakening our immune systems, cooling our metabolisms, and feeling like failures as we helplessly watch our weight yo-yo up and down over the years. We experience severe frustration and discouragement because we ultimately feel as if we can successfully manage every aspect of our lives *but* our own body weight. The feeling that we can't even control something as basic as our own bodies carries over into our daily lives, making us feel broken. Finally, we simply give up and spend the last decades of our lives being overweight, struggling with obesity-related degenerative illnesses such as high cholesterol, hypertension, heart disease, and Type 1 or Type 2 diabetes. We become complacent, accepting that things are never going to change for us.

The truth is, it doesn't have to be that way. Getting lean and physically conditioned, and having more than enough energy to sustain us through the toughest day, does not result from starving ourselves or eating reduced-calorie, "healthy" foods—or exercising to extremes. It comes from learning to keep ourselves properly fueled by eating and exercising appropriately for our metabolic type.

■ The Three Nutrient Groups

There is a great deal of confusion in many people's minds about what constitutes a fat, a protein, and a carbohydrate. Let's begin by clearly defining these terms.

Protein

The body uses protein for tissue repair. The first category of protein foods are those that are animal derived. These include foods such as fish, turkey, chicken, eggs, and steak. They are *complete proteins*, meaning that they contain a complete profile of all the amino acids humans need to build and repair muscle tissue. The leanest animal protein is fish. The next leanest is turkey or chicken (white meat is leaner than dark meat). Red meats have a variety of fat content. The leanest beef cuts are flank, filet mignon, London broil, and round. The fattier beef choices are porterhouse, rib-eye, and T-bone. If you are choosing ground beef, be aware that it always has a relatively high-fat content. If you want ground beef, it is always best to have your flank, filet, London broil, or round ground at the market or butcher. If you want a leaner ground, mix in some turkey breast.

Protein substitutes. People do not realize that many of the foods that they believe are adequate protein substitutes are *primarily* utilized by the body as carbohydrate because they are starch based. These include foods such as soy or whey products, nuts, legumes, foods processed from bulgur (such as Garden Burgers), or combination foods eaten together, such as rice and legumes. If you are a vegetarian and do not choose to eat animal protein, you need to be careful to ingest a wide enough profile of protein substitutes to receive the full range of amino acids to repair muscle tissue.

Dairy. Another category of food commonly used as a protein substitute is the group of foods that include dairy products. While many people consider dairy to be a protein, the body will utilize it first as lactose, a milk sugar. Therefore, people who believe that they can get sufficient protein in their daily diet from eating dairy products are misinformed. Another important consideration is that nearly all adults have an inherent inability to utilize dairy products and are, therefore, lactose intolerant. Aside from possibly elevating cholesterol and triglyceride levels (even in individuals who are fat-and-protein-efficient), a diet rich in dairy products such as butter and cheese is going to create digestive difficulties, including gastritis, colitis, irritable bowel disorder, esophageal reflux, abdominal cramping, and abnormal amounts of phlegm.

Fat

The body uses fat as an energy source. There are two basic types of dietary fat, saturated and unsaturated. Saturated fats, which are solid at room temperature, are found in all types of animal proteins and dairy. Unsaturated fats, which are liquid at room temperature, are found in nut and vegetable oils. Some EPA (essential phospholipid acid) fish oil fats, even though they are animal derived, are also unsaturated and have numerous health benefits. Salmon is a good example. Regardless of your metabolic type, it is a good idea to eat fish at least three times a week.

At present, our culture has become obsessed with the concept of fats. A great deal of misinformation exists about them that has actually caused us to gain weight, not lose it. Often fat has blanket classifications, such as "bad fats" (saturated), the fats that "cause" cholesterol elevation; and "good fats" (unsaturated), those that are more easily utilized as an energy source and "do not cause cholesterol." However, any information about fat should always be assessed in the context of how well your specific metabolic type utilizes fat, protein, and carbohydrate. Simply following the metabolic type–specific menu plans I have designed for you later in the book will take care of all of your worries about fat choices, regardless of your metabolic type.

Carbohydrate

The body uses carbohydrate as an energy source by converting it to sugar. There are three basic different types of carbohydrates. The first, *fibrous carbohydrates,* includes vegetables. Vegetables have a fairly low caloric value but help to promote digestion. The second, *starchy/complex carbohydrates* are used, primarily, as an energy source. They can be broken down into two further categories—single ingredient and multi-ingredient. Single-ingredient carbohydrate includes foods such as white and brown rice, oatmeal, potatoes, yams, and corn. Multi-ingredient carbohydrate includes breads, cakes, pasta, crackers, and cookies. Although multi-ingredient carbohydrates are more convenient food choices, since so many of them are prepackaged, it is always better to choose a single-ingredient carbohydrate, even though they may require more preparation time. The reason for this is that single-ingredient carbohydrates are not processed foods, nor are they made with sugar and yeast. **Foods with yeast, such as many types of bread, should be avoided because yeast is one of the most infectious bacteria in existence and promotes many types of illnesses.** Many people are yeast-sensitive and don't even know it. The third type of carbohydrate, the *simple-sugar carbohydrate,* includes any carbohydrate that contains simple sugars such as fructose or sucrose. This category also includes single-ingredient and multi-ingredient foods. Fruit is an example of a single-ingredient simple-sugar carbohydrate, and candy is an example of a multi-ingredient simple-sugar carbohydrate.

■ The Three Metabolic Types

To understand what constitutes "appropriate" or "inappropriate" food choices for the individual, you first need to understand what I mean by metabolic type. There are three basic types that each utilize different percentages of fat, protein, and carbohydrate: (1) *Fat-and-Protein Efficient,* (2) *Carbohydrate Efficient,* and (3) a rare third type, *Dual Metabolism,* which evenly utilizes foods from all three groups. All three types are evenly distributed across gender lines.

Fat-and-Protein-Efficient Type

The most physically resilient of all metabolic types is the **fat-and-protein-efficient** individual (74 percent of the population). This person digests nutrients from these two food groups more efficiently than carbohydrate by converting fat into lipids for energy and utilizing protein for efficient tissue repair. The correct food program for this metabolic type should reflect this capacity. In other words, this individual utilizes chicken, fish, turkey, steak, and eggs (fats and proteins) more easily than bread, oatmeal, pasta, and candy (carbohydrates). This metabolism should ideally eat a diet consisting of 50 percent protein, 25 percent fat, and 25 percent carbohydrate. Because of this type's ability to digest and utilize protein, his or her body becomes strong quickly and carries a lot of lean muscle tissue. Therefore, this individual's primary exercise should be weight training (75 percent), with some cardiovascular exercise (25 percent). Cardiovascular exercise is difficult for the fat-and-protein-efficient individual as this type has such a low cardiovascular threshold and has a physique that is thick and muscular.

While you can't always tell someone's metabolic type by appearance, this kind of individual, whether male or female, usually has a muscular, blocklike shape and will gain muscle evenly over his or her entire body. The downside of this is that when this type becomes fat, he or she also tends to gain weight evenly over the entire body. Since this metabolism does not hoard fat in a specific place, many of these individuals do not realize how overweight they have become. Because of the ease with which this individual digests and utilizes fats, this person is less likely to develop illnesses such as high cholesterol and heart disease, and their HDLs (good cholesterol) will usually be higher than average. And, therefore, the LDLs (bad cholesterol) will tend to be lower than average. On the other hand, when this person is improperly nourished, their triglycerides can rapidly elevate to acute levels, causing a predisposition toward diseases such as hypoglycemia, hyperglycemia, and Type 2 diabetes.

Carbohydrate-Efficient Type

The carbohydrate-efficient person (23 percent of the population) easily digests and utilizes foods from this group (brown and white rice, breads, cereals, grains, pasta, fruits, vegetables, and so on) and has a strong, stable insulin (blood sugar) response. The appearance of this type is generally tall and thin. This individual's elevated carbohydrate intake enables him to excel at endurance exercises and sports. Ideally, this type's primary exercise program should include all types of cardiovascular activities (75 percent), with some secondary weight training (25 percent). While the ideal food program for this metabolism should consist of only 20 percent protein and 12 percent fat, this type should eat a tremendous amount of carbohydrates, 68 percent. This individual carries less muscle mass than the fat-and-protein-efficient type and has a metabolism designed for endurance and great aerobic capacity. While it is difficult for this type to build a lot of bulky muscle, they excel at activities that require stamina, such as long-distance running, bicycling, and basketball. When a carbohydrate-efficient individual gains weight, the body will most likely have a disproportionate appearance, with relatively thin face, arms, and legs, and large abdomen, hips, and buttocks. Because of the ease with which this metabolism utilizes all sugars, they will be less likely to develop blood-sugar-related illnesses such as Type 2 diabetes and more likely to develop problems related to elevated cholesterol involving low HDLs and elevated LDLs if the food program is too high in protein and fat.

Dual-Metabolism Type

The rare **dual metabolism** (3 percent of the population) can digest and utilize all three food groups with equal efficiency. This metabolism results from a combination of genetic factors and environmental activities throughout a lifetime. This food program should be equally divided between fats, proteins, and carbohydrates, and the ideal exercise program for this type should consist of 50 percent cardiovascular and 50 percent weight training. Given the proper dietary and exercise regimen, this type has a body that combines both strength and endurance. A person with a dual metabolism has an athletic V-shaped appearance, with wide shoulders, narrow hips, and evenly distributed muscular mass. When someone with a dual metabolism gains excess weight, this person will gain it equally in all parts of the body.

This metabolic type is the most sensitive of all three metabolisms, yet the most responsive when fed correctly. Since this metabolism requires a balance of all three nutrients to be efficiently fueled, it is always adversely affected when trying to follow popular diets, as most of the current weight-management programs on the market are either high-protein or high-carbohydrate in design. When improperly fed, it will hoard fat more rapidly than all other metabolisms. But when fed the correct balance of carbohydrate, protein, and fat, this type responds fastest.

While metabolism is partly a product of environment—for example, many professional athletes and their children have the super-efficient dual metabolism—most of the factors that influence metabolic type are genetic. In other words, whatever foods were plentiful in the part of the world that one's ancestors came from are most likely the kinds of foods that a person can most easily digest. People who live in cold, harsh northern climates tend to be fat-and-protein-efficient since their bodies need large amounts of these food groups to stay warm and active. In fact, Eskimos, before their contact with outsiders, ate a diet made up almost entirely of fat and protein, yet had no heart disease whatsoever since their bodies were so well adapted to efficiently digesting and utilizing these energy sources. On the other hand, people who inhabit tropical or equatorial regions are carbohydrate-efficient. Their bodies are designed to function best on what is at hand—predominantly grains, vegetables, fruits, and legumes.

Of course, since most of us are a genetic mix of ancestors from many parts of the world, discovering one's metabolic type takes a bit of investigating.

■ Discovering Your Metabolic Type

There are two basic methods for determining your metabolic type. The first and most accurate way is through what doctors refer to as a *full lipid study.* This information, found within your blood, is the most accurate method to determine your metabolic type, offering specific numeric data that can be charted and studied as your health improves through proper nutrition and exercise. Another way to assess your health history and your family's health history is through a questionnaire provided in this chapter. The old adage, "The apple doesn't fall far from the tree," holds true in this regard. If your parents, grandparents, and siblings suffer from certain types of illnesses, such as heart disease or diabetes, this will tell you something about what types of food someone with your genetic background can efficiently utilize, and the kinds of diseases to which you may be genetically predisposed.

Identifying Metabolic Type Through Blood Screening

The most accurate way to determine your metabolic type is through blood screening. Your metabolic type is based upon the evaluation of five numerical figures taken from a full lipid profile panel, easily obtained from your doctor:

High-Density Lipid Protein, or HDL. This is what is known as the "good," or protective, cholesterol. You can think of HDL as the garbage collector of the blood stream. If small amounts of plaque

A Word About How to Interpret One's Total Cholesterol Level

Ideally, for performance purposes, your total cholesterol should be 100 plus your age. Not many people will have this figure, however, because we live in a society where the average food choices contribute to higher cholesterol levels. The medical community has set a desired standard for total cholesterol of 200 or below. This is used as a general rule to indicate whether or not you are within the range that is considered healthy.

If your total cholesterol is between 200 and 239, it is considered borderline high. But the true factor that reflects whether or not you should have concerns about your health is the ratio between total cholesterol and your HDL. If your total cholesterol is 236, but your HDL is high, doctors will have fewer concerns about your health.

A cholesterol level above 240 is considered high. How much concern you should have about that figure, however, depends upon factors that cause coronary heart disease, or what doctors refer to as *CHD*. A "definite CHD" would include either a previous heart attack or a heart-rhythm disorder such as angina. CHD risk factors include:

■ male gender
■ a family history of premature heart attacks or sudden death before the age of 55 in a parent or a sibling
■ cigarette smoking—more than 10 a day
■ hypertension/high blood pressure
■ an HDL level less than 35
■ diabetes
■ history of stroke
■ severe obesity

If you have two or more CHD risk factors with a total cholesterol level of 200 to 239, you should take steps to lower your total cholesterol and raise your HDL through activities such as proper nutrition and exercise.

Keep in mind, also, that having a good total cholesterol number does not automatically mean that you are eating the proper foods for your metabolic type. One client shared her concern with me about her 72-year-old uncle. While his total cholesterol was only 168, four points less than his age, he had struggled for decades with an HDL between 20 and 25mg/dl (milligrams/deciliter of blood). During the periods when he faithfully performed cardiovascular exercises daily, which is supposed to increase HDL, he was puzzled that his HDLs never seemed to rise. His problem was that he had a fat-and-protein-efficient metabolism but had been so concerned about watching his diet that he ate too many carbohydrates for his type and did not ingest enough fats and proteins to support the elevation of HDLs. He was also wasting muscle tissue because he was undernourished.

have been laid down in your blood vessels, when you have enough HDL, you will be able to dissolve them and utilize this plaque as an energy source.

Low-Density Lipid Protein, or LDL. This, conversely, is known as the "bad" cholesterol, the type that collects in your blood vessels as plaque and clogs them if too much of it is present in your blood stream, or if there is not sufficient HDL to counteract it. Your LDL can be found by taking your total cholesterol and subtracting the sum of your HDLs plus your triglycerides divided by five.

$$\text{LDL} = \text{Total cholesterol} - \left(\text{HDL} + \frac{\text{triglycerides}}{5} \right)$$

Total Cholesterol, or TC. This is calculated by adding your HDL plus your LDL plus your triglycerides divided by five.

$$\text{Total cholesterol} = \text{HDL} + \text{LDL} + \frac{\text{triglycerides}}{5}$$

Ratio Between Your Total Cholesterol and Your HDL. The average male has a 3.5-to-1 ratio. The average female has a 4.5-to-1 ratio. The average athlete has a 2.1-to-1 to a 2.8-to-1 ratio. The lower the ratio, the more efficient your metabolism will be at utilizing fats as an energy source and proteins for tissue repair.

$$\frac{\text{Total Cholesterol}}{\text{HDL}}$$

Triglyceride Level. Triglycerides appear in the blood immediately after a meal. Under normal circumstances, triglycerides are stripped of their fatty acids as they pass through various tissues, especially adipose (beneath the skin) fat tissue and skeletal muscle. In this way, they are converted into a stored form of energy that is gradually released and metabolized between meals according to the energy needs of the body. We all know how carbohydrates satiate appetite and how great they taste, and how quickly we can become addicted to them. Unfortunately, if you are insulin sensitive and ingest too many carbohydrates for your metabolic type, your triglyceride level will elevate. When this happens, you become predisposed toward diseases such as diabetes, hypertriglyceridemia, hyperglycemia, or hypoglycemia, and even alcoholism.

Armed with an understanding of the basic vocabulary of blood chemistry and a full lipid profile obtained from your doctor, you can fill in the Blood Work Profile and use it to begin to identify your metabolic type in the table Metabolic Type by Blood Profile.

Blood Work Profile
Gender
Weight
Age
Total cholesterol
HDL
LDL
Ratio
Triglycerides

Step 1: Look at the first column in the chart on the following page. Are your numbers within the ranges of *three* of these *four* categories: HDL, ratio, total cholesterol, and triglycerides? If so, you have the rare dual metabolism. If not, go to Step 2.

Step 2: Look at the second column. Are your numbers within the ranges of any *two* of these *three* categories: HDL, ratio, and triglycerides? If so, you are carbohydrate-efficient. If not, go to Step 3.

Metabolic Typing by Blood Profile

	Dual Metabolism	Carbohydrate-Efficient	Fat-and-Protein-Efficient
MALES			
HDL	Above 45	Below 45	Above 45
LDL	100–130	Above 130	Below 100
TC	145–260	Below 240	Below 200
RATIO	3.0–5.0	Above 3.5	Below 3.5
TRIGL	60–110	Below 110	Above 140
FEMALES			
HDL	Above 45	Below 40	Above 55
LDL	100–130	Above 180	Below 110
TC	160–240	Below 240	Below 200
RATIO	Below 3.5	Above 5.0	Below 4.0
TRIGL	Below 110	Below 100	Above 140

Step 3: Look at the third column. Are your numbers within the ranges of any *two* of these *three* categories: HDL, ratio, and triglycerides? If so, you are fat-and-protein-efficient. If not, go to Step 4.

Step 4: If your HDLs are below 45, your triglycerides over 140, and your LDLs over 130, it is likely that your body is extremely out of balance nutritionally and you will not fall into any of these categories. You need to see what happens to your body after following a good, consistent food program for four weeks; in this case, the dual metabolism food program. This program will give you an equal amount of all nutrients, allowing your body to stabilize and rebalance itself. Then go have your blood test done again and follow the steps above to reassess yourself. At that time, it is likely that you will end up either as a dual metabolism or a fat-and-protein efficient metabolism.

Identifying Metabolic Type Using the Personal-Health and Family-History Questionnaires

The following health questionnaires are the ones used by my clients around the world to assess their metabolic type. I also use them with great success on my website (www.pfcnutrition.com) and with my phone clients. In Metabolic Typing Questionnaire 1, you will check off either "Yes" or "No."

Metabolic Typing Questionnaire I		
Do you have any of the following diseases?		
	Yes	No
Alcoholism		
Diabetes, Type I (juvenile onset)		
Diabetes, Type 2 (adult onset)		
Do either of your parents have any of the following diseases?		
	Yes	No
Alcoholism		
Diabetes, Type I (juvenile onset)		
Diabetes, Type 2 (adult onset)		

If you answered yes to any of the questions above, you are automatically fat-and-protein-efficient. This type of metabolism is the only one that can develop diseases related to blood sugar because fat-and-protein-efficient individuals have difficulty efficiently utilizing carbohydrates as energy.

If you answered no to all of these questions, continue on to Metabolic Typing Questionnaire 2. You will notice that some of these questions also pertain to your parents and your grandparents. Since you might be too young to have developed some illnesses such as heart disease and adult-onset diabetes, which often result from the cumulative effect of years of inappropriate nutrition, it is important to fill in the blanks referring to other family members. If you aren't sure, take the time to find out as much information as you can. Your parents' and grandparents' disease patterns can represent a scenario of your own future health profile if you continue to eat inappropriately for your metabolic type.

Some clients are not sure what constitutes heart, liver, and kidney disease, so let me give you some basic guidelines:

Heart disease includes any condition related to atherosclerosis or arteriosclerosis. One example would be a heart attack related to the buildup of plaque in your circulatory system or the degeneration of your arteries. If you, your parents, or your grandparents have had a heart attack or surgeries to insert an angioplast or a stent in the veins or arteries of their heart, those would be clear indications of heart disease.

Conditions that *do not* constitute heart disease would include mitro-valve prolapse, heart murmur, congenital defects of the heart, weakening of the heart due to rheumatic fever, or the thickening of the heart muscle due to sleep apnea. For example, one client's father died of a heart attack at the age of 35. However, this attack was caused by an episode of Quinzey's disease, a viral infection that had weakened his heart earlier in life.

I define kidney disease as any condition resulting in elevated urea levels resulting from poor kidney function; for example, kidney stones. Since proper kidney function is closely related to factors such as appropriate protein intake, the health and efficiency of your kidneys is closely tied in to appropriate nutrition. Kidney disease does not include bladder infections.

Liver disease is closely related to the processes by which insulin is produced, regulated, and utilized in the body. Therefore, poor liver function would be a clear indication that you and your family cannot easily utilize sugars if you or they are ingesting an excessive amount of carbohydrate for your metabolic types. Liver disease would not include cirrhosis of the liver.

None of these questions are cancer related. If you have had cancer in any of the organ systems listed in the questionnaire, your answer will be zero.

To get your total score for Metabolic Typing Questionnaire 2, simply add up the point values for each answer. Keep in mind that some of your answers will be zero (0), meaning that you do not have any problems in that area. For example, if your sleep is "restless," your answer will be "+3," but if your sleep is "restful," your answer will be "0."

If your score is very low, meaning that you are within one or two points of another metabolic type, it would be a good idea to go and have your blood work done. Since HMOs and insurance plans often have strict criteria for ordering blood work, it might be difficult to

Metabolic Typing Questionnaire 2

	Points
Is your sleep:	
Restful (+0)　　Restless (+3)	
Do you get food cravings?	
Yes (+0)　　No (−4)	
If yes, your cravings are most commonly (do *not* answer if "No" to cravings)	
French fries, buffalo wings, or cheese quesadillas (+2)　　Cookies, candy, or ice cream (+4)　　A juicy steak (+2)	
How many times do you urinate during the night?	
One or two (+0)　　Three or more (+2)	
Do you have night sweats or chills?	
Yes (+1)　　No (+0)	
Which of the following three body types best describes you? **If you are presently overweight, which one described you in your prime?**	
Sturdy, stocky frame that builds strength easily with exercise (+2)　　Natural V-shape body, particularly when exercising regularly (+0)　　Long and lean; difficult to build muscle (−2)	
Which activities are more comfortable for you?	
Strength activities (weight lifting, power yoga, etc.) (+2)　　Endurance activities (jogging, cycling, etc.) (−4)　　Both equally comfortable (+0)	
Can you speak while jogging without feeling strained?	
Yes (−2)　　No (+0)	
Total Points:	
How many grandparents are affected by the following diseases?	
Diabetes, Type 1 (juvenile onset)　　# of grandparents × (+3)	
Diabetes, Type 2 (adult onset)　　# of grandparents × (+3)	
Total Points:	

Please indicate which diseases affect you. Also indicate how many parents or grandparents are affected, and multiply that number times the number in parentheses. For instance, if 2 of your grandparents had gout, 2 × (−2) = −4.

You	Your parents (how many?)	Your grandparents (how many?)	Points
Gall stones			
(−5)	# of parents × (−3)	# of grandparents × (−2)	
Glaucoma			
(+3)	# of parents × (+2)	# of grandparents × (+1)	
Gout			
(−5)	# of parents × (−3)	# of grandparents × (−2)	
Heart attack or heart disease			
(−5)	# of parents × (−4)	# × (−3)	
Kidney disease			
(−3)	(−1)		
Liver disease			
(−3)	(−1)		
Stroke			
(−1)	(−1)		
		Total Points for This Section:	
		Grand Total of Points:	

get your doctor to do this without your being ill. If this is the case, you can have this done for a minimal cost at your local Red Cross or any other health service or organization that offers cholesterol testing. The type of blood panel you should ask for is a full lipid profile.

After you have finished the questionnaire, use the following criteria to determine your metabolic type. Add together all the positive numbers and all the negative numbers from the questions you answered. If you answered no to any category, count that as a zero. If your total number is positive, you are fat-and-protein-efficient. If your total number turns out to be negative, you are carbohydrate-efficient. If your total number is zero, you have a dual metabolism.

Even if you have already typed yourself using your blood panel, I suggest that you still answer these questions, as they will provide even more valuable information about your current state of health, your hereditary health risks, and how well your food patterns are working for you. For example, you might discover that you don't sleep as well as you should at night, or that you always have low-grade or serious digestive problems. That tells you something important about whether your state of health, your quality of life, and your current food choices are working for you. Sometimes you become so used to feeling bad that you no longer notice, because not feeling good seems "normal." Since this book is about becoming aware of how you feel emotionally and physically so that you can use nutrition and exercise to create a vibrant state of health and well-being, you must start by accurately assessing the state of your nutritional health, and continue to expand upon this information in subsequent chapters.

After completing this questionnaire, a client named Peter realized that he might have potential hereditary health risks since *both* his parents suffered from problems with their blood sugar, and his mom had developed Type 2 diabetes. Discovering that he was fat-and-protein-efficient, the type that does not utilize carbohydrates efficiently, Peter asked me if his family history automatically meant that he was doomed to develop blood sugar problems. I explained to him that eating a food program appropriate for his type—50 percent protein, 25 percent fat, and 25 percent carbohydrate—and doing appropriate exercise would ensure that his insulin response remained stable.

Now that we have determined your metabolic type, let's see where you currently stand healthwise.

■ Body Composition

When most people think about how much they weigh, they think in terms of pounds on a scale. While scale weight tells you something about your health, it is more important to determine body composition; that is, how many pounds of fat you carry in relation to pounds of muscle (lean weight). Your body fat compared to body weight is your body fat percentage.

This number is a very important tool in determining your health and well-being, as there are healthy and unhealthy percentages of body fat for each person's frame. The following table will give you an idea of your current condition.

Body Fat Percentage		
Level	**Men**	**Women**
Excellent, very lean	<11	<14
Good/lean	11–14	14–17
Average	15–17	18–22
Fair/fat	18–22	23–27
Obese	22+	27+

You may have read that as a person ages body fat will inevitably rise. Many body fat tables in doctors' offices or in gyms reflect this by listing higher levels of "healthy" body fat for people in their forties, fifties, and sixties. Contrary to popular opinion, you are not doomed to a higher body fat percentage just because you are getting older and undergoing hormonal changes such as menopause. Increased body fat is primarily related to improper nutrition and hydration, lack of exercise, and health decay. Of course, it is less likely that at age 60 you would have a body fat percentage of 14, but getting older does not mean that you must be resigned to "automatically" developing higher body fat, regardless of how you eat and exercise.

A number of the criteria that doctors currently use to measure one's health can be deceiving. These include scale weight and cholesterol levels. For example, I have a 47-year-old client who is 5 feet 8 inches tall and weighed 158 pounds when she first came to see me. While she knew she was overweight, she wasn't obese according the definitions laid down by the widely used height-and-weight tables developed by the Metropolitan Life Insurance Company. At 192, her total cholesterol was within the normal range, and her HDL level was great at 70. But her body fat percentage was a whopping 34.5 percent! Even though she *looked* fairly solid, and no one would have said she was obese, her high fat percentage made her *technically* obese in the area where it counted most—body composition.

Since fat is four times the volume of muscle, I always tell clients that their goal should not necessarily be to lose scale weight, but, ultimately, to "take up less room in the room." If muscle weighs more than fat, a person should strive to weigh as much as possible per square inch, but to have fewer total square inches. The scale can't tell someone how much fat or lean muscle his or her body is carrying.

■ Calculating the Ratio of Your Body Fat to Lean Muscle

Some fitness experts downplay the value of body composition, putting more emphasis on other measurements, such as the Body Mass Index. But I find that the fat-to-lean-muscle ratio is one of the most important physical indications of internal health. If the client I mentioned above whose body fat was 34.5 percent had not been accurately measured, she would not have known her high level of risk for developing obesity-related illnesses as she aged. Ultimately, as this unhealthy trend continued, her cholesterol would have climbed as well, adding to the decay of her health.

There are several techniques for calculating your body composition. I'll discuss some of the most accurate and available techniques in case you want to have this procedure done by a trained technician, but I have found that a relatively simple at-home test also gives good results.

The test I am including here falls under the category known as *anthropometric measurement,* which assumes that body fat is distributed at various sites on the body, such as the hips and waist, and can be measured there to provide a fairly accurate picture of overall body fat. (Muscle tissue is also localized at certain parts of the body, such as the biceps, forearms, and calves.) This test has a plus or minus error rate of 5 percent. To take this test, use a cloth measuring tape and get out your pen, paper, and calculator.

To have a clear understanding of the amount of *pounds* of body fat versus lean muscle tissue that you carry, multiply your total weight times your percentage of body fat. For example, if you weigh 200 pounds and your body fat is 25%, you have fifty pounds of fat on your frame:

200 lbs. × .25 (% body fat) = 50 lbs. of fat

If you subtract your body fat in pounds from your total weight, your answer will be the amount of pounds of lean tissue that you carry:

200 lbs. − 50 lbs. of fat = 150 lbs. of lean muscle

Knowing how many pounds of body fat versus lean muscle you have should increase your motivation to make a body composition

At-Home Body-Fat Test for Males

Step 1: Taking Measurements

1. Height in inches_____
2. Hips in inches_____
3. Waist in inches_____
4. Weight in pounds_____

Step 2: Determining Your Percentage of Body Fat

1. Multiply your hips (inches) _____ × 1.4 = _____ minus 2 = _____ (A)
2. Multiply your waist (inches) _____ × 0.72 = _____ minus 4 = _____ (B)
3. Add A plus B = _____ (C)
4. Multiply your height (inches) _____ × 0.61 = _____ (D)
5. Subtract D from C, then subtract 10 more: C − D − 10 = _____ %

Your answer will be your approximate body fat percentage, if you are a male.

At-Home Body-Fat Test for Females

Step 1: Taking Measurements

1. Height in inches_____
2. Hips in inches_____
3. Waist in inches_____
4. Weight in pounds_____

Step 2: Determining Your Percentage of Body Fat

1. Multiply your hips (inches) _____ × 1.4 = _____ minus 1 = _____ (A)
2. Multiply your waist (inches) _____ × 0.72 = _____ minus 2 = _____ (B)
3. Add A plus B = _____ (C)
4. Multiply your height (inches) _____ × 0.61 = _____ (D)
5. Subtract D from C, then subtract 10 more: C − D − 10 = _____ %

Your answer will be your approximate body fat percentage, if you are a female.

change. Some clients who come into my office have a body fat percentage as high as 50 percent. If that person weighs in at 240 pounds, he is carrying around 120 pounds of dead weight. No wonder he feels tired! On the plus side, I always tell such a client that he is already an athlete since he is able to carry around so much weight daily. If he can do something as physically difficult as that, then following my program should be easy.

On the other hand, an athlete who also weighs 240 pounds but whose body fat is 7 percent is carrying 16.8 pounds of fat and 223.2 of lean muscle. That's why it is so easy for him to move around on a daily basis. Consider what the energy level of this type of individual must be compared to your own.

When a client begins my program, he will repair muscle tissue and lose pounds of fat. After years of not receiving proper nutritional support, it is likely that what lean muscle he has will not be in a healthy state of repair. At the beginning of any correct food program, as muscle tissue starts to repair itself, it will start to weigh a bit more. Meanwhile, as body fat, which is four times the volume of muscle, is released as energy, a person will start to watch the inches melt off. Before he knows it, his clothes will be looser and he will be taking up less room in the room.

■ Other Body-Composition Tests

If you prefer to have a body composition test conducted by a trained technician, other options, in order of price and accuracy, include *hydrostatic weighing, bioelectrical impedance,* and *skinfold measurement with a caliper.*

Hydrostatic Weighing

Although it is the most expensive, costing between $100 and $150, hydrostatic weighing is currently considered the gold standard of body composition tests. This technique is based upon the assumption that the density and specific gravity of muscle is greater than that of fat. For this reason, lean tissue should sink in water and fat tissue should float. By comparing a test subject's mass measured while under water with his mass measured while out of water, a technician can calculate your body composition rather accurately, within plus or minus 3 percent of your true body composition. You can usually find a facility for hydrostatic weighing at a local university, hospital wellness center, college, health club, or fitness center.

Bioelectrical Impedance

This composition test is based on the fact that lean tissue, because of its higher water content, is more conductive of electrical current than fat tissue. A technician attaches a bioimpedance meter to the subject's hands and feet and passes current through the body via electrodes. The more lean tissue a person has, the greater his or her conductive potential. As with hydrostatic weighing, there is a plus or minus 3 percent margin of error, if done correctly.

These days, with the advanced technology available, even some bathroom scales are equipped with bioelectrical impedence devices that can measure body fat. Unfortunately, these scales can measure you only vertically and are generally not very accurate. It is much better to have this test done by an expert with proper equipment.

Skinfold Measurement with a Caliper

This is the most convenient method for measuring body fat since it is low cost (about $5 to $15) and is readily available at your local hospitals, physical therapy centers, health clubs, schools, universities, and through the offices of exercise physiologists and dietitians. The assumption behind this test is that subcutaneous body fat is proportional to overall body fat. Therefore, the ratio of body fat to lean muscle can be calculated by measuring anywhere from four to eight sites of skin thickness and plugging the numbers into a mathematical formula. This test has an error rate of plus or minus 5 percent, depending upon the skill of the technician administering the test. The most accurate tests are done with Skindex computerized skinfold calipers. There is a larger margin of error for tests that use manual calipers.

■ The Two Main Reasons for an Inefficient Metabolism

We have all experienced the frustration of not being able to keep ourselves thin and lean, no matter how hard we try or how much weight we lost on our last diet. The great majority of people have metabolisms that are functioning far below normal but don't know what to do about it. One widespread fitness myth is that some people have naturally "slow" metabolisms and others have naturally "fast" metabolisms. We often hear statements like these: "She eats like a bird and just keeps gaining weight" or "He eats like a horse but he's skinny as a rail." The fast- or slow-metabolism theory is even reinforced in some of the most popular diet books, leading people to conclude that metabolic rate is due to heredity, God's will, or just the luck of the draw. This is simply not so. There are two basic (and very real) reasons why metabolisms become slow, and they both stem from inefficient fueling.

The first reason is inconsistent eating habits that cause blood sugar to yo-yo up and down. The result is an irregular nutrient pattern, eating habits controlled by mood and event, and weight gain. Ideally, people should maintain consistent blood sugar levels by eating either a meal or a snack every two to four hours. Most of us, because of our busy lifestyles, significantly undereat, eating only two meals a day, or eat at such widely spaced intervals that our blood sugar goes up and down like a yo-yo. We also eat very inconsistently. One day we eat oatmeal for breakfast, the next day a piece of fruit, the next day we skip breakfast, the following day we have cold pizza or a leftover piece of birthday cake, the next day we eat a granola bar, and so on. The body never knows what kind of fuel it will get—so no wonder it hoards fat. This, by the way, is the reason almost *any* diet plan people follow will initially cause them to lose some weight, because, after years of catch as catch can, the body is finally experiencing a consistent eating pattern. The body isn't constantly in a state of emergency, trying to survive by hoarding fat.

The second reason for developing an inefficient metabolism is our natural tendency to become less active as we get older. When we are children or college-age adults, we are constantly on the move—running, playing, going out for team sports in school and in college. For that reason, we burn up everything we eat (and we eat a lot!) with little left over to store as fat. When we get older, we become deskbound or spend too many hours in front of the TV. Exercising the body is no longer part of our daily lives but turns into an activity that we must *schedule*—a workout at the gym, or a bike ride, or ball game with a friend. Much of the time, we are so busy that it is easy to relegate exercise to the lowest position on our daily priorities list.

■ The Three Internal Metabolic Thermostats

Metabolic efficiency is governed by three internal thermostats: (1) *the metabolic thermostat,* which uses calories as heat energy units; (2) *the hydration thermostat,* which uses water to create a consistent temperature pattern internally; and (3) *the insulatory thermostat,* which stores fat below the skin. It is important to understand how each of these three internal metabolic thermostats works because they ultimately regulate how efficiently the body utilizes caloric heat to provide our bodies with nutrients for energy and tissue repair. When they are *not* working efficiently, the result is weight gain in the form of body fat.

The Metabolic Thermostat

This thermostat controls caloric heat patterns. To see how it works, you need to understand three things:

- Metabolism is a function of heat.
- The definition of a calorie is a heat-energy unit.
- Fat converts to a lipid for energy only in a hot place.

To create enough heat to release fat effectively as energy, you need to establish a consistent caloric heat pattern. This means figuring out how many calories you must ingest daily to bring your metabolism to peak efficiency. Most people don't understand the crucial importance of maintaining an optimum heat pattern through proper food intake. When you start a new food program, it takes a total of forty-eight hours to create enough consistent internal caloric heat to establish metabolic efficiency.

If you are consistent with your food program, your body will maintain its caloric temperature and your body fat will drop. If, because of a particular mood or event, you undereat or skip a meal, you will have undermined your caloric-management system for that day—your body will lack sufficient calories to efficiently utilize fat and repair muscle tissue. Having lost that day, you will need an additional forty-eight hours to get back on track with your current food program. That means a total of three days lost: the day that you got off track and the two days that it will take you to re-establish metabolic efficiency through being consistent with your food program. If you undereat twice in one week, you will have lost the entire week.

Food programming is like a business in which you are trying to maintain a high level of performance in order to develop the physique and energy you want. As with any successful business, it requires a management system to which you hold yourself accountable. To fuel your body efficiently, you must eat your foods consistently throughout the day.

Water: The Hydration Thermostat

Most people don't really understand the importance of proper hydration. Since our bodies are composed of 70 percent water, this all-important nutrient is critical for everyday functioning. Water serves a number of purposes:

■ Water enables nutrients to get to cells. For example, a minimum of 3.8 grams of water is needed to utilize 1 gram of carbohydrate. If you are insulin resistant, that number can potentially double.

■ Water is essential for maintaining proper blood viscosity (density and balance of nutrients) within the vascular system.

■ Sufficient hydration creates the proper balance of salts and biles to extract toxins in the form of waste products from the body.

■ Water helps to ensure a good electrolyte balance. Muscular strength and coordination are directly related to proper hydration. Just try running or playing any sport without drinking water beforehand. You will discover that your body will not respond as efficiently or with as much coordination as it does when hydrated.

■ Water controls body temperature. Acting as a thermostat, water allows the body to regulate temperature through perspiration and sweat as the body relates to the environment. With proper hydration, the body maintains a temperature that allows for optimum performance and the regulation of fat and carbohydrate use. Lack of water will cause the body to regulate its temperature in an alternative way by hoarding fat, using its insulatory thermostat. This is just one of the many ways the body uses adaptation to ensure survival. Remember, though, the more your body has to adapt to survive, the less it can focus on performance, energy, and physique.

Ideally, the amount of water necessary for proper hydration is one ounce of water per one pound of body weight. For example, a person weighing 160 pounds should drink 160 ounces (twenty 8-ounce glasses or about three 1.58-quart bottles) of water a day. This may seem like a lot, but you will be surprised at how easy it is to adjust to this amount. If you begin your day with a few glasses, have a few with every meal, and carry a bottle of water with you, staying properly hydrated will become an easy part of your routine. You will also notice that your body feels better when you drink enough water and that you actually experience mild discomfort or thirst when you are underhydrated.

There is a lot of controversy among medical practitioners about correct water intake. For years, the standard advice given by doctors has been to drink eight 8-ounce glasses of water per day. However, when you look at how widely people vary in size and weight, it makes no logical sense to conclude that every single person has the same daily water requirement and should drink the same amount of water every day!

Keep in mind that the coffee, tea, and diet soda that you drink—which contain caffeine, tannins, and other chemicals that the body must process—are not the same as pure water and should not be included as part of your total water intake, and may at times, because of caffeine content, produce an adverse diuretic effect.

Sometimes a client will ask me if it is possible to overhydrate. I tell them, "I've explained to you the rule of proper hydration. That's the number that is medically, scientifically, best suited for someone with your particular body weight. When it comes to drinking more, simply use common sense." Drinking twice as much water will *not* give you twice the benefit. But if it is a hot day and you have just had a strenuous workout in the gym, played tennis for an hour, or jogged two miles, your body will undoubtedly require a bit more water that day to replenish itself and rebalance your electrolytes. On physically active days, when you are perspiring more than usual, pay attention to your level of thirst. Something you should *not* do, however, is come to the end of your day, realize that you have had only a third of your daily water intake, and quickly drink three more quarts right before going to bed. If you do this, you will have a very uncomfortable night's sleep!

The Insulatory Thermostat

If your daily intake of water is too low, your body then moves to the third internal thermostat, the insulatory thermostat. Water acts as a heat regulator to control your core body temperature, helping you to maintain the proper internal temperature for optimal functioning. **If you do not drink enough, your body will automatically adapt the survival strategy of storing fat subcutaneously to act as insulation in order to maintain a constant core temperature. Even if your food program is completely on target, if your water intake is low, you will still hoard fat.** On the other hand, if you are drinking the correct amount of water daily, and cheat a bit on the foods, you will still continue to drop body fat. That clearly shows the sensitivity of this third metabolic thermostat. The insulatory thermostat is a survival mechanism that is used when your body experiences trauma and needs to adapt in order to survive.

■ Examples of Eating for Your Metabolism

Over the years, it has never failed to thrill me to see the phenomenal changes that occur in people's bodies, self-esteem, sex lives, and health whenever they begin eating and exercising for their metabolic type. I have seen people transform themselves from depressed, exhausted, obese individuals, hiding under baggy clothing, into confident men and women who are filled with energy, lean and fit, and proud to show off their bodies to the world.

As my clients drop pounds, inches, and clothing sizes, they tell me heartwarming stories about improved marriages and relationships, and that they inspire greater respect from their colleagues and from the world at large because, through proper weight loss and metabolically appropriate dietary regimens, they now feel more confident and in control of their lives.

To show how metabolic typing works, here are stories of three different individuals who represent the three metabolic types: fat-and-protein-efficient, carbohydrate-efficient, and the dual metabolism. While their stories might sound exceptional, they are actually very typical of the types of dramatic changes that occur in people's lives and bodies when they learn how to fuel their metabolisms efficiently.

Case History: Jessica, a Fat-and-Protein-Efficient Metabolism

Jessica has a fat-and-protein-efficient metabolism, which means that she is able to most easily digest and utilize fats and proteins. A 41-year-old entrepreneur, Jessica came to see me because her energy levels were so low she could barely make it through the day.

At 5 feet 4 inches tall and 131 pounds, Jessica was not obese. Her total cholesterol was 197, within the normal range, and she had a great HDL of 70, demonstrating her body's ability to efficiently utilize animal protein and fat. Her problem was with her triglycerides, which were 456. "The doctors had always told me I had perfect cholesterol. In fact, my HDL and LDL ratio, at 2.8, was considered athletic. However, my triglycerides were through the roof." The "normal" serum triglycerides range is between 35 to 165 mg/dl, so Jessica's number was dangerously high.

Jessica's main problem was that she did not know how to eat the right kinds of foods to properly fuel herself. "Since I was always exhausted, I constantly ate junk food and carbs—cookies, pizza, whole bags of pretzels, hunks of cheese and bread, chocolate brownies—to keep myself going during the day. I thought eating carbohydrates was the right thing to do because fats are not good for you, right?" Since her metabolism was fat-and-protein-efficient, Jessica was only making her problem worse as her energy peaked and crashed all day long from the sugar she was ingesting. Her high triglyceride levels were also making her vulnerable to developing diabetes. The excess sugars she couldn't utilize were stored as fat, and Jessica's body fat percentage had climbed to 38.15%

Like many people, Jessica spent a significant amount of time in the gym and in exercise classes, but she wasn't using the right food program to give her the nutritional support she needed to create changes in her physique. "I never knew I was too undernourished for my body to take advantage of all that exercise. Even though I thought I was eating a lot, I wasn't eating consistently, so I wasn't ingesting enough calories."

Within two weeks of eating a food plan tailored for her fat-and-protein-efficient metabolism, Jessica's triglycerides had dropped into the normal range. "I felt as if I woke up from a long, hazy journey, as if I had been living with a film of exhaustion over my eyes for years. Suddenly, the world looked bright again, and I felt energized and inspired."

As the weeks went by, Jessica began to see even more transformations. "My posture, strength, and endurance improved. When I finally began getting enough protein, my body fat dropped to 24 percent, a loss of 14 percent in just eight weeks. I had been ashamed of my high body fat and felt relieved and happy to see such a great change."

Jessica's story clearly shows what can happen to a person when she begins eating for her metabolic type. At the end of that eight-week period, her triglyceride levels had dropped to 95, her weight was a lean and toned 126, her total cholesterol level was 176, her HDL had climbed to an amazing 79, and her LDL had dropped to 78. Her ratio of total cholesterol to HDL was a healthy 2.2.

"Before I started Phil's program I was actually dreading my vacation plans—kayaking in the Caribbean with my husband. The idea of living in a bathing suit made me shudder. In fact, the mere idea of shopping for a suit was depressing. After only two months of eating right for my metabolic type, my body changed shape so dramatically that I strutted around in my bathing suit with total confidence and pride."

Case History: Bob, the Carbohydrate-Efficient Metabolism

When Bob, a 42-year-old man, first came to see me, he was lethargic and suffered from bloating and constipation. His body temperature went up and down, and sometimes he would find himself feeling hot and sweaty in the middle of a business meeting. Bob was afraid that this embarrassing sweatiness was making him look nervous, unprepared, and unsure of himself.

Bob's exhaustion and the negative effects it was having on his life was the main reason he had come to my office. "I couldn't seem to drum up any enthusiasm for my job anymore, and I was scared that I was losing my edge. It was the same at home. Half the time, I was too tired to even go out on the weekends. This was getting to be a real problem between me and my wife, who is very extroverted and has a lot of friends. She said I was turning us both into hermits."

Over the last five years Bob, who is 5 feet 11 inches had gained 40 pounds and now weighed 230. His body fat, which was at 31 percent, reflected that gain. He had lost about 15 pounds six months before on the Atkins Diet but had gained it all back. "Even after I quit the diet, which was making me feel sick, I still tried to stay away from carbohydrates such as bread, pasta, potatoes, and rice, and tried to eat a lot of protein. From what I'd read, carbohydrates made people fat, so why should I eat them?" Bob's blood work reflected this. His HDLs, at 25, were so low that he didn't have the capacity to utilize the fats and proteins he was ingesting. His LDLs were 200. His triglycerides were in the mid-normal range at 80, indicating that he had a high capacity to utilize carbohydrates.

I explained to Bob that, on a high-fat and -protein diet, foods he could not efficiently digest and utilize, all he was doing was laying down plaque, elevating his cholesterol levels, and running the risk of heart disease. After we had reviewed his current food program, I removed the heavy fats and proteins he was eating consistently throughout the day and gave him protein only at two meals—4 ounces at lunch and 8 ounces at dinner. I also suggested that he eat proteins that are low in fats, such as fish and chicken.

After three months on the correct food program for his metabolic type, Bob had fantastic results. His weight dropped to 197 pounds, his HDLs elevated to 39, his LDLs had dropped to 125, and his body fat to 16 percent. His triglycerides remained stable at 80. "The other day someone I hadn't seen in six weeks told me how great I looked. He didn't just say it once, he said it over and over, 'Man, what are you doing to yourself? You look fantastic!' And he's not the only one. My sister flew in from New York last week, and she said she'd really been worried about me and had been trying to work up the courage to tell me I needed to lose weight.

"What I'm most happy about is my marriage. My wife, Alley, and I have been together for ten years, and all the fizz had gone out of our marriage. But now she can't stop telling me how much she loves the 'new me,' and our sex life is the greatest it's ever been. We just got back from our second honeymoon in Hawaii. Best of all,

Alley has started Phil's program, and I can already see the results. We've both decided that we're going to take it to the limit."

Case History: Joy, the Dual Metabolism

Joy is a classic example of a dual metabolism, an individual who can utilize fats, proteins, and carbohydrates with equal ease. Her family history also reflects this ability—only one person in her immediate family has ever had any heart or blood sugar diseases, indicating that most of her closest relatives have no difficulty efficiently utilizing fats, proteins, and carbohydrates. Joy was 47 years old, weighed 158 pounds, had a body fat of 34.5 percent and a total cholesterol level of 192.

Joy was shocked to find out that her body fat was so high. "Since I walked an hour a day, every day, and ate what I considered to be a 'healthy' diet of organic vegetables, soy, dairy, and seafood, I had expected that number to be much lower. Realizing where my body had gotten to just blew me away."

As I assessed Joy's current food patterns, I discovered two important nutritional issues. First, she was not eating for her metabolic type. Her medical questionnaire and blood work clearly showed that she had a dual metabolism, which requires a diet of 33.3 percent fat, 33.3 percent protein, and 33.3 percent carbohydrate. But her typical daily meals consisted of toast with butter and half an avocado for breakfast; a large salad of raw vegetables, cheese, and a half can of tuna or salmon for lunch; a late-afternoon scone; and a piece of fish or chicken for dinner with a tossed salad or one vegetable. Joy was trying to eat a healthy, organic, semivegetarian meal because that was what she thought was good for her. But the truth was, she needed more protein and carbohydrates for breakfast and lunch to help her repair muscle tissue and to give her the energy she needed. By 4:00 in the afternoon, she would usually feel so exhausted that she'd go out to Starbucks and have a maple scone and a cup of coffee, just to get her through the rest of the day.

Second, when I added up Joy's daily calories, I discovered that she was 650 calories below what she needed to efficiently fuel her metabolism. In other words, her metabolic rate was only functioning at 66 percent of its full capacity. This was one of the primary reasons Joy was hoarding fat, because her metabolism was cool.

Joy had danced and been very athletic throughout her twenties and thirties, but her life had become more sedentary in her forties. Improper fueling of her body, especially lack of sufficient protein to repair her body after her daily sessions of aerobic activity, had caused her to lose 9 pounds of muscle over the years. This could be seen in her poor posture. She simply didn't have enough muscle to support her skeletal structure and hold herself upright. Also, as the athletic dual metabolism, Joy needed 50 percent of her exercise program to be weight training. At that time, she was doing no strength training at all. Initially, I asked her to stop all exercise for the next two weeks so that her body would have a chance to repair itself as she began to increase the amount of calories of fat, protein, and carbohydrates in her food program. "At first it was scary to eat all that food, but I immediately noticed a difference in how I felt. I had tons of energy throughout the day and never bottomed out. When Phil finally told me to start exercising again, I noticed that my lower back, which used to hurt when I worked out, began to feel stronger. That had been a problem since I'd hit my forties."

For the last five months, Joy has been following the appropriate food-and-exercise plan for her dual metabolism. Her current weight is 136 pounds, which means that she has lost 22 pounds of scale weight. In terms of body composition, however, she has actually lost 26.7 pounds of fat and gained 5.8 pounds of muscle since her body fat percentage has dropped 14 points to 20.5 percent. "What is really amazing to me is how low my cholesterol and triglycerides have become. I started out in the normal range, with good HDLs, even though I knew my ideal total cholesterol should be 100 plus my age. I never dreamed, however, that I would do *better* than the ideal. After five months on his program, I have a total cholesterol of 137, an HDL of 66, a ratio value of 2.1:1, triglycerides at 52, and blood glucose of 84. That's better than perfect for a dual metabolism and, according to Phil, I'm as internally healthy as a person can get. I'm just amazed. I never thought I could be so healthy and fit.

"Although I'm still working on getting my body fat percentage lower, I can't believe how wonderful my body looks to me in the mirror every day. I realize that I'd just given up, thinking that putting on an extra ten pounds each decade was a natural part of aging. What really floored me, however, was buying a dress for my cousin's wedding. I used to wear a size twelve, so I took a size ten into the dressing room. It was too big, so I went out and got a size eight. *That dress size was too big.* I tried on a six, and I couldn't believe the sexy woman who was staring back at me in the dressing room mirror.

"I've always been an attractive woman, and I'd feared getting older, even though I kept telling myself that it was okay as long as the inner person had substance. But since I've been on Phil's program, I realized that I am no longer afraid of getting old because I know I can do it with strength, grace, beauty, and health. And that means everything to me."

These are just three examples of the thousands of people that have discovered a leaner, healthier, more confident self on my program. People like Jessica, Bob, and Joy are the reason I get out of bed in the morning, because I love to watch people's lives transform physically, emotionally, and spiritually as they learn to eat and exercise to fuel their unique metabolisms. So, what would you rather do? Watch your weight yo-yo up and down over the years as you alternately starve yourself and gain back the weight? Or would you rather eat well, always feel full, and watch yourself getting healthier and stronger every week? You decide.

■ Playing the Genetic Cards You Were Dealt

In general, I find that the female clients who come to me for nutritional coaching want to be thin and lean, and the men want to be muscular and lean. These results are not always possible, however. I tell each of my clients, "You have been dealt certain genetic cards. There is a lot you can do with those cards, but you cannot develop a body type that you do not possess. Instead, strive to do the best you can with what you have. Most of the time, I promise that you'll find that pretty darn amazing."

For example, I often find that my carbohydrate-efficient male clients want to develop more muscularity but feel frustrated when they can't "bulk up." The reason for this is that the carbohydrate-efficient type has a naturally leaner body that does well at endurance activities like running and swimming. If this kind of person is willing to do a tremendous amount of focused weight training, he might put on a good deal of muscle, but, under normal circumstances, he will always look more like a Dennis Quaid than an Arnold Schwarzenegger.

If a carbohydrate-efficient woman or one with a dual metabolism wants to look thin and willowy, she can successfully achieve that goal. But women who are fat-and-protein-efficient will find this difficult because their bodies naturally want to develop muscle tissue for a physique that is strong and robust. When working with women who have this predisposition, I always tell them, "These are the genetic cards you were dealt. They represent a specific metabolic framework, and we have to do the very best we can to develop the type of physique you want, but within this framework."

For the most part, I tend to work somewhat differently with my fat-and-protein-efficient female clients than I do with fat-and-protein-efficient men. With the guys, the sky's the limit regarding how much muscle they want to add to their body. And, of course, there are some women who also really like that look—they, too, want to be very muscular and athletic-looking. But most of my female clients would rather be as svelte as possible. In order to accommodate their goal, I control their physical development within the framework of their genetic metabolic structure, coaching them weekly about their physique and structural reality.

The fat-and-protein-efficient woman will seldom be able to develop a waiflike look, but she can still become svelte. Gillian Anderson and Kirstie Alley are fat-and-protein-efficient. Both women have muscular, athletic physiques that are also very sensual, strong, and beautiful. Many shorter women with stockier arms and legs are fat-and-protein-efficient. This physique, when properly fueled and given an appropriate exercise regime, will be tremendously appealing and athletic.

If you aspire to have the look of a *Cosmopolitan* magazine cover girl, know that there is beauty in every metabolic type. Each has its own distinctive look. If you are fat-and-protein-efficient, you may never have the long sinewy legs of a runway model. But know that you can maintain a great deal of muscularity with incredible athletic vitality, which would obviously look great on the cover of any magazine. If you are carbohydrate-efficient or dual metabolism, know that you cannot truly have that more muscular look, but you will be able to develop a long willowy physique that also looks beautiful. In my experience, it is always much better to be who you really are—to work within the framework of your genetics to develop the body that you were born with and to find beauty in it. Strive to be the best and the healthiest you can be.

■ When Thin People Feel Too Fat

One type of individual who suffers from an inaccurate body image is the person (usually a woman) who believes that she is always overweight no matter how thin she is. This person sees fat where none exists. She usually perceives herself as very "fit" because she exercises a lot. But her limbs may actually look twiglike because she does not eat enough of the proper nutrients to correctly repair her muscle tissue. She is one example in a group of thousands who display symptoms of eating disorders such as anorexia or bulimia. Eating disorders, especially among young people, are increasingly common. It is estimated that as many as 10 to 15 percent of adolescent girls and young women suffer from them.

A client named Judith is a fitness model with a dual metabolism. She came to my clinic for nutritional coaching because she needed my help to get rid of those "pockets of fat" that her rigorous exercise program could not eradicate. Judith was extremely physically fit, and there was not an ounce of fat on her body. What she called fat were actually small folds of skin that were just that—skin. But she was so obsessed with getting rid of these perceived imperfections that she sought my help.

Judith's inaccurate perception of her body as fat has narrowed the hallway of her life so much that she has become imprisoned within her food choices. When she is not modeling, Judith does nothing but take naps in the afternoon and exercise in the gym. She follows a strict six-meal regimen, meticulously measured. She spreads these minimeals throughout the day so that she has just enough energy to function. Sometimes she allows herself two ounces of tuna before she goes to bed.

If someone says to Judith, "God, you look thin," she answers, "But I eat six times a day." When they ask her what she eats, she says, "I eat fish, steak, and chicken." And she does. But her portions are so small that they don't give her anywhere near the nutritional support she needs to keep her metabolism efficient and her performance levels high. All she does is model, exercise, and nap—she does nothing extraneous.

Another version of Judith would be the individual who is so obsessed with the fad lifestyles portrayed in fashion magazines that her eating pattern is always based on the calorically restricted diets of popular models. In her attempt to achieve a high-fashion look, she may eat only a salad with a little protein once a day. This growing nutritional trend in the U.S. leads to innumerable accounts of health decay and even death each year.

The difficulty with getting these clients to understand that they are malnourished is that they usually consider themselves to be experts on nutrition. In these cases, when I coach them I preface my statements about health and food programming with remarks such as, "As I'm sure you know, . . ." or "You probably had this happen before. . . ." To some degree, these individuals are nutritionally educated and well read on the subject of dieting. They usually *appear* very physically fit, and involve themselves in a lot of health-conscious activities and choices, such as drinking lots of water and avoiding sweets. Yet they are rapidly wasting muscle tissue in their quest for leanness because their portions are too small. My job is to help them make that quantum leap into the idea that one must eat more food to maintain health and optimum weight. I re-educate them about what an athletic female body looks like, versus a body that shows signs of wasting muscle tissue. Have you ever seen those women at the gym who are very slim, but the legs sticking out of their gym shorts look almost frighteningly thin? They usually have no calf muscles to speak of and so little fat in their arms and legs that their muscles look wiry and sharply delineated. That kind of physique is not healthy, athletic, or attractive.

3. Creating a Youthful Future

Eating for Your Metabolic Type

Like everything in life, from running a business to running a home, successful food programming is about coming up with an effective daily *management system*. Learning how to eat for your metabolic type may take a certain amount of paying attention to your meal patterns, but it will soon become just another one of your daily routines, one that will make all others easier to manage, causing you to be a more effective individual. The results that you will see within weeks—weight loss, greater energy and performance levels, fewer moods swings, and better sleeping patterns—will inspire you to continue. The implementation of this plan within your life can truly help you to achieve the youthfulness and longevity all of us seek.

Unlike fad diets that leave you feeling hungry, nutritionally restricted, and irritable, the Turn Up the Heat Program will leave you satisfied and full. As one of my clients, a man in his late forties named Craig, told me, "I don't like to think of myself as dieting. For me, that occurs as a whole world of deprivation about things I can't have. I don't like to think about my life that way. But your program isn't a diet. It's a designed way of eating and living that works for me. It provides a great deal of personal empowerment."

In this chapter I will coach you on how to set up your Foundation Food Program for your metabolic type. This will be accomplished in four easy-to-follow steps:

1. Determine the average amount of calories you eat per day.
2. Establish a caloric number representative of your active basal metabolic rate (ABMR), the amount of calories you need to support your normal body functions and daily activities. Using these two caloric amounts, you will then be able to:
3. Determine at what caloric temperature your metabolism currently functions and how far you are from your ideal metabolic temperature of 100 degrees (ABMR). This will enable you to:
4. Establish a daily caloric intake that will stabilize your metabolism, match your metabolic type, and act as the foundation for future weekly food patterns.

Once you have established your Foundation Food Program, I will show you how to move forward from week to week, adjusting your food choices as your body changes and your metabolism heats up, becoming more efficient at burning fat as energy and utilizing nutrients appropriate for your metabolic type.

Initially, as you calculate your correct daily caloric intake, chances are you will discover that currently you are actually ingesting fewer calories than needed to properly repair and maintain your body and reduce body fat. I will show you how to use the charts provided in part II of the book to gradually raise your caloric intake of foods specific to your metabolic type until you have increased your metabolic efficiency to 100 percent (100 degrees). At this point, the amount and type of calories you are ingesting will accurately match your active basal metabolic rate, and all of your physiological processes will be operating at peak efficiency. When this happens, you will be able to lose weight by burning excess body fat and be able to repair and build lean muscle. As we shall see later, there is a very small portion of the population whose metabolisms are *more* efficient than 100 degrees—bodybuilders or elite athletes who carry a *much* higher percentage of lean muscle on their frame than the average person. But for most of us, 100 percent metabolic efficiency (100 degrees) is our ultimate nutritional goal.

Your Foundation Food Program (first week's menu) will not be too calorically different from your current food program. It is primarily designed to stabilize your metabolic temperature and eating patterns. It was not designed for substantial weight loss. Future weekly dietary protocols will be built upon this foundation. These later weeks will move you toward the proper percentages and amounts of foods you should ingest daily for your metabolic type. The result of this will be fat loss, muscular repair, improved digestion, better sleep, stable moods, and increased energy.

It is unsafe and unhealthy to move directly from your current eating habits into a radically different program suited for your metabolic type. Your body would naturally resist such a drastic restructuring, and the results would be digestively and metabolically traumatic. For example, if you are fat-and-protein-efficient, ideally 50 percent of your calories should be protein to keep your body in optimum condition. But if for the last ten years you have been eating a mostly vegetarian diet containing a high percentage of carbohydrate foods, such as breads, cheese, rice, pasta, and potatoes, and only 25 percent protein, you couldn't suddenly increase your protein intake to 50 percent and still remain healthy. Your body would have difficulty adjusting to this 100 percent increase in protein and would possibly develop conditions such as constipation, gastritus, gall stones, exhaustion, restless sleep, difficulty in concentrating, anxiety, and mood swings. If you suddenly went on a high-protein, low-carbohydrate diet such as the Atkins program, the results would be the same. Your body would resist this drastic nutritional shift and experience the symptoms described above.

Instead, your food programs will gradually change weekly, at first resembling a caloric structure not unlike your current food pattern. As each week passes, the new menu structures will more closely resemble your metabolic type and ideal caloric scenario. These patterns will shift weekly, in 10 to 15 percent increments calorically and nutritionally.

As your body responds to these food programs, you will not only lose scale weight but you will also see your body composition change. You will gain lean muscle and lose fat. Since fat is four times the volume of lean muscle tissue, your goal will be to weigh as much as you possibly can per square inch, but to take up fewer square inches of space. In other words, to "take up less room in the room."

Remember, this food program is not about "always being right." It's about doing the best you can, paying enough attention to your food plan to improve weekly. If you attempt to follow this program to the best of your ability, you can do no wrong. The simple effort of making good choices about the foods best suited for your metabolic type, and trying to eat them consistently, will be a breakthrough from your old nutritional habits. It will teach you to take responsibility for the food choices you make and to remember that you need to stay well fueled to lose weight. Once you have worked with this food program for a few weeks, you will find that even your "worst" eating days are better than your "best" days under your old eating habits.

■ Step 1: Calculating Your Average Caloric Intake

This section will teach you to calculate how many calories you are currently eating during an average day. First, you will need to keep track of everything you eat over the course of three days. It is best if you choose two weekdays and one weekend day because people often eat differently on the weekends. To calculate the caloric content of what you eat, pay attention to your portion sizes, write down the content of your restaurant meals, and read the caloric values on the labels of any packaged foods you choose. Don't forget to keep track of things such as salad dressing, butter, and mayonnaise. Most of us eat these foods in small amounts, but they can significantly contribute to caloric content.

Photocopy the following chart and use it to record what you eat for three days. To find the caloric value of each food, use appendix A in the back of the book or buy an inexpensive pocket-size calorie counter. When you are finished, calculate the average of these three days to get a more accurate account of your normal caloric consumption.

■ Step 2: Calculating Your Active Basal Metabolic Rate

Next, you'll calculate your resting basal metabolic rate (BMR)—this is the number of calories your body needs to complete all of its complex functions, such as digestion, breathing, and the circulation of your blood each day. To find your resting BMR, divide your body

Add up your calories for each of the three days and then divide by 3 to get an average. **Here is an example:**

Day 1 Total Calories = 1,357
Day 2 Total Calories = 1,315
Day 3 Total Calories = 1,823
Grand Total = 4,495

4,495 Calories ÷ 3 = 1,498 (Daily Caloric Average)

DAY #

Name of Food	Quantity	Calories
	Total Calories:	

Day 1 Total Calories = _____
Day 2 Total Calories = _____
Day 3 Total Calories = _____

Grand Total = _____ ÷ 3 = _____ (Your Daily Caloric Average) weight in pounds by 2.26. Then multiply that number by 24 and round off your answer to whole numbers.

Here is an example:

Body Weight: 160 lbs. ÷ 2.26 × 24 = 1,699 = (Resting BMR)

Your Body Weight: _____ lbs. ÷ 2.26 × 24 = _____ (Your Resting BMR)

The figure above represents the number of calories your body would need if you were to lie in bed all day without moving a muscle (that is, your *resting* basal metabolism).

Your active basal metabolic rate (ABMR) is a higher number that takes into account your resting BMR in addition to your daily *activity* level—walking, driving, shopping, exercising; all of these movements raise your daily caloric expenditure. To calculate your ABMR, use your resting BMR and your gender.

Here is an example for males:

A Resting BMR of 1,699 × 1.15 = 1,954 (Active BMR [Equal to 100°])

Males: Your BMR: _____ × 1.15 = _____ = Your Active BMR

Here is an example for females:

A Resting BMR of 1,699 × 1.1 = 1,869 (Active BMR [Equal to 100°])

Females: Your BMR: _____ × 1.1 = _____ = Your Active BMR

■ Step 3: Determining Your Current Metabolic Temperature

The relationship between your current average daily caloric intake (step 1) and your Active Basal Metabolic Rate (step 2) is a very important aspect in determining your metabolic efficiency. Remember, calories are heat-energy units, and your metabolism is a function of that caloric heat. Metabolic efficiency is the ability to effectively use fat as an energy source and repair muscle tissue.

Although we have been talking about a goal of 100 percent (100 degrees) metabolic efficiency, in actuality we will use a temperature scale of 0 to 150 degrees. I designed the metabolic temperature scale this way because *it is possible to have a core metabolic temperature over 100 degrees if you are an athlete or bodybuilder who has an exceptionally low body fat percentage and a greater than average amount of lean muscle.* These individuals require additional caloric heat to adequately fuel and repair muscle tissue, requiring their daily caloric intake to be over and above their ABMR. Later, I will show you how to calculate the amount of calories needed to fuel this type of metabolism.

To complete step 3, review the average number of calories you currently consume daily (as you calculated in step 1). Compare this number with your body's ideal daily caloric needs, known as your "ideal metabolic temperature," or Active Basal Metabolic Rate, which when represented as a temperature is 100 degrees. When you are consistently consuming a number of calories that matches your ABMR, you are at 100 degrees. At this point you are burning fat and repairing muscle tissue efficiently.

In step 2 you calculated a caloric amount that represents your ABMR. This figure is the amount of daily caloric heat your body ideally needs to utilize fat efficiently and to repair muscle tissue. In order to use fat as energy and to reduce body fat correctly, your daily caloric intake should ideally equal calories equivalent to your ABMR. When this occurs, you are ingesting sufficient caloric heat daily to support a metabolic temperature (100 degrees) that can efficiently burn body fat as energy.

It is possible to metabolically function above your ABMR (100 degrees) and continue to burn fat, as is the case with numerous athletes who carry a great amount of muscle tissue to support their physical needs and exercise requirements. This additional muscle tissue requires an increased amount of caloric heat to properly fuel and repair it. The amount of additional calories ingested daily varies from athlete to athlete, depending upon his or her lean muscle mass.

In the rare case that you are actually overeating—ingesting calories over and above your ABMR—and are not an athlete, this program will adjust nutrient percentages to create a more efficient metabolism that will enable weight loss and tissue repair, and guide you toward your correct adjusted daily caloric intake.

Discovering your current metabolic temperature is a critical aspect of understanding your current metabolic efficiency. A daily caloric intake of less than 100 degrees of your ABMR indicates a suppressed metabolism. A daily caloric intake that represents 79 degrees or less will result in an acutely suppressed metabolic condition. The cooler your metabolic temperature, the less efficient your metabolism. When you are consuming a number of calories that match your ABMR, your metabolism is functioning at 100 degrees, and at this point, it is burning fat efficiently.

To calculate your current metabolic temperature, divide your three-day caloric average by your ABMR and multiply it by 100 degrees. See the table below.

Here is an example:

Three-Day Caloric Average:	Active 1,245 ÷ BMR: 1,699 × 100° = 73°	Current Metabolic Temperature
Three-Day Caloric Average: _____ (Current Caloric Temperature)	Active ÷ BMR: _____ × 100° = _____	Current Metabolic Temperature

At 73 degrees the individual above is operating at about three-quarters of his metabolic efficiency. How did you turn out? Place yourself on the scale below to visually measure your current metabolic temperature.

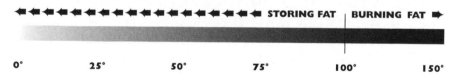

If your metabolic temperature is below 100 degrees, your metabolism is suppressed. Of course, the lower your number, the more severely suppressed your metabolism is. Obviously, if your metabolic temperature is in the lower ranges, your body is storing fat, not efficiently burning it. Remember, any temperature below 80 degrees is considered acutely suppressed.

■ Step 4: Creating Your Food Programs and Determing Your Metabolic Scenario

At this point, you know four things: (1) your metabolic type, (2) your current daily caloric intake, (3) your Active Basal Metabolic Rate (ideal caloric intake to reach a metabolic temperature of 100 degrees), and (4) your current metabolic temperature. This is all the information you need to begin your food programming.

There are five metabolic scenarios described below. You will recognize yourself in one of these. Simply follow the instructions given and you will be able to easily identify your caloric level and your first week's menu, your Foundation Food Program.

Metabolic Scenario 1: Metabolic Starvation (Fewer Than 1,200 Calories Daily)

If your three-day caloric average is less than 1,200 calories, then you have, through the years, developed such an adversarial relationship with food that you have starved your metabolism. At this low caloric intake, you are hoarding fat and wasting muscle tissue to an extreme degree. The coping mechanisms you have chosen to manage your current food plan have perhaps caused the development of behaviors that are leading you toward an eating disorder. To begin repairing the damage done to your body and your metabolism, you will need to start with a daily caloric intake of approximately 1,200 calories. Therefore, your Foundation Food Program will begin at Level 1, Week 1 for your metabolic type. (See part II, page 145, if you are fat-and-protein-efficient; page 203, if you are carbohydrate-efficient; or page 267, if you have a dual metabolism.)

In this particular scenario, your metabolism could heal rapidly. So if at any time you experience excessive hunger, immediately elevate yourself to the appropriate week of the next level.

Metabolic Scenario 2: The Severely Suppressed Metabolism (79 Degrees or Below, But Above 1,200 Calories Daily)

This scenario will be the one that fits the majority of readers since most people are eating far fewer calories than needed because they have been restricting their foods for many years in hopes of losing weight.

If your current metabolic temperature is 79 degrees or below, your metabolism is severely suppressed. Because you are eating fewer calories than you should, your body has ensured its survival by reducing its metabolic heat and establishing a new, lower (cooler) metabolic temperature. Since your body interprets your insufficient or inconsistent caloric intake as a sign of impending starvation, it has cooled itself metabolically and, therefore, adapted in order to make due with as few calories as possible, choosing to store calories as fat rather than to burn them. You will need to gradually consume more calories until you have created sufficient metabolic heat to raise your core temperature to 100 degrees. You will also need to drink the appropriate daily amount of water for your current body weight to enable you to more efficiently utilize your calories as heat-energy units. These two actions will help your body begin to burn its stored fat.

When your current metabolic temperature is 79 degrees or below, it is too cool to use the caloric value of your ABMR as a nutritional starting point. Eating this amount of extra calories would adversely affect your metabolism, which would not be able to efficiently utilize that much food. Instead, you should elevate your average daily caloric intake by an increment of 10 percent and use this as your starting point. To do so, take the three-day average caloric intake you calculated in step 1 and increase that number by 10 percent. Based on this number:

■ depending on your metabolic type, go to your appropriate food plan in part II: page 145 if you are fat-and-protein-efficient; page 203 if you are carbohydrate-efficient; and page 267 if you have a dual metabolism;
■ find your appropriate caloric level within that section (the range closest to your three-day average caloric intake increased by 10 percent);
■ begin your program at week 1 of that level.

A client named Pete, who is fat-and-protein-efficient, had a severely suppressed metabolism of 75 degrees. We found that his three-day average caloric was 1,500 calories. Because his metabolic temperature was so low, we could not use the caloric value of his ABMR as a nutritional starting point. Instead, we increased his three-day average caloric intake by 10 percent to 1,650 calories. We then looked up this number in the fat-and-protein-efficient food program on page 145 and found the caloric level closest to it in Level 4. The first week of Level 4 then became his Foundation Food Program.

Metabolic Scenario 3: The Moderately Suppressed Metabolism (80 to 99 Degrees)

If your metabolic temperature is between 80 and 99 degrees, your metabolism is suppressed, but not acutely so. The closer you are to a temperature of 99 degrees, the closer you are to eating the right amount of calories for your weight. Therefore, to find the appropriate caloric level for your Foundation Food Program, you will not need to significantly increase the number of calories you are eating daily (as you would if your metabolism were severely suppressed.) Instead, start with the caloric number of your ABMR, previously calculated in step 2. Then:

■ depending on your metabolic type, go to your appropriate food plan in part II: page 145 if you are fat-and-protein-efficient; page 203 if you are carbohydrate-efficient; and page 267 if you have a dual metabolism;
■ find your appropriate level (the caloric range closest to your current caloric ABMR);
■ begin your program at week 1 of that level.

The final two scenarios described here are for people who are more fit than the average individual and already have a relatively well-structured food program, yet wish to refine and improve their nutritional rigor by eating correctly for their specific metabolic type.

Metabolic Scenario 4: Your Metabolism Is Already Operating at Full Efficiency (100 Degrees)

If your metabolic temperature is 100 degrees, your metabolism is not suppressed. In other words, it is functioning at 100 percent of its efficiency. Finding the appropriate caloric level for your Foundation Food Program will depend upon your specific physique goals. Therefore, you will choose one of the following:

(1) If you wish to maintain your current lean weight and reduce pounds of body fat, you will start with the actual caloric number of your ABMR. Doing this will enable you to maintain your current lean weight and drop unwanted body fat because you will be eating the appropriate *types* of fats, proteins, and carbohydrates needed for your metabolic type.

(2) If, however, you wish to reduce body fat while *adding* more lean muscle to your frame, simply add an additional 10 percent to your caloric ABMR if you are female, and an additional 15 percent if you are male, and then find your appropriate level:

■ depending on your metabolic type, go to your appropriate food plan in part II: page 145 if you are fat-and-protein-efficient; page 203 if you are carbohydrate-efficient; and page 267 if you have a dual metabolism;

■ depending upon your goal, either find your appropriate level (the caloric range closest to your current caloric ABMR, or the caloric number that is 10 to 15 percent higher than your ABMR, depending upon whether you are male or female);

■ begin your program at week 1 of that level.

Metabolic Scenario 5: When Your Metabolism Is Extremely Efficient (Over 100 Degrees)

Your metabolism is not suppressed. In fact, if your metabolic temperature is *above* 100 degrees, you are one of those rare individuals who consistently eats more calories than mathematically indicated by your ABMR. This means that, based on physique averages, chances are you carry more muscle tissue than most people do—either because of your genetic makeup, the athletic activities in which you are involved, or both. Therefore, you will simply gradually adjust your food program to meet the correct percentages of fat, protein, and carbohydrate for your metabolic type. As you follow the personalized food program, you will definitely begin to feel full and satisfied, while also experiencing the numerous health benefits of nutritional balance.

If your current metabolic temperature is over 100 degrees, you cannot use your ABMR because the calories you are eating right now to support your high percentage of muscle mass exceed your ABMR. Therefore, you should:

- depending on your metabolic type, go to your appropriate food plan in part II: page 145 if you are fat-and-protein-efficient; page 203 if you are carbohydrate-efficient; and page 267 if you have a dual metabolism;
- find your current three-day average caloric intake, previously calculated in step 1;
- use that figure to find your appropriate level (the caloric range closest to your current three-day caloric average);
- begin your program with week 1 of that level.

Important Points in the Turn Up the Heat Program

How often does your menu change? Once you have established your level and Foundation Food Program, as determined by your specific metabolic type and scenario, your basic menu pattern will change each week (not each day). Your food program will teach your body daily nutritional consistency by providing your metabolism with appropriate meal patterns that will stabilize your caloric intake, creating the efficient use of caloric heat. Evenly spacing meals throughout the day will help to stabilize correct metabolic processes that will aid in tissue repair, weight loss, and energy.

Your menu patterns will change every seven days because it is necessary to adjust and/or increase your weekly caloric intake to match your body's change in composition (body-fat reduction). This dynamic aspect of the food plan will keep your weight and body composition from reaching a plateau. This problem is frequently seen with static food protocols that do not change from week to week.

Frequency of eating. You will be eating five to seven meals per day and should never go more than three and a half hours without a meal. This consistency will help your body to burn fat as fuel instead of storing it.

Do not skip meals. It is vitally important that you (1) do not skip any meals, (2) eat all of the food exchanges listed in each meal, and (3) eat your meals in the proper order. That is why the meals are numbered. For example, if it is lunchtime (Meal 3) and you realize that you have not had your midmorning snack (Meal 2), eat the snack before you eat lunch, even if it means that only five minutes separate those two meals. It is *always* better to eat your food than to skip a meal. While it is best to eat consistently spaced meals, sometimes a busy lifestyle does not accommodate this food scheduling. If you can, consistently space your meals throughout the day. If your lifestyle does not allow this, plan your meals as well as you can, but remember to eat *every meal, every day*. You do not want your appetite to control your food pattern; let your food pattern control your appetite. If you eat only when you are hungry, this will cause inconsistencies in your food programming because you will often find yourself eating when you are too hungry to make wise choices. Remember, the purpose of your meals is to act as fuel to provide you with nutrients to enhance performance and physique.

Week 2: Remove breads containing yeast from your menu. After your first week it is important to either decrease or, preferably, remove all multi-ingredient bread products containing yeast and sugar combinations from your food plan. Remember, carbohydrates break down into sugars in your digestive tract. Yeast—the most invasive and infectious bacteria you can ingest—feeds on sugar, causing low and inconsistent blood sugar levels. This results in low energy levels, poor digestion, and inconsistent use of fats, proteins, and carbohydrates. While carbohydrate-efficient individuals handle bread with yeast much better than fat-and-protein-efficient individuals and the dual metabolism, it is still a wise nutritional choice to avoid all yeast-based bread products if possible. Even though breads containing yeast and sugar are listed in the Turn Up the Heat Food Exchange List in appendix B, as a general rule, *do not eat any of these after the first week*. Instead, choose pita bread, tortillas, and various other types of flat breads that do not contain yeast (or contain very low amounts of yeast).

Treat day. Sometimes, especially during the first few weeks of the program, you may find that the craving for an old favorite food, such as chocolate cake, can become overwhelming or obsessive. For that reason, I allow clients to set aside one day a week (the same day every week) to become "treat day." If, for example, you choose Saturday as your treat day, make sure that you eat all of your regular foods for that day and drink all of your water, but allow yourself to have those donuts, brie cheese, or pepperoni pizza you have been dreaming about. Just knowing that you can enjoy your favorite food one day per week, without guilt, will make it easier for you to stay on the program the other six days. You will also find that, as time goes by, you probably won't need a treat day anymore because the cravings you had for certain foods either wane or you no longer wish to have the digestive difficulties you experience after eating them. It's all about knowing that you are free to make choices.

Reassessment. Every four weeks, based on your new body weight, you will reassess your metabolic temperature for improvement and a possible shift in your caloric level. To reassess, simply use the caloric amount from whatever week you are currently in as your daily caloric average and use the formula below. This frequent caloric reassessment, based on changing body weight, enables this food program to be dynamic, not static.

There are a total of eleven levels, with Level 1 as the calorically lowest level and Level 11 as the calorically highest level. Generally speaking, the more food you consume, the higher your level. When I speak of moving up a level, I mean moving to a higher caloric level, for example, from Level 4 to Level 5. When I speak of moving down a level, I mean moving from a higher caloric level to a lower caloric level, for example, from Level 8 to Level 7. Refer to the bullet points below for *when* to change levels.

Step 1: New Resting BMR

**Your Current
Body Weight:** _____ lbs. ÷ 2.26 × 24 = _____ **(Your Resting BMR)**

Step 2: New Active BMR

Males: Your BMR: _____ × 1.15 = _____ = **Your Active BMR**

Females: Your BMR: _____ × 1.1 = _____ = **Your Active BMR**

Step 3: Current Metabolic Temperature

Three-Day Caloric Average:	**Active + BMR:**		**Current Metabolic Temperature**
_____	_____	× 100° = _____	

Based on your new metabolic temperature and ABMR, one of three things should happen. You will:

- ■ Move down a caloric level if you have lost sufficient body weight.
- ■ Stay in the same caloric level if your scale weight has not changed. If you have been faithfully following the program for that four-week period, this usually indicates an even shift between the body fat you have lost and the lean muscle you have gained. Although the scale remains generally the same, you will notice that you take up less room in the room, and that is truly more important than scale weight.
- ■ Move up a caloric level (1) if you are experiencing food cravings or (2) if you have gained enough lean muscle weight to have slightly elevated your scale weight. You do not have to get your ratio of body fat to lean muscle tested to know when you have gained lean muscle. You will easily be able to tell if your clothes are looser or you find yourself taking in your belt a notch or two. Increased strength and muscularity are also signs of this, too. Someone who is eating and exercising appropriately for his or her metabolic type will see significant changes in the space of one month.
- ■ Move up another caloric level if, upon re-evaluation, you find that your metabolic scenario has shifted to the next higher scenario, indicating that your metabolic temperature is now closer to 100 degrees. If this takes place, that is an indication that you have gained a significant amount of muscle tissue while losing body fat. Therefore, you will need to ingest a greater amount of calories to support this newly developed, metabolically active tissue.

When you move up to a higher caloric level, or down to a lower caloric level, always continue to progress through the weeks. For example, if you have completed four weeks in one level and, upon reassessing, need to move up to a higher caloric level, or down to a lower caloric level, always begin with Week 5 of that level. If you need to move up or down a level after completing Week 8, always begin with Week 9 of the next highest or lowest caloric level. The reason for this is that the further you progress through a twelve-week pattern, the more each week's food program becomes suited to the specific needs of your metabolic type.

If you find yourself finishing out a complete level of twelve weeks, you simply reassess as usual and begin with Week 1 of the appropriate twelve-week caloric level, either a new one or the one you are currently in, depending upon the results of your reassessment.

If food cravings persist or you are experiencing unusual hunger after two weeks at your level, it is all right to re-evaluate yourself at that time. Under such circumstances, I recommend that you elevate to the next higher level (and begin at Week 3 of that level). This will provide your body with more calories daily to use as fuel and help you to control your cravings. However, don't forget, you *must* re-evaluate yourself every four weeks.

Your goal is to reach a caloric intake that brings you as close as possible to 100 degrees (or over, if your metabolic profile fits scenario 4 or 5).

■ The Four Categories of Food

As you look through the Turn Up the Heat Food Exchange List for your food program (appendix B, page 341), you will find the foods you will be eating listed according to the following four categories: Vegetables, Fruits, Breads, and Meat. I explain each category below:

Category 1: Vegetables

Vegetables are *fibrous carbohydrates* with very few energy-source calories. Therefore, including these important foods in your program will not significantly increase your caloric intake. But vegetables do add vital micronutrients, minerals, and fiber to your diet that promote a healthy digestive process. If you are still hungry after a meal, you can eat extra servings of vegetables, but make sure to finish all your other foods. Some examples of vegetables include spinach, tomato, and lettuce. Quantities in the Food Exchange List pertain to raw vegetables. So, in other words, if you are allowed 1 cup of asparagus, measure that cup *before* cooking. Steaming vegetables is best for your digestion. Restrict vegetables such as broccoli, cauliflower, carrots, and any vegetable with a waxy (paraffin-coated) skin (like cucumbers) if you have a sensitive stomach or are prone to difficult or inconsistent digestive tendencies such as irritable bowel disorder or gastritus.

Category 2: Fruits

Fruits are a *simple carbohydrate*, making them an energy-source food. Unlike complex carbohydrates, which offer a long-lasting, starch-based source of energy, fruits, which contain the simple sugar fructose, offer a quick, less stable energy source. Examples of fruits include bananas, apples, oranges, and berries. It is best to avoid juices and dried fruits since they are extremely high in sugar content compared to a single serving of fresh fruit.

Much has been written about the glycemic index of fruits, cautioning people to avoid high-glycemic fruits such as bananas and pineapples. In my experience, this is nutritionally irrelevant. In reality, all portions of fruits, as listed in the Food Exchange List, are approximately within 10 to 20 calories of each other and will be utilized by the body in exactly the same way. In other words, they are nutritionally and calorically equal.

Category 3: Bread

When you see the word "bread" listed in the menu plans in this book, it refers to starch-based *complex carbohydrates*. This type of carbohydrate produces a slow rise in blood sugar and is considered a long-term source of energy, compared to simple carbohydrates such as candy or fruit.

Subcategories of "Bread" include (1) starchy vegetables such as potatoes, winter squash, and corn; (2) beans and legumes such as kidney beans and peas; (3) yeast-bound breads, such as bagels or sandwich breads; (4) no- or low-yeast multi-ingredient breads such as pita or levash; (5) cereals such as corn grits and oatmeal; (6) pastas such as spaghetti or rice noodles; (7) grains such as white and brown rice or bulgar wheat.

Category 4: Meat

Meat includes all foods in which most of the calories come from protein. Foods found in the meat list promote tissue repair and supply the body with dietary fats that are used as an energy source. The best protein choices are eggs, fish, poultry, and beef since the amino acid profiles of these foods are the same as that of human muscle, enabling them to efficiently repair and build muscle tissue. Meats have varying amounts of fat, with fish as the leanest and beef as the fattiest. You should only consider foods such as soy protein, tofu, and beans as an item from the meat category if you are a vegetarian, since the body will process these foods first as a complex carbohydrate (an energy food source) before it utilizes them as a protein (a tissue-repair food source).

Nuts form an additional subcategory within the meat list. Most of the calories in nuts come from protein and fat. The fat found in nuts is unsaturated and, therefore, is an important part of your food program. Eating the amounts of nuts prescribed in your food program provides your body with essential fatty acids for energy while satisfying hunger. Subcategories of nuts include foods such as nut butters, oils, and avocados. Watch quantities when eating nuts. Put them in measured baggies so you don't eat more than prescribed. Buy only natural or organic nut butters since most commercial nut butters have other ingredients and large amounts of sugar added to them.

The Turn Up the Heat Allowable Food Exchange List (appendix B) lists all the foods by category and subcategory. It also lists them by portions, or "exchanges." What this means simply is that one type of food within a category can be exchanged for another. For example, an apple can be exchanged for an orange; they are the same kind of food—a fruit/carbohydrate—found in the same food category, "the fruit list," and contain approximately the same amount of calories. Two ounces of swordfish can be exchanged for one ounce of chicken or beef, ⅓ large bagel for one slice of whole wheat bread, 1 cup of asparagus for 3 cups Romaine lettuce, and so on. Obviously, an exchange *may or may not* be what you would consider a serving. For example, if an ounce of chicken is labeled as "1," you may need from 4 to 12 *exchanges* of chicken to make up one *serving* of chicken for a meal. How many exchanges you will need per meal will be indicated in your weekly menu plan.

As we have seen above, you will use the three food plans in part II to choose the menu plan that is associated with your metabolic type—fat-and-protein-efficient; carbohydrate-efficient; or the dual metabolism. There are eleven caloric levels within each metabolic type, and twelve weeks within each level, but, keep in mind, you do not need to complete all twelve weeks within each level before you move on (to a different level as indicated by your four-week evaluation). The level at which you find your food plan will depend upon your current metabolic temperature and its appropriate metabolic scenario, which you will reassess only once per month. It only takes one minute of math to know *exactly* what your metabolic temperature is. Since this dynamic food program changes every week, you will *never* plateau. You will *always* be burning fat, building lean muscle, increasing your energy, and lowering your cholesterol and triglyceride levels, and improving your health.

Case History: Bill, a Fat-and-Protein-Efficient Individual

To understand how this works, let's take a look at the case history of a client named Bill. Since Bill had an acutely suppressed metabolism (below 79 degrees), his scenario represents the one that most readers will follow.

When Bill first came to me for nutritional coaching, he was 33 years old, 5 feet 11 inches tall, weighed 270 pounds, had a triglyceride level of 285, a total cholesterol level of 188, an HDL of 36, and LDL of 98, and a ratio of 5.2. His body fat percentage was 36.15 percent, which meant that he was carrying 97.6 pounds of fat and 172.4 pounds of lean muscle. He didn't feel healthy and wanted help with the weight problem that he had struggled with all his life.

Bill was a classic case of a fat-and-protein-efficient individual who ate almost no protein except for an occasional steak or piece of fish. Since his diet consisted mostly of carbohydrates, a nutrient type he could not efficiently utilize, his body fat and triglycerides were at dangerously high levels. As a child, Bill had always had a weight problem. All his life the message he had been given was, "Stay away from fats." Ironically, a low-fat diet was the *worst* type of food program for a person like him. When he limited his protein and focused on nonfat, high-carbohydrate foods, he wasn't getting the nutrients he needed to stay metabolically healthy, let alone reduce his scale weight and body fat.

During the day Bill felt sluggish. The mood swings he experienced reflected the insulin highs and lows he encountered from eating meals that were mostly composed of carbohydrate, which, of course, converted to sugars. By 3:00 or 4:00 in the afternoon, he was exhausted and found it hard to concentrate on his work. At night, he slept poorly, often averaging less than six hours of restless sleep.

Sometimes he would experience muscle cramping in his legs, which would awaken him in the middle of the night. Bill drank a maximum of 3 glasses of water per day, meaning that he was severely underhydrated most of the time and that his body did not have enough water to efficiently utilize fats, proteins, and carbohydrates, or maintain a core temperature pattern without hoarding unwanted fat for insulation.

I'm going to take you through the first five weeks of Bill's food program to show you how he (1) established his Foundation Food Program, and then (2) moved through the food levels for his metabolic type.

Step 1, Calculating Caloric Average: When I did a three-day breakdown of Bill's caloric intake to get an average, I observed that there was a wide discrepancy between his weekday and weekend eating patterns. On an average Monday through Friday, Bill's typical meal plan was a slice of whole grain bread in the morning with some orange juice, salad and pasta for lunch, an occasional afternoon snack of a candy bar, and usually either more pasta with some vegetables or a slice of pizza for dinner. On the weekends he would eat fewer meals but *much* larger quantities of food. He would routinely enjoy huge restaurant dinners with his girlfriend, including appetizers, wine, and calorie-rich desserts, including his favorite chocolate cheesecake.

Taking all of this into consideration, Bill had a caloric average of 2,190.

Step 2, Calculating Active Basal Metabolic Rate (ABMR): The next thing I calculated was Bill's resting metabolic rate, using the following formula:

Bill's Body Weight: 270 lbs. ÷ 2.26 × 24 = 2,867 (Bill's Resting BMR)

Using Bill's resting BMR, I then calculated Bill's active BMR by multiplying 2867 times 1.15 since he is a male:

Bill's Resting BMR: 2,867 × 1.15 = 3,297 (Bill's ABMR)

This number represented Bill's ideal current caloric intake for his weight (to reach 100 degrees).

Step 3, Determining Current Metabolic Temperature: To find Bill's current metabolic temperature, I divided his caloric average by his ABMR and took that number times 100 degrees:

Three-Day	Bill's Initial
Caloric	Metabolic
Average: 2,190 ÷ ABMR: 3,297 × 100° = 66°	Temperature

At 66 degrees, Bill's metabolic temperature was severely suppressed (Metabolic Scenario 2) because it was below 80 degrees.

Step 4, Determining the Foundation Food Program: Since Bill's metabolism had cooled and he was eating over a thousand calories less than his ideal amount, it would have been metabolically traumatic to suddenly increase his daily calories dramatically. Instead, I increased his current daily average caloric intake by 10 percent to find the number of calories he needed for his Foundation Food Program:

2,190 Calories (Bill's Average) × 10% = 219 Calories (Increase Necessary)

2,190 Calories + 219 Calories = 2,409 (Approximate Calories of Foundation Food Program)

In Bill's case, he will go to the chapter for the Fat-and-Protein-Efficient Food Program on page 145 and look under the column entitled Caloric Range of Level. There he will find his appropriate level. Based on the above equation and Bill's metabolic scenario, he is looking for a range that includes the caloric number 2,409. This number falls within the Level 8 range of calories. I have copied the chart below so that you can follow Bill's process:

Therefore, Week 1 of Level 8 will be Bill's Foundation Food Program. I have suggested some foods for the actual exchange amounts to show you how this works. I am also including some condiments (low-calorie salad dressing), flavor enhancers (lite syrups and lite or all-fruit jams), and items such as ½ cup nonfat milk per day from the Free Foods List found in appendix C. You are allowed specific portions of these free foods daily and should use them to make your meals more enjoyable and flavorful.

Level	Caloric Range of Level
1	Under 1,200
2	1,201–1,365
3	1,366–1,480
4	1,481–1,685
5	1,686–1,805
6	1,806–2,180
7	2,181–2,330
8	2,331–2,450
9	2,451–2,765
10	2,766–3,065
11	3,066 and up

Level 8, Week 1

Bill's Foundation Food Program: 2,452 calories per day

Meal 1: 1 medium bagel, ½ cantaloupe, 2 eggs, 1 tablespoon all-fruit jam (3 Bread exchanges, 1 Fruit exchange, 2 Meat exchanges, 1 Free Food)

Meal 2: 1 apple, 1 tablespoon peanut butter (1 Fruit exchange, 1 Meat exchange)

Meal 3: 1½ pitas, 4 ounces turkey, 3 cups romaine lettuce, 1 tablespoon low-calorie salad dressing (3 Bread exchanges, 4 Meat exchanges, 1 Vegetable exchange)

Meal 4: 1 plum, ⅛ cup almonds (1 Fruit exchange, 1 Meat exchange)

Meal 5: 1 cup watermelon, 2 ounces turkey (1 Fruit exchange, 2 Meat exchanges)

Meal 6: 1 baked potato, 1 tablespoon nondairy butter, 8 ounces salmon, 2 cups cooked spinach, 3 cups salad, 1 tablespoon low-calorie dressing (3 Bread exchanges, 8 Meat exchanges, 2 Vegetable exchanges)

Meal 7: 2 pears, 2 cups popcorn (2 Fruit exchanges, 2 Bread exchanges)

Notice that although Bill was eating a good deal more protein than he was before, the carbohydrate content of the meals for Week 1 was still very high. That was because Bill had been ingesting such a large number of carbohydrates to begin with. To simply drop his carbohydrates to 25 percent, the ideal amount for a fat-and-protein-efficient individual, would have put a strain on Bill's organs, metabolism, digestion, and elimination, possibly causing metabolic trauma.

The second week, we kept Bill's food program exactly the same but removed all multi-ingredient bread products that contained yeast and sugar. Yeast is a fat-and-protein-efficient individual's worst enemy.

Level 8, Week 2
2,452 calories per day

Meal 1: 1½ cups of oatmeal, ½ cup nonfat milk, ½ banana, 6 egg whites (3 Bread exchanges, 1 Free Food, 1 Fruit exchange, 2 Meat exchanges)
Meal 2: 1 peach, ⅛ cup cashews (1 Fruit exchange, 1 Meat exchange)
Meal 3: 1 cup rice, 8 ounces tuna, 1 tomato (3 Bread exchanges, 4 Meat exchanges, 1 Vegetable exchange)
Meal 4: 1 apple, 1 tablespoon peanut butter (1 Fruit exchange, 1 Meat exchange)
Meal 5: 1 nectarine, 2 ounces turkey (1 Fruit exchange, 2 Meat exchanges)
Meal 6: 1½ cups corn, 8 ounces chicken breast, 1 cup green beans, 1 cup asparagus, 1 tablespoon nondairy butter (3 Bread exchanges, 8 Meat exchanges, 2 Vegetable Exchanges)
Meal 7: 2 large shredded wheat biscuits, 3 cups strawberries (2 Bread exchanges, 3 Fruit exchanges)

For the third week of Bill's food program, we kept the exchanges for Meals 1 through 4 the same (varying the foods, of course, using the Food Exchange List in appendix B). For Meal 5, we increased his Meat exchanges to 3 and kept his Fruit. For Meal 6, we halved his Bread exchange, allowing him ½ cup of rice (or ½ potato or ½ yam). Meal 7 stayed the same. (Notice in Meal 3 that 4 Meat exchanges is equal to 8 ounces of tuna because 2 ounces of tuna is equal to 1 exchange, as found in your Food Exchange List in appendix B.)

By this time, Bill's body had begun to adapt, utilizing a greater amount of protein and fewer carbohydrates. By decreasing his daily carbohydrate intake, we also began to stimulate a more efficient use of fat metabolism. By getting rid of simple sugars, we forced his body to feed off of its fat stores as an energy source.

The increase in Bill's water intake produced dramatic results as well. He began to look better as the texture and tone of his skin improved. His energy began to soar as the nutrients he was ingesting began to move more efficiently through his body. Bill's water intake (weighing 270 pounds, he was consuming 270 ounces of water a day) also helped greatly in utilizing sugars and fat as energy.

Level 8, Week 3
2,401 calories per day

Meal 1: 1½ cups bran flakes, ½ cup nonfat milk, 1 cup raspberries, 2 eggs (3 Bread exchanges, 1 Free Food, 1 Fruit exchange, 2 Meat exchanges)

Meal 2: 1 apple, 1 tablespoon peanut butter (1 Fruit exchange, 1 Meat exchange)

Meal 3: 1 cup rice, 8 ounces shrimp, 1 cup zucchini (3 Bread exchanges, 4 Meat exchanges, 1 Vegetable exchange)

Meal 4: 1 apple, 1 tablespoon peanut butter (1 Fruit exchange, 1 Meat exchange)

Meal 5: 1 cup grapes, 2 ounces turkey, ⅛ cup almonds (1 Fruit exchange, 3 Meat exchanges)

Meal 6: ½ cup rice, 8 ounces flank steak, 1 cup asparagus, 3 cups green salad, 1 tablespoon low-calorie salad dressing (1½ Bread exchanges, 8 Meat exchanges, 2 Vegetable exchanges, 1 Free Food)

Meal 7: 2 cups applesauce, 2 large shredded wheat biscuits (2 Fruit exchanges, 2 Bread exchanges)

At Week 4 we kept the exact same food pattern, except that in Meal 6 we added an extra vegetable and increased his Meat from 8 to 10 ounces, and removed the Bread from Meal 7 so that it would be fruit only.

Level 8, Week 4
2,407 calories per day

Meal 1: 1½ cups oatmeal, 1 grapefruit, 2 eggs (3 Bread exchanges, 1 Fruit exchange, 2 Meat exchanges)

Meal 2: 1 cup grapes, 1 tablespoon peanut butter (1 Fruit exchange, 1 Meat exchange)

Meal 3: 1 cup kidney beans, 8 ounces tuna, 3 cups romaine lettuce (3 Bread exchanges, 4 Meat exchanges, 1 Vegetable exchange)

Meal 4: 1 apple, ⅛ cup almonds (1 Fruit exchange, 1 Meat exchange)

Meal 5: ½ cantaloupe, 4 ounces tuna, ⅛ cup cashews (1 Fruit exchange, 3 Meat exchanges)

Meal 6: ½ yam, 10 ounces chicken breast, 1 cup summer squash, 1 cup asparagus, 3 cups salad (1½ Bread exchanges, 10 Meat exchanges, 3 Vegetable exchanges)

Meal 7: 2 cups applesauce (2 Fruit exchanges)

By Week 5 it was time for Bill to re-evaluate his metabolism to see if he should stay in Level 8 or make a level shift. By then Bill had lost 27 pounds and weighed in at 243. Plugging in his new weight and his three-day caloric average (taken from Week 4 of Level 8), we once again calculated his metabolic temperature:

243 lbs. ÷ 2.26 × 24 = 2,580 (Bill's Resting BMR)

(Resting BMR) 2,580 × 1.15 = 2,967 (Bill's Active BMR)

Three-Day			**New Current**
Caloric		**Active**	**Metabolic**

Average: 2,407 ÷ BMR: 2,967 × 100° = 81° Temperature

As you can see at this point, Bill's metabolism was no longer severely suppressed. In fact, at 81 degrees, he now falls into a higher and more efficient metabolic category, Metabolic Scenario 3, the moderately suppressed metabolism, which has a temperature range of between 80 and 99 degrees. Since this scenario instructs the reader to find their level by beginning with their caloric ABMR, Bill will now use that number, which is 2,967. If you look at page 145, you will see that Bill has elevated his level and now falls into the caloric range of Level 10. Not only has he lost 27 pounds of weight, he has added a significant amount of muscle that requires more calories to fuel and repair it. At this point, Bill will start with Week 5 of Level 10.

Why does he not simply go to Week 1 of Level 10? Remember our rule on page 77: when you move up to a higher caloric level (or down to a lower caloric level, as the case might be), always continue to cycle *forward* from your current week. In Bill's case he is moving from Week 4 of Level 8 to Week 5 of Level 10. The reason for this is that each consecutive week is more suited to the needs of your metabolic type. If Bill had gone back to Week 1 of Level 10, he would be returning to a week that is primarily designed to stabilize and balance caloric patterns and create a foundation food program. When

Bill reaches Week 8 of Level 10 and conducts his next four-week metabolic assessment, he will then continue onto *Week 9* of whatever level is then appropriate for the changes he has undergone in weight loss, metabolic efficiency, and body composition. Movement is always *forward* until a twelve-week cycle has been completed. When Bill is completely finished with his first twelve weeks, however, he *will* be returning to Week 1 of whatever level is now appropriate for him.

As Bill moves through Level 10, the caloric values of each week will continue to cycle up and down, as they did in Level 8. This cycling is an integral part of the food program since it ensures that the program is dynamic, matching your body's changing caloric needs as your weight and body composition change and keeping your weight loss from reaching a plateau.

To successfully follow this metabolic nutrition program, you must trust the system's mathematics, understanding that each of your reassessments will clearly show your next nutritional step. Be as consistent with the weekly food programs as possible. But remember, do not be unreasonably harsh on yourself if you slip up. Just keep drinking all of your water and get back on track as soon as possible. Know that following this program will become only easier with time and that the results will be well worth your effort.

Bill is only one of the thousands of clients who have seen phenomenal results on this program. His first week alone, he lost 6.75 pounds. Four months later, as of the writing of this book, his weight has dropped to 210 and his body fat to 16 percent. That means that he is now carrying only 33.6 pounds of fat and 176.4 pounds of lean muscle. In other words, Bill has *lost* 64 pounds of fat and gained 4 pounds of lean tissue. His total scale weight loss is 60 pounds. His total cholesterol has dropped to 180, his HDL has risen to 69, his LDL is 90, his triglycerides are 104, and his ratio is 2.6.

Bill told me, "I have tons of energy and feel like a 22-year-old." He sleeps soundly every night and is more productive at work. The change is evident in more ways than one—since his weight loss, he has purchased a brand-new wardrobe. Most important, he got rid of his "overweight past" by making a point of throwing away all his "fat clothes."

Bill is a classic example of a person who does not need to perform a great amount of exercise in order to lose weight. For the last four months, he has been walking only an hour a day, four or five times a week. But he has gotten so excited about the changes in his body that he now wants to do more. Recently, he asked me to design a gym workout program for him so that he can build some muscle.

Overall, Bill's weight loss averages out to be 15 pounds per month, about 4 pounds per week. Since many people have heard the rule of thumb, "You should lose only between 1 and 2 pounds a week if you want to remain healthy," you may be questioning this number. The truth is, the only time this much weight loss is unhealthy is if you are starving off muscle and hoarding fat on an ultra-low-calorie food program. Keep in mind that when Bill begins exercising in the gym, his scale weight loss will slow a bit. He will continue losing fat, but he will now be actively building additional lean muscle. At present, Bill is eating more than 2,700 calories a day, which includes 20 to 22 ounces of lean protein. He is certainly not starving himself.

■ Keeping a Nutrition Journal

To help my clients stay faithful to their food programs, I ask them to keep a daily food journal. I have included a blank one below for you to copy and use. Notice that there is a space for your water intake, since drinking your water is a very important part of this program. There is also a section at the bottom, "Notes," where you can record measurements and other details—the amount of weight and inches you are losing, how much you are exercising, and what issues come up for you daily as you change your food patterns, including energy level, sleep, moods, and digestion.

Daily nutritional journaling will provide a powerful tool to help you maintain your menu compliance. It will serve as a written history of your weight-loss journey, documenting the numerous emotions, activities, newly created habits, obstacles, solutions, and improved health and quality of life you are creating. It will prove to be an exceptional record of your extraordinary commitment to the improvement of your health, performance, and physique.

Nutrition Journal

Date:

Meal 1, Time: Water:

Meal 2, Time: Water:

Meal 3, Time: Water:

Meal 4, Time: Water:

Meal 5, Time: Water:

Meal 6, Time: Water:

Meal 7, Time: Water:

Notes:

Rate yourself from 1–10 in the following areas:

Sleep

Digestion

Moods

Energy

Activity and Exercise

■ Helpful Tips

In my clinic, I pass out tip cards to help my patients make wise nutritional and lifestyle choices, and to cope with food situations when they are eating away from home. I have included a few of those here to serve as useful guides.

General Tips

- Plan to eat meals at approximately the same time each day. This will increase the efficiency of the body's digestive process.
- Prepare your foods in advance and store them for easy access. For example, make a large portion of white or brown rice and keep it in the refrigerator.
- Always use your food diary. This helps you to visualize your patterns of eating and to stick to the program.
- Try not to eat while engaging in other activities, such as reading or watching television. This will allow you to focus on your meal and will further help you to avoid overeating.
- Try not to go into the kitchen at any time other than mealtime. Avoid temptation.
- Pin your list of goals to the refrigerator. This ought to stop you from reaching in there.
- Don't skip your meals. Remember that your body requires fuel and your food is it.
- Try not to eat late at night. But it is better to eat late at night than not to eat all of your daily food.
- Keep cut-up vegetables readily available. We can't always control our munchies, but we can control what we choose to munch on.

Healthy Tips for Eating Out

- Choose restaurants that offer a variety of foods that fall under your meal plan.
- Before going out, try eating a snack to avoid overeating.
- Ask that all food be prepared without oil or butter.

■ Order vegetables steamed.

■ When eating Chinese food, ask for no MSG because of high salt content.

■ Ask for sauces and dressings on the side.

■ Request nonfat salad dressings.

■ Use salsa on salads and baked potato.

■ Ask for steamed white or brown rice.

■ Order grilled or broiled chicken or fish.

■ Use mustard instead of mayonnaise.

■ Order water instead of iced tea or diet soda.

■ Ask that all chicken be prepared skinless.

SAFE CHOICES

■ Grilled chicken salad with nonfat dressing.

■ Grilled lean fish with steamed vegetables and steamed rice.

■ Salad bar (pick fresh vegetables without cheese or croutons) and a plain baked potato.

To be successful in this program, all it takes is your willingness to be coachable and to realize that weight loss and body changes take time. This food program is not about "being perfect." If you attempt to follow this program to the best of your ability, you can do no wrong. The simple effort to make good choices about the foods best suited for your metabolic type, and trying to eat them consistently, will be a breakthrough from your old eating habits. It will teach you to take responsibility for the food choices you make and to remember that you need to stay well fueled to lose weight and live an active, healthy life. Once you have worked with this food program for a few weeks, I guarantee that you will never want to go back to your old way of eating. As one of my clients told me recently, "Honestly, who would want to stop feeling and looking this good?"

4. Quickstart

A 2- to 3-Week Program to Maximize Your Weight Loss

Even when you understand all the benefits that eating for your metabolic type provides, there are times when life throws you a curve ball. Sometimes, following an initial evaluation, a client will say to me, "Following your program makes perfect sense to me. I can easily see the logic of eating the appropriate percentages of fat, protein, and carbohydrate for my particular metabolism, and I understand how the cycling of menus each week will keep me from plateauing as I set my goals for losing weight and body fat. But I have one big problem. In two weeks I will be attending my high school reunion [substitute *wedding, family reunion, yearly awards dinner for my job,* and such others], and I really need to lose some weight fast. Is there anything you can do for me in the short term?"

Fortunately, there is something I can do. Although diets involving caloric deprivation are not healthy over the long term, you can Quickstart your metabolism for two or three weeks to achieve an immediate weight-loss goal—from 5 to 8 pounds and up to 2.5 percent body fat each week. This is significantly more than you will be losing on your regular food program. After that, however, to remain healthy, you must start your food program designed for your metabolic type.

Quickstart is a strict food-management program that requires you to be very focused on your daily menus and exercise patterns. As long as you feel comfortable with this strict format, it will enable you to drop considerable weight and body fat in a short period of time while still achieving consistent energy patterns. To understand how Quickstart works, let's take a look at a client of mine named Mary.

Case History: How Mary Got Her Quickstart

Like many of my clients, Mary had been on about five other diets before coming to my office at the recommendation of a friend. At 5 feet 7 inches, Mary weighed 184 pounds with a body fat of 34.7 percent. Since she had been told that drinking too many fluids would cause bloating, she chose to restrict her water intake, drinking only two 8-ounce glasses of water per day. She was amazed when I told her that she could automatically drop 5 pounds just by drinking the proper amount of water (1 ounce per 1 pound of body weight daily).

Mary had been struggling with a weight problem since she was a little girl. Over the years, she developed a very adversarial relationship with food because she felt as though it was the cause of her obesity. She felt broken and was tired of being embarrassed about her size. Mary has a lot on her plate. She has a husband and two children, a household to run, and has been holding down a stressful job. For years, she had been putting her own health, physique, and performance levels on the back burner so that she could make time for everyone else. As a result, she now found her health and fitness in a state of decay, making her feel even more ashamed of her weight and extremely sensitive about her appearance.

For several years, as part of her strategy to lose weight, Mary had been consistently undereating. At our first meeting, Mary described her eating habits to me. She always skipped breakfast and numerous other meals as well. Her lunchtime meal usually consisted of a Chinese chicken salad (lettuce, cabbage, 2 ounces of chicken chunks, cashews, water chestnuts, grated carrots, and lite salad dressing). By late afternoon she felt so exhausted that she had to go to Starbucks for a double café mocha to give herself a much needed boost. A few times a week she would grab 8 to 10 chocolate-covered expresso beans to increase her energy level. In the evening, because she was so wiped out, she would take the easiest possible route to cook for her family. She would pick up a loaf of Italian bread (which she didn't eat), tear open a bag of prewashed lettuce, and cook a pot of pasta with marinara sauce. She justified this to herself by saying that pasta was good for her because it was low in fat and she was trying to stay on a low-fat diet. Ironically, this was her worst possible choice. Mary has a dual metabolism, requiring a balance of fats, proteins, and carbohydrates. The removal of any one of these nutrients from her diet, or a lack of nutritional balance, would cause excessive, unwanted weight gain.

Her beverages of choice were coffee during the day and diet soda at night to satisfy her need for something that tasted sweet. Her water intake was, at best, two 8-ounce glasses per day.

Mary was completely frustrated since she was combining her low-fat, low-calorie diet with forty-five minutes of cardiovascular exercise five days a week—and still not losing any weight. I explained to her that the reason for this was (1) her low water intake, (2) her low caloric heat patterns, and (3) eating inappropriate nutrient amounts for her metabolic type.

Mary was thrilled to know that she had the most responsive of the three metabolic types, the dual metabolism, which would make it easy for her to bring her metabolic temperature up to 100 degrees. But she looked dejected and somewhat agitated when I began explaining to her how the program worked. Noticing this, I asked her what was wrong.

She said, "This is all great news, and I understand how much your food program is going to help me—and I really want to do it. But it's not going to solve my immediate problem."

"What's your immediate problem?" I asked.

Looking embarrassed, Mary said, "My youngest sister is getting married in three weeks and I'm going to be her matron of honor. But I've done something rather foolish. She lives in another state so, when she called to ask for my size and measurements three months ago, I lied and said that I was two sizes smaller. I was sure I could drop the weight in three months, but I haven't been able to, no matter how hard I've tried.

"I understand what you're saying about eating for your metabolic type, and it all makes complete sense, but doing all this great nutritional stuff won't get me out of this jam I've gotten myself into. Is there any way I can drop some pounds quickly in a healthy way? At this wedding I'm going to see family members and people from my hometown that I haven't seen in decades, and my weight is at an all-time high. My parents have always been very judgmental about my weight, and I do not want my excess body fat to be the topic of their conversations."

I explained to Mary that there was a quick and healthy way to lose weight, but she would have to understand that (1) there were rules that she needed to strictly follow, and (2) she should not stay on the program for more than three weeks. Upon completion of the three weeks, she should begin her Foundation Food Program for her metabolic type. Mary looked greatly relieved, and we began setting up her Quickstart program right away. . . .

■ The Quickstart Basic Plan

There are five basic steps to Quickstart:

1. Completely remove from your diet all multi-ingredient carbohydrates containing yeast and sugar, such as cake, cookies, breads, bagels, and muffins.
2. Remove all starchy carbohydrates, such as potatoes, rice, yams, sweet potatoes, corn, and pasta, from the evening meal. Evening is a time when you do not need carbs for energy. Consume only vegetables (fibrous carbohydrates) and fish for dinner, unless you are allergic to fish (see below).
3. Stabilize your caloric intake with the correct food program, according to gender (see below).
4. Elevate your water intake to the amount that is appropriate to your weight—1 ounce of water to 1 pound of body weight. Even if your food choices aren't perfect the first week, the increased water alone will cause you to lose approximately 5 pounds in the first week.
5. Maintain your current exercise program at a level that is comfortable for you. Don't attempt to overdo the exercise. Since you are dropping starchy and complex carbohydrates from your food plan, you will be consuming very restricted amounts of energy-source foods. Therefore, you won't have the energy for a challenging workout regimen.

The Quickstart plan is the same for everyone, regardless of your metabolic type. Below are three weeks of Quickstart meal plans (with some suggestions for food choices) for both females and males. You can use the Turn Up the Heat Allowable Food Exchange List in appendix B for appropriate exchanges. Keep in mind that all meats or fish should be grilled or broiled, not fried, and prepared without oil or butter. Peanut butter should be "all natural" (peanuts only), and preferably organic, since peanut crops are heavily sprayed with pesticides and fungicides. In the menus where fish is listed for the evening meal, do not substitute other exchanges, unless, of course, you are allergic to fish. In that case you should substitute a boneless chicken breast or white meat turkey—never red meat.

Fish has the least fat of any other protein source, so eating it for your evening meal will help support your Quickstart program weight loss. Regardless of the type of fish you choose (some are listed as 1 ounce per exchange and others are listed as 2 ounces per exchange, depending on fat and caloric content), for the Quickstart program eat only *4 ounces* of fish at lunch and dinner if you are female and *8 ounces* (at dinner only, 4 ounces at lunch) if you are male.

Avoid eating vegetables such as cauliflower, carrots, and broccoli. These are the most difficult vegetables to digest—more so if you suffer from any form of irritable bowel disorder or colitis—and they are likely to cause bloating, digestive discomfort, and constipation. The best choice of vegetables to enhance digestion are steamed spinach, asparagus, zucchini, summer squash, and tomatoes. Salads (raw) should never be eaten alone, only as an accompaniment to other vegetables, which should be eaten steamed. The food choices listed in parenthesis are only suggestions. For variety, use the food exchange list found in appendix B, keeping in mind the food-choice restrictions outlined above.

Avoid food shopping when hungry. Never go grocery shopping when you are hungry. This has become the waterloo of more clients than I can list.

Possible Side Effects and What to Do About Them

Since Quickstart is a strict food-management program that demands your complete attention, there are some potential side effects or emotional states that might pop up for you during your fourteen to twenty-one days on the program. Many of these suggestions are simply common sense and require only that you take care of yourself and be aware of your emotional and physical states.

QUICKSTART PROGRAM FOR FEMALES		
	Week 1	**Week 2**	**Week 3**
Meal 1	B2 (1 cup oatmeal)	B2 (1 cup oatmeal)	B2 (1 cup oatmeal)
	F1 (orange or banana)	F1 (orange or banana)	
Meal 2	F1 (apple)	F1 (apple)	V1 (2 cups raw celery)
Meal 3	B 1½ (½ cup rice) M4 (4 oz. chicken breast or 4 oz. fish) V1 (2 cups steamed spinach)	M4 (4 oz. chicken breast or 4 oz. fish) V2 (1 cup steamed tomato and 1 cup summer squash)	M4 (4 oz. chicken breast or 4 oz. fish) V2 (2 cups summer squash and 3 cups salad with 1 tblsp. low-calorie dressing)
Meal 4	F1 (orange)	V1 (2 cups raw celery) PB1 (1 T peanut butter)	V1 (tomato)
Meal 5	M4 (4 oz. fish only) V3 (1 cup zucchini, 1 cup asparagus, 1 cup salad)	M4 (4 oz. fish only) V3 (1 cup asparagus, 1 cup steamed tomato, 3 cups salad)	M4 (4 oz. fish only) V3 (1 cup zucchini, 2 cups steamed spinach, 3 cups salad)
Meal 6	F1 (mixed berries)	0	0

B = Bread List, M = Meat List, F = Fruit List, V = Vegetable List

Lack of energy. If you find yourself feeling tired in the afternoon, try to schedule a break or some downtime. If you have a choice about when to begin the Quickstart program, choose a two- or three-week period where you do not have a lot of stressful demands placed upon you or a lot of activities scheduled. If you need to begin Quickstart immediately to get ready for a wedding or family event two or three weeks from the present, don't overload yourself with unnecessary responsibilities. As much as possible, try to kick back and give yourself a break.

Sugar cravings. Whenever you remove carbohydrates from a food plan, you might possibly experience some kind of sugar craving. I always tell my clients, "You can overcome the urge for sugar by eating a few grapes or a couple of pieces of frozen pineapple or banana. Another good strategy is to make flavored ice by filling an ice cube tray with Kool-Aid sweetened with NutraSweet." One client of mine told

QUICKSTART PROGRAM FOR MALES

	Week 1	Week 2	Week 3
Meal 1	B3 (1½ cups oatmeal) FI (orange or banana)	B3 (1½ cups oatmeal) FI (orange or banana)	B3 (1½ cups oatmeal)
Meal 2	FI (apple)	VI (2 cups raw celery) PBI (1 tblsp. peanut butter)	VI (2 cups raw celery)
Meal 3	B3 (1 cup rice) M4 (4 oz. chicken breast or 4 oz. fish) VI (1 cup summer squash)	B1½ (½ potato) M4 (4 oz. chicken breast or 4 oz. fish) V (2 cups steamed spinach)	M4 (4 oz. chicken breast or 4 oz. fish) V3 (1 cup summer squash, 1 cup asparagus, and 3 cups salad with 1 tblsp. low-calorie dressing)
Meal 4	VI (2 cups raw celery) PBI (1 tblsp. peanut butter)	VI (2 cups raw celery) PBI (1 tblsp. peanut butter)	VI (2 cups raw celery) PBI (1 tblsp. peanut butter)
Meal 5	M8 (8 oz. fish only) V3 (1 cup zucchini, 1 cup asparagus, 3 cups salad)	M8 (8 oz. fish only) V3 (1 cup asparagus, 1 cup zucchini, 3 cups salad)	MI (1 hard-boiled egg)
Meal 6	FI (mixed berries)	0	M4 (8 oz. fish only) V3 (1 cup zucchini, 1 cup steamed tomato, 3 cups salad)

B = Bread List, M = Meat List, F = Fruit List, V = Vegetable List

me she made a cup of Good Earth Tea when she craved something sweet. It has absolutely no sugar in it, but contains stevia, an herb with a very sweet taste.

Anxiety and being quick-tempered. When a person goes on a low-calorie food plan, he or she often experiences heightened levels of anxiety and quick-temperedness. Part of this is because of the lower levels of sugar in your blood stream from eating fewer carbohydrates and calories and from the stress of having to pay more attention to your foods than you ever have before.

There are several things I can suggest to alleviate anxiety and feeling quick-tempered. First, when you know you are about to say something angry or sarcastic, take a few deep breaths, count to ten, and think before you speak. Make sure that you get at least seven, preferably eight, hours of sleep every night—lack of sleep will make you less able to handle your emotions. Sometimes a person will feel anxious when everything around them seems to be moving too fast. Close your office door for five minutes and take a breather, or find a quiet place to settle down for a few minutes so that you can find your mental balance again.

When you feel on edge, take a moment to tell yourself that this food plan is your choice and that you are doing the very best you can. No one is forcing you to do it. You have chosen this aggressive type of food plan because you know the rewards will be great. Also remember that this won't last forever. It's just for two or three weeks. Then you can begin the food program for your metabolic type and your anxiety levels and irritability will subside.

Increased muscle soreness. You may notice that your muscles feel a bit sorer than usual after exercising because you don't have as much food as you usually do to repair them. Again, realize that this is only temporary and that you have the option of pulling back your level of exercise for a couple of weeks if you want to.

■ How Did Mary Do?

Mary stayed on her Quickstart program faithfully, drinking even more water than required and sticking with her schedule of walking. When she came in for her evaluation at the end of three weeks, Mary was ecstatic to discover that she had lost 22 pounds and that her body fat had dropped 7 percent. She looked and felt great. At 162 pounds, she was confident that she could now fit into that bridesmaid's dress. When she came back from the wedding, she was beaming. "Everyone told me how great I looked. I think it was one of the best weekends of my entire life. And I didn't lose control of myself and eat everything in sight, as I was afraid I'd do. I'd worked too hard to ever let myself go like that again." Mary was so fired up from her Quickstart results that she could hardly wait to start her 12-week metabolic food plan.

Like Mary, you may find yourself in a situation where you have to lose weight quickly for an important event in your life. Quickstart is not meant to be a long-term food program, but if you are willing to give it your all, you will be amazed at how rapidly you can drop weight without compromising your health. If you've been struggling with fad diets that never quite deliver on their promises, know that Quickstart can easily give you the boost you need to get over the initial hump of weight loss. Quickstart is designed to provide a healthy jumping off point to a leaner, more energetic, and more attractive you.

So, enjoy that event you are getting ready for, be proud of your newfound physique, and get ready to see your health and vitality soar as you get started on your regular metabolic food program in the weeks to come.

5. Maintenance

Allowing Your Metabolism to Mature

Once you have reached your weight-loss and physique goals, where do you go from there? You have two choices: One is to set a new goal, as many of my clients do. For example, I have a client with whom I've been working for several months. At this point, she is 5 feet 8 inches, weighs 140 pounds, and her body fat ratio is 24 percent. Her current goal is to weigh 135 pounds and have 18 percent body fat. But when she reaches that goal, she may decide that she wants to continue her reduction program and add weight training so that her body fat is 16 percent. Or she may decide that she would like to weigh a bit less than 135, which she could easily do with additional dynamic food programming, without compromising her health.

Upon completing the twelve-week protocol, if you decide that you want to lose more weight, then you should once again re-evaluate your metabolic temperature and choose the appropriate metabolic scenario. If necessary, you should adjust your level (see page 76 for instructions on when to change levels). Whatever level you find yourself in, start with Week 1 and keep cycling through the twelve weeks until you reach your new weight-loss goal. If you decide that you want to intensify your workout to create a more muscular physique, you need to recalculate your metabolic temperature and move up a level to support your body's additional caloric and protein requirements for the development of additional muscle tissue.

However, if you get to Week 12 of a level and feel that you are exactly where you want to be, then you will keep Week 12 as your *permanent* food program.

Since it will take ninety days for your metabolism to mature, the next three months will be crucial for establishing the dietary foundation for your lifetime nutritional maintenance program. During this time, because you will be following the same menu pattern every week, you will learn more about how your body reacts to certain food choices you make and how much flexibility you can build into the pattern without sacrificing its quality and purpose.

Most important, this ninety-day maturation period involves learning how to make good nutritional choices. Say, for example, that you are fat-and-protein-efficient, and that the dinner menu for your maintenance program does not allow starchy carbohydrates such as rice or potato. However, you have decided that you really want to enjoy a juicy steak with a baked potato this evening. That potato for supper is not going to make or break your metabolic balance, but you should also know that a wise nutritional choice would be to eat fish and vegetables only for dinner for the next three days. The same would be true if your evening snack is a piece of fruit, but you decide one night that, instead, you want a piece of apple pie as a snack. For the next week, you need to be very strict about your other food choices and not "bend the rules" for a while. And remember that these sorts of "treats" should be the occasional fun and joyous exceptions, not the rule.

When adding in a food that is not on your program, it's also important to adjust the contents of your meal so that all of your other food choices are as healthy as possible. For example, if you decide you want to have a dessert after your dinner, be aware that fish and steamed vegetables would be the healthiest nutritional choice for your evening meal. Don't have a potato as well as a dessert—that would be an excessive amount of carbohydrates. This sort of nutritional awareness will help to ensure your metabolic efficiency.

Do keep in mind that it is important to stay within your food choices as much as possible during this ninety-day period. This will not only help your metabolism to mature, it will also make you more resistant to menu inconsistencies. Be honest with yourself about what nutritional choices you are making and learn how to own them and their consequences. At the end of ninety days, you will continue with the maintenance program. This will ensure that your weight and energy levels will remain constant. Of course, if you decide to (1) lose more weight or (2) add more muscularity to your frame, you can always reassess and cycle through another twelve weeks in the appropriate level (see page 76).

■ What Happens If You Go Off the Program?

Sometimes in life you face situations where you are undergoing intense stress or emotional trauma. You lose a loved one or a job, or face a family crisis. Even though these are the very situations in which it would most benefit you to stay on your food program—since good nutrition will give you the physical, emotional, and mental stamina to weather the hard times—sometimes you just won't have the strength to do so. The result could be unwanted weight gain.

When that happens, don't beat yourself up or assign blame. Just know that you have your original twelve-week program to fall back on. Maybe in the past when you gained weight, then returned to your old diet, you did so with a sense of failure. "Well, I did it again, went off my diet. Boy, I have no self-control at all." Now things are different. You know that you have the nutritional tools to help you get right back where you want to be in the areas of weight, health, and performance. Just begin at Week 1 of your appropriate menu level and cycle on through all twelve weeks. If you have reached your goals by the time you complete Week 12, simply continue with that week as your maintenance program.

There might also be times during your maintenance program when you suspect that you have been "cheating" a lot and not being truthful to yourself about your food choices. At that time, it's good to check in with yourself by using the "Statements for Self-Evaluation," which I have designed for that purpose. If you don't feel satisfied with your results, then you may want to cycle through your twelve-week program again to help get yourself back on track nutritionally and metabolically. Start a new food journal to keep track of your water intake, food choices, patterns, and consistency.

How to Use the "Statements for Self-evaluation"

Rate each statement on a scale of 1 (poor) to 5 (excellent), depending on how satisfied you are with that aspect of your food programming, workout, or general daily performance. A score of 76 to 100 points indicates that you are doing all right. If your score is 41 to 75 points, it's time to cycle back through your twelve weeks again. If your score is 40 or below, chances are you are experiencing unwanted weight gain, low or inconsistent energy patterns, or less than optimal health. If so, it's time to get back on track and reclaim your health, vitality, and physique.

If you do need to cycle back through your twelve weeks, make sure that you faithfully resume keeping your food journal. Once

Statements for Self-evaluation

		Points
1.	I am eating all the foods prescribed on my daily menu.	
2.	I am eating all my foods at the correct time.	
3.	I am not skipping any of my meals.	
4.	I enjoy the foods I am eating.	
5.	I am using my exchange list and do not eat foods that are not on it.	
6.	I faithfully measure all my foods.	
7.	I have digestive difficulties, such as constipation, diarrhea, bloating.	
8.	I am drinking all my daily water.	
9.	I am taking all my supplements.	
10.	I like the way I feel.	
11.	I like the way my body looks.	
12.	I have a great deal of energy and my performance level is high.	
13.	My sleep is restful.	
14.	My stress levels are low.	
15.	I am emotionally stable.	
16.	I feel satisfied with the way I cope with friends, colleagues, and family members.	
17.	I have a good attitude.	
18.	I am doing resistance exercises on a regular basis.	
19.	I am participating in aerobic activities on a regular basis.	
20.	My workouts feel satisfying.	
	TOTAL:	

you've drifted from your food protocol, it becomes easier to be less honest with yourself about what you are actually eating. You might have been telling yourself, "What I ate today [or didn't eat] wasn't really that bad." After all, if you throw away the candy bar wrapper, it's as if that candy bar never really existed. But when you are diligent about writing down everything that you eat, you must face the absolute truth about the integrity of your food choices and how they affect your performance and energy levels. Re-establishing your level of awareness by weighing yourself once a week, taking stock of how your clothes fit and whether you are bloated or having digestive difficulties, and noting the consistency of your energy levels and moods are all key to regaining your metabolic efficiency.

■ What Happens Nutritionally If You Add a Significant Amount of Exercise to Your Lifestyle?

You may reach a point in your life where you decide that you want to set new fitness goals to increase your lean muscle and body mass. To accomplish this, you begin stepping up your workout routine. For example, if for the past six months your regular pattern has been to exercise three times a week, and now you decide that you would like to increase the frequency of your exercise to five to six times per week, your protein intake must increase. If your protein intake remains static, you will likely find that you feel "weaker" in the gym because of the additional energy this intensified workout regimen requires. You will now need additional caloric support for muscle repair and movement.

Remember, the only food that repairs muscle is protein, so you will need to do one of two things: Either increase your protein intake per meal by 2 ounces (if you are male) and 1 ounce (if you are female); or, if you feel that you are making significant changes in your metabolism and percentage of lean muscle, you can review chapter 3 and re-evaluate your metabolic efficiency. You may find yourself at the same level, but if you sense food cravings or unusual hunger, or you are disappointed with the increase in your strength, then elevate to the next caloric level to promote more energy and muscular development.

■ The Unique Characteristics of Each Metabolic Type

Since your ninety-day metabolic maintenance program does not change calorically from week to week, which means that you will be eating the same general meal patterns and number of calories each day, it will give you an opportunity to really understand the finer points of your individual metabolism—and how to be creative with your food choices.

Each metabolic type has its particular sensitivities to foods and vulnerabilities to disease. People with a fat-and-protein-efficient metabolism have the greatest sensitivity toward sugars. For that reason, if they do not maintain appropriate nutritional balance, they become vulnerable to diseases such as diabetes, hypoglycemia, and hypertriglyceridimia (acute elevation of their triglyceride levels). If you are fat-and-protein-efficient, your ninety-day maintenance program will give you an opportunity to discover the degree of sensitivity your body has to sugars. This information will ultimately affect your carbohydrate choices. On the other hand, when properly fueled, the fat-and-protein-efficient metabolism has the greatest resistance to disease of any other metabolic type because the body's immune system is protein-based and these individuals eat the greatest amount of protein.

If you have a carbohydrate-efficient metabolism, the opposite situation exists. You can easily digest and use carbohydrates, but your body can utilize only a relatively small daily intake of protein (20 percent). If you are carbohydrate-efficient, be very conscientious about ingesting all of your protein requirement daily. In other words, never skip *any* of the protein in your meals. Ingesting enough protein is especially important for the support of your immune function. Remember, the immune system is protein-based. Falling short of your daily caloric allotment of protein will cause you to become more vulnerable to possible infection or disease because of immune system decay. Consistently eating the proper amount and type of protein is especially crucial for maintaining a high quality of life into your elder years. If carbohydrate-efficient, eating too much protein, especially if it has a high fat content, will cause an elevation of LDL cholesterol. For this reason, you should always choose lean protein, such as fish, chicken, or turkey breast. Compared to the fat-and-protein-efficient metabolism, you might have difficulty utilizing protein such as red meat or pork, which are higher in saturated fats.

If you have a dual metabolism (easily able to utilize all three nutrients—fats, proteins, and carbohydrates), you will be gifted with wonderfully balanced health. Since 33.3 percent of your daily nutritional intake is protein, you will not be as generally susceptible to disease as the carbohydrate-efficient individual, and less susceptible to diseases related to sugar sensitivities found in the fat-and-protein-efficient individual.

But, your metabolism is also the most sensitive and responsive to your choices, meaning that if you drift from your metabolic maintenance program, you will see adverse results much more quickly than the other two metabolic types. During your ninety-day maintenance program, it is especially important that you pay attention to your food choices and the correct balance between your nutrients. Since your metabolism is so sensitive and responsive, it is easier for you to rapidly gain body fat if you eat an inappropriate balance of fat, protein, and carbohydrate.

Of course, the good news is that your extremely responsive dual metabolism makes it easier for you to get back on track if you gain weight or stray from your food program because it is also the most efficient of the three metabolic types in terms of rapid body fat loss and composition change in partnership with appropriate nutritional patterns.

■ General Supplementation

Any nutritional program is greatly enhanced by appropriate supplementation. Below you will find a chart describing the basic functions of the most commonly taken vitamins, minerals, and other nutritional supplements. Although the amount and types of supplementation vary from person to person, depending on your individual goals and health and exercise needs, I generally recommend the following basic maintenance program:

   ■ A good multivitamin-multimineral combination taken twice daily—with your first meal in the morning and with lunch—to act as a shield against infections and to help prevent stress.

- A multimineral complex of calcium, magnesium, and zinc citrate with vitamin D, taken at bedtime, to reduce muscular spasms and cramping, to nutritionally support the strength of your skeletal system to avoid osteoporosis, and to help you relax and sleep at night.
- Liquid L-carnitine to stimulate the use of fat as energy. Although this supplement comes in capsules, it is most efficiently utilized in a liquid form in a glycerin base.
- A combination of the minerals chromium polynicotinate (unlike chromium picolinate, this supplement contains niacin, the intrinsic factor for the utilization of chromium) and vanadyl sulfate to create more efficient glucose tolerance to enhance the use of carbohydrates as an energy source. This combination is especially good for people who have a predisposition toward diabetes or other sugar sensitivities. They allow the body to tolerate more efficiently the use of glucose as an energy source.
- Whey protein powder and colostrum to enhance immune function and support tissue repair.

While a qualified salesperson at your local health food store can recommend a high-quality brand of vitamins, be aware that there is a difference between pharmaceutical-grade vitamins and vitamins that are only FDA approved. Pharmaceutical vitamins are manufactured using the same guidelines as prescription drugs; each capsule is within 1 percent of the ingredients you see listed on the label. There can be as much as a 20 percent variance in vitamins that are merely FDA approved. If you do decide to purchase your vitamins locally, always buy capsules as opposed to tablets since this usually ensures a somewhat higher level of quality. (For additional information on supplementation and how many supplements to take for your body weight, you can go to my website at www.pfcnutrition.com.)

■ Helpful Tips for Metabolic Maintenance

I have a number of tip cards that I give to clients who come to my clinic. These are designed to serve as a quick reference guide of helpful strategies for maintaining consistency on the food program. I am including some of these tips here to give you some quick and easy guidelines to help keep your performance on track.

QUICK REFERENCE GUIDE
FOR MAKING HEALTHY FOOD CHOICES

Meats (Proteins)	Breads (Complex Carbohydrates)	Vegetables (Fibrous Carbohydrates)	Fruit (Simple Carbohydrates)
Tuna	Potato	Summer Squash	Apple
Yellowtail	Yam	Cabbage	Apricots
Salmon	Sweet Potato	Mushrooms	Banana
Halibut	Rice, White	Tomatoes	Grapefruit
Swordfish	Rice, Brown	Cucumber	Pineapple
Chicken	Shredded Wheat	Onions	Blueberries
Turkey	Bran	Green Beans	Blackberries
Lean Steak	Oatmeal	Asparagus	Strawberries
Eggs	Corn Tortillas	Carrots	Cantaloupe
Tofu	Corn	Spinach	Watermelon
Whey Protein	Pasta	Zucchini	Nectarines
Soy Protein	Butternut	Cauliflower	Oranges
Almonds	Squash	Broccoli	Peaches
Peanut Butter			Pears

AVOID: Foods high in sugar, yeast breads, cream sauces, oils, butter, deep-fried foods

Cooking and Flavoring Tips

- Be creative in seasoning your foods. Use a lot of spices and powders to create tasty dishes.
- Avoid salt in your cooking.
- Use all-fruit spreads to add flavor to hot cereals and breads.
- Use nonfat plain yogurt instead of mayonnaise.
- Trim away excess fat and skins from meat, poultry, and fish.
- Use cooking sprays such as Pam rather than regular oils.
- Use nonstick frying pans, pressure cookers, steamer baskets, and roasting racks to cook foods. These tools help to separate fats from foods during the cooking process.

Behavioral Tips

- Make a scheduled time in your daily routine to exercise. Following a consistent pattern will ensure success.
- Don't eat out of boredom, depression, or negative emotions. Although this can be difficult, be aware of these times in order to break your patterns. Get involved in other activities that are more constructive and positive.
- Lose weight for yourself. Don't do it for someone else. Hold yourself accountable for all aspects of your program.
- Set realistic, short-term goals so that you quickly see results.
- Take charge of your attitude. Don't let others make decisions for you.

6. Uncovering the Body You Were Born With

Exercise Programs for Your Metabolic Type

One of the greatest benefits of following a nutritional program for your metabolic type is how it enhances the physique changes you experience as you exercise. Just as the three metabolic types each have different nutritional needs, they also have different exercise requirements. The fat-and-protein-efficient metabolism, with its ability to utilize large amounts of protein to build and repair muscle tissue, excels at strength training, so this metabolic type should follow an exercise program that emphasizes weights and uses cardiovascular activity as its secondary exercise. The long-and-lean carbohydrate-efficient person is able to utilize the large quantities of carbohydrates he ingests as an energy source and, therefore, naturally excels at endurance exercises. This type of individual will do best at cardiovascular training, with weight training secondary. The versatile dual metabolism, which evenly combines strength and endurance, will experience the greatest physique changes when following a workout program equally divided between weight training and cardiovascular exercise.

In this chapter, I have designed three basic workouts that are tailored to the unique exercise needs of each metabolic type. I offer these programs as a guide to help you enjoy your workouts and to receive maxim health and physique benefits from them.

▪ The Importance of Exercise

While it is true that you can lose weight and gain lean muscle just by following a food plan for your metabolic type, combining proper nutrition with a metabolically appropriate exercise program provides important and substantial benefits. It imparts vigor and efficiency to all organs and secures and maintains the healthful integrity of all their functions. Exercise aids in the correction of postural alignment and recovery from injuries, improves the tone and quality of muscle tissue, and stimulates the processes of digestion, absorption, metabolism, and elimination. It also strengthens blood vessels, the lungs, and the heart, resulting in the improved transfer of oxygen to the cells and increased circulation of the vascular and lymph systems. Added benefits are a sharper mind, and a body that radiates energy and balance.

The key to succeeding at any type of exercise is a strong will and a sincere desire to improve one's physical condition. It is important to have an exercise program that fits individual metabolic needs and capacities. A beginning fitness program should be challenging but not overly strenuous. But since the body will adapt to a particular level of exercise, just as it does to a static eating program, your workout should gradually increase in difficulty as your endurance improves, taking on a dynamic pattern. Your fitness program may contain many different forms of physical activity: sports, workouts in the gym or at home, cardiovascular exercises, classes in yoga or kickboxing. As long as you stay within the parameters of exercising for your metabolic type, described in this chapter, you can pick the ones you enjoy. Most important, work out regularly and maintain a metabolically appropriate food regimen.

Remember: Exercise does not create changes in your physique, it only creates the *potential* for physique changes. Workouts (exercise) systematically break down muscle tissue. The food you eat afterward is what repairs those muscles and completes your physique change. In the long run, exercise without proper nutritional support often does more harm than good. For example, if you don't ingest sufficient protein, your body will cannibalize its own muscle tissue in an effort to nourish itself. If you create a balance between exercise and nutrition, you will not only build a leaner, more muscular, and attractive physique, you will also optimize your health, stamina, and performance levels.

■ If You Are a Stranger to Exercise . . .

Some readers of this book may have never consciously exercised before, or may be severely deconditioned. Ultimately, for overall conditioning, if you haven't exercised in years, can't get to a gym, or have physical restrictions that make it difficult for you to work out with weights, then I suggest that you do some form of cardiovascular work. This type of exercise strengthens your heart and lungs; reduces stress; elevates HDLs and reduces LDLs, if your foods are correct; and helps to keep you young. A cardio workout routine can fit into the busiest of schedules. You can walk during your lunch hour, bike with your kids after work or run while they bike, go hiking with the whole family, among many other activities. Once you get started, your cardiovascular routine can be expanded into many popular classes, including Tae-Bo, kickboxing, spinning, martial arts, or any of the varieties of aerobics classes.

If you do only one form of cardiovascular exercise, however, I suggest that you choose walking. This is by far the most effective conditioning exercise for anyone, at any age. Ideally, you should walk a minimum of 40 minutes, 5 times a week. But if you have become so deconditioned that you can walk only 10 minutes in the beginning, then do that. In the weeks to come, increase your walking time by five minutes per week as you gain strength and aerobic conditioning. In just a few short weeks, you will be walking an hour at each cardiovascular session.

You can take yoga classes. This form of isometric exercise will stretch and condition your body, improve the function of all your internal organs, increase the efficiency of your circulatory and endocrine systems, and reduce stress. There are a variety of yoga classes for almost any need: yoga for pregnancy, yoga for back problems, heat yoga for added stretching, ashtanga yoga (a powerful type of yoga for building strength).

■ The Benefits of Progressive Weight Training

Regardless of your metabolic type, a certain portion of your workout will consist of progressive weight training in order to strengthen the musculoskeletal system. The benefits of weight training include increased muscle fiber size and density; increased muscle contractile strength; and increased tendon, bone, and ligament tensile strength. Exercising with weights will give the body a greater physical capacity, a more efficient metabolic function, and a decreased risk of general injury.

Physical Capacity

The most obvious benefits of a well-balanced strength-training program can be seen clearly in the changes that occur in your physique. The result will be a leaner, firmer, and fitter appearance due to the decreased amount of body fat and the addition of healthy muscle. Since lean muscle mass will slowly decrease if strength training does not continue, it is important to find a comfortable training regimen and to upgrade whenever you feel your body has adapted and needs greater intensity to create additional physique changes.

If you perform resistance exercises (weight training) regularly, you can expect to see dramatic changes in your strength. The American Council on Exercise states that previously untrained men and women gain about 2 to 4 pounds of muscle and 20 to 40 percent more strength after only two months of regular exercise. It does not matter at what age you begin exercising. You can start reaping great benefits from exercise *at any age*, even if you have never exercised before in your life.

If you decide to exercise with your children, however, do not permit them to begin training with weights or performing resistance exercises until the age of twelve. At that time the body's epithelial plates (growth plates at the ends of the bones that grow outward as the bones lengthen) have matured enough for the body to support weighted movements as long as the young person maintains proper posture and full range of motion. Before the age of twelve, children should concentrate on developing balance and stamina in a diverse array of sports and athletic activities of their choice.

Metabolic Function

Exercise increases the ratio of lean muscle to fat and improves metabolic efficiency. Simply put, there are basically two types of biological tissue: functional and nonfunctional. Muscle tissue is an active tissue, meaning that it can efficiently utilize caloric energy from stored fat to create movement. Fat tissue is nonfunctional—it burns no calories because it *is*, in and of itself, a fuel for the activation of the body's functional tissue.

The activation of muscle tissue releases metabolic heat as energy. The more muscle tissue you have, the more caloric heat required to create muscular movement and, therefore, the higher your metabolic temperature. Conversely, if you stop exercising, muscle tissue will atrophy, causing a decrease in metabolic function and temperature.

■ Cardiovascular (Aerobic) Exercise

Types of exercise that strengthen the cardiovascular system are known as aerobic modalities. This includes activities such as walking outside or on a treadmill; jogging; using an elliptical trainer; step classes; riding a road, stationary, or recumbent bicycle; swimming; skipping rope; using a Stairmaster or versa climber; hiking; taking an aerobics exercise class; or stadium stair climbing.

Since the heart is a muscle, it, too, must be exercised regularly. Cardiovascular exercise helps to decrease the risk of disease to your heart and circulatory system by helping to decrease risk factors such as excess weight or obesity, and to increase levels of HDL ("good" cholesterol) and lower your LDL levels ("bad" cholesterol). Cardiovascular exercise increases the body's ability to utilize fat and to consume oxygen. Endurance activities such as walking, trail hiking, jogging, and bicycling have proven beneficial in reducing the disease risk or symptoms for Type 1 and Type 2 diabetes and high blood pressure (hypertension). They have also been shown to improve pulmonary conditioning in women, both during and after pregnancy. People who achieve aerobic fitness generally have more stamina, which translates to less fatigue and fewer risks for certain types of injuries. Cardiovascular exercise will give you a deeper, more restful sleep and enable a more efficient use of nutrients.

The Proper and Safe Way to Do Cardiovascular Exercises

There are three phases of aerobic exercise: the warm-up, the aerobic phase, and the cooldown. Each phase has a specific purpose and each applies to all levels, from the beginner to the advanced.

The Warm-up. The first phase, lasting 5 to 10 minutes, prepares the body for vigorous exercise. It gets the blood circulating, gets oxygen into the muscles of the body, and enables you to become mentally focused. Correct stretching movements are important because they increase flexibility and reduce the risk of injury. Your warm-up should be a combination of smooth, controlled stretching and rhythmic limbering exercises. For example, never bounce when you are touching your toes or doing any other kind of stretching movement. Short, jerky movements give your muscles a confusing mixed message of rapid stretching and contraction. Instead, concentrate on elongating your body and breathing into all of your stretches in a controlled and relaxed way. Never overstretch, especially if your body type is naturally extremely limber. In other words, never "lock" your joints or extend a muscle beyond its joint capacity. If you do overstretch, you will experience pain and discomfort. Allowing your knees and elbows to be slightly bent at all times (a "soft lock" position) will preserve your joints and muscles from unnecessary wear and tear while stretching.

Rhythmic limbering exercises also increase the flexibility of your ligaments, tendons, and other soft tissue, causing muscular extension and preparing your muscles for the more strenuous exercises ahead. Examples of some warm-up exercises include arm circles, small kicks, knee lifts, touching your toes, and any exercise that involves the movements of the bones and joints. Perform all these movements at a moderate pace, in a smooth and controlled fashion with an even cadence.

The Aerobic Phase. There are a variety of exercises that qualify as aerobic by causing an increased demand for oxygen over an extended period of time. We mentioned several of these above. Whichever you choose, start slowly and increase the intensity of the activity until you reach a pace that your body can endure for an extended period of time. Depending upon your level of fitness, the length of your aerobic workout will range from 15 minutes for beginners, 30 to 45 minutes for intermediates, to 1 full hour for those who are advanced. You will know that you are performing at the proper level of intensity if you are able to speak without discomfort or without gasping for air. This is called assessing your perceived exertion level. Maintain an even breathing pattern at all times, inhaling through your nose and exhaling through your mouth.

Because your body will adapt to doing the same type of activities, try to vary the kinds of aerobic exercises you are performing to ensure that your body will continue to change and grow stronger. Changing exercise modalities will also help to maintain your interest in cardiovascular activity.

The Cooldown. This phase provides a transition between a vigorous aerobic workout and less aerobically taxing exercise. A cooldown, which consists of a light activity such as walking on a treadmill, should last between 2 to 5 minutes. Allowing your heart rate to decrease gradually and without stress will reduce the risk of dizziness or fainting.

Some basic tips for maximizing your cardiovascular workout and minimizing injury include the following:

■ Always wear proper footwear. Invest in a good pair of shoes that are designed to support your feet and minimize jarring to your spine and joints during ballistic movements. Enlist the help of a qualified salesperson in a local store that specializes in sports footwear. Since there is a big difference between shoes used primarily for walking, shoes for jogging, shoes for hiking, and so on, be specific about the kind of activity you will be doing while wearing the shoes. Take your time and walk around the store to make sure the shoes are a comfortable fit and that your toes aren't banging against the front of the shoe. In fact, it's often wise to buy a shoe that is a half or full size bigger than your daily street wear to allow for maximum comfort during vigorous aerobic activity. You can fill up any remaining space in the shoe with one or two pairs of good athletic socks made of natural fibers that allow your foot to "breath" and to provide extra cushioning. I recommend Thorlo double-padded athletic socks. If you know you will be running or hiking up and down hills, this cushioning and foot support is especially beneficial.

■ Always wear loose, comfortable clothing that will allow your body's heat to escape during vigorous exercise. In colder weather, wear layers that you can take off as your body begins to warm up.

■ Stretch before performing cardiovascular or any type of exercise to ensure that your body is warmed up. Also stretch out afterward.

■ Make sure that you drink water throughout your workout to keep yourself hydrated. This will enhance your endurance capacity, keep your muscles from cramping, and help to maintain proper electrolyte balance in your system. It will also help to stabilize your body temperature. You should be able to consume 1.5 liters (50.7 ounces) of water during 1 hour of cardiovascular activity.

■ If you experience severe shortness of breath, wheezing or coughing, chest pain or tightness, severe muscle pains or cramps, or dizziness or nausea while involved in cardiovascular activities, stop immediately and rest for 10 to 15 minutes. If these symptoms do not disappear after resting, call you doctor immediately.

■ Normal reactions to cardiovascular activity include a faster heart rate that is not uncomfortable, mild or moderate perspiration, quicker breathing rate, and tender muscles that might last a day or two.

Exercising at the Proper Aerobic Intensity

There are two ways to ensure that you are exercising with the proper aerobic intensity—exerting yourself enough to get your heart pumping above its normal rate at rest yet still somewhat below its maximum rate.

Use the "Perceived Exertion" or "Talk Test." This means that you should always be able to carry on a conversation while you are walking, jogging, bicycling, and so on. If you find that you are exerting yourself so much that you gasp for air when you speak, then you need to reduce the intensity of your aerobic workout.

Use Your Target Heart Rate for Training. The second way to ensure that you are exercising at the proper level of aerobic intensity is to calculate your maximal heart rate. This will allow you to identify your appropriate target heart rate for aerobic exercise. Knowing your target heart rate zone will help you maintain an aerobic intensity that is appropriate for consistently using fat as energy during exercise. If your heart rate falls below your target zone, you are not working intensely enough to use fat as energy. If it goes above your target zone, you are working too hard, causing your body to use more carbohydrates than fat as energy. The latter will stimulate your cardiorespiratory system (your lungs and oxygen uptake) more than your cardiovascular system (your heart and your blood transport system).

An easy way to calculate your target heart rate zone for aerobic exercise is to use the following "220 minus age" formula.

■ **Step 1:** Subtract your age from 220.
■ **Step 2:** Multiply that number times 70% (.7) to get the low end of your range.
■ **Step 3:** Multiply that number by 80% (.8) to get the high end of your range.

Example: A 40-Year-Old Man

(220 – 40 [age])	180
(70%—low intensity range)	× .7
(70%—lower limit exercise heart rate)	126
(220 - 40 [age])	180
(80%—upper intensity range)	× .8
(80%—upper limit intensity range)	144

Target heart rate = 126–144 beats per minute

To see if you are within this range, immediately after exercising take your pulse for 6 seconds and multiply that number times 10. If that number is *below* your lower target heart rate range, you need to exert yourself more. If that number is *above* your upper target heart rate range, you need to reduce your intensity.

Another way to accurately keep track of your heart rate while exercising is to purchase a heart monitor that fits around your wrist like a wristwatch. You can purchase this device at your local sporting goods store.

The following chart shows the target heart rate zone for ages 10 through 85.

Age	Maximal Heart Rate	Target Heart Rate Zone Ranges		
		Low 70%	Ideal 75%	High 80%
10	210	147	157	168
15	205	144	154	164
20	200	140	150	160
25	195	137	147	156
30	190	133	143	152
35	185	130	139	148
40	180	126	135	144
45	175	123	131	140
50	170	119	127	136
55	165	116	124	132
60	160	112	120	128
65	155	109	116	124
70	150	105	112	120
75	145	102	109	116
80	140	98	105	112
85	135	95	101	108

A common question clients ask me is if their maximal heart rate can be increased through achieving a greater fitness level. In other words, can a person who is 40 eventually become so aerobically conditioned that he or she is exercising at the heart rate of someone who is 30? In reality, no. Scientifically, your target heart rate for your age is simply the place where your body burns fat most efficiently. If you exceed that number, you are no longer using fat as an energy source. Therefore, *your goal is not to exercise at a higher heart rate, but to increase the level of intensity that it takes for you to reach your target heart rate.* For example, initially when you begin using an exercise bike you discover that level 1 is too easy for you but that you can reach your target heart rate through the amount of exertion required on exercise level 2. But a month later, after your fitness level has improved, level 2 on the bike is so easy for you that you can't get your heart rate into your target zone. So you have to move up to level 3.

When exercising aerobically, your goal will always be to intensify the level of your workout, not the range of your heart rate.

■ The Basics of Weight Training

If you have never lifted weights before, you are about to discover what an enjoyable activity weight lifting can be and how easy it is to learn routines best suited for your specific metabolic needs. One of the best things about weight training is that you can start at any level and continually move up to higher levels—and always get results. If you are already familiar with weight lifting, the workout guidelines in this chapter should help you to maximize your workout for your metabolic type.

When choosing a gym, make sure that the gym has a wide variety of free weights and machines that are easily adjustable for your height and physique type. If you have never lifted weights before, you may wish to hire a personal trainer initially to show you how to lift safely and correctly use the various machines and free weights. In choosing a trainer, there are certain qualifications you should look for. Make sure that your trainer has either college-level degrees in physiology, kinesiology, or physical therapy and/or certifications from organizations such as the National Academy of Sports Medicine, the American College of Sports Medicine, the American Counsel on Exercise, the International Fitness Professionals Association, or the Aerobics and Fitness Association of America.

Below, I have included three basic programs—divided between weights and cardiovascular activities—specifically tailored for the three metabolic types. Whatever your goals or level of experience, you will find helpful instruction here.

For years I have created and documented a wide variety of workouts for my clients, based on a variety of weekly training schedules designed to fit easily into even the busiest of lifestyles. Within the following pages you will find workouts designed for each metabolic type. I have also included an Exercise Log so that you can keep track of your weight-training workouts and record your progress.

As you go through your program, use the following guidelines as your "coach":

> ■ Always make sure to spend 5 to 10 minutes warming up and stretching prior to lifting. A stationary bike or a treadmill are great choices for a quick warm-up. Be sure to spend 3 to 5 minutes on the bike or treadmill after lifting to facilitate your cooldown process.

▪ Always drink plenty of water while exercising. Carry a large bottle with you as you move from machine to machine. Drink water in between your sets as necessary to stay well hydrated. You should be able to consume 1.5 liters of water (50.7 ounces) within a 1-hour workout.

▪ Follow the ABCs of training listed below. Weight training helps to improve posture and to shape, tone, and strengthen muscle tissue more effectively than any other form of exercise. As your body develops muscular shape and strength, your spine will be more securely supported by the surrounding muscles. This weight training effect is called postural stability. The benefits of weight training can be seen in improved posture, muscularity, and muscular strength and endurance. To fully achieve all these benefits always make certain that:

1. You are positioned in the machine correctly or, if you are using free weights, that you are correctly stabilizing proper joint alignment and posture.

2. Never compromise your form, stability, alignment, or posture to increase the pounds being lifted. Injury and poor posture are almost certain to be the result. You will become significantly stronger by maintaining proper position and form during your lifts, even with light weights. Keep safety in mind and never handle more weight than your body can stabilize.

3. Complete all repetitions for each set. If the weight becomes heavy, stop the set, reduce the weight, and continue until the set of repetitions is complete. If you have any questions about how to use the machines in your gym or how much weight you should be lifting, ask a trainer. Don't risk injuring yourself.

▪ The exercises within each workout program are to be performed in order. Each exercise works a particular muscle or group of muscles from a specific angle and in a particular order. The workouts are designed to systematically exhaust the muscle(s). Start at the top of your workout sheet with the first exercise and work your way through. Complete the sets and repetitions for each exercise and record your weight increments in the appropriate spaces in the Exercise Log.

▪ As with any exercise program, it is always best to slowly familiarize yourself with the workout protocols. To ensure the correct muscular adaption for this new activity, perform only one or two sets at most, per exercise, for the first two or three workout sessions. This will help ensure that your muscles can safely adjust to the exercises listed in your program. The following day after exercising you should experience slight muscular tightness or soreness, but nothing so extreme that the soreness limits your muscular range of motion or any involvement in your regular daily activities. Based on your soreness and comfort level with the exercises, you may increase the number of sets for each exercise.

■ Once you've gotten to the point where you can complete the entire workout program, track your progress for approximately 4 to 6 weeks in your Exercise Log. At that point, evaluate your program, document your improvements, and upgrade your workout by consulting with a trainer at your gym, visiting an online training website, or consulting a good weight training book. (See page 126 for suggestions.) Exercise programs should change every four to six weeks—the body will eventually adjust to any regimen and will require variations in exercises, sets, and repetition schemes to promote continual change in physique and strength. Of course, if you simply get bored with your routine, change it—never let boredom cause you to stop weight training.

■ To ensure the proper documentation of your results, I have included a Monthly Body Measurements Chart and a Body Weight and Composition Chart. At the end of each exercise program, I have also included a log for your weight and cardiovascular workouts. These charts are designed to be interactive. Use them to establish a written history of your progress.

I recommend that anyone considering an exercise program should consult his or her doctor first and, if necessary, complete a full physical examination. It is always best to notify all of your health professionals about any choices you are making in regard to fitness, nutrition, and change of lifestyle.

■ Keeping Track of Your Body Weight and Composition

Because you'll be losing fat and firming up your lean body tissue, your scale weight will not tell you the entire story of your progress. The best way to keep track of how much actual fat you are losing is by keeping track of lost inches. The following body measurements should be taken with a tape measure every three weeks. Make sure to measure the same area of each body part each month. If possible, I recommend that you have someone else do the measuring.

Neck—Measure around the middle of the neck.
Chest—Measure around the chest at the nipple line.
Upper arms—Measure around the upper arm.
Hips—Measure around the hips at the mid-buttock area.
Waist—Measure the smallest circumference below your rib cage and
   above your navel.
Thighs—Measure around the middle of the thigh.
Calves—Measure around the middle of each calf.

Date

Body Part	Day 1	End of Week 3	End of Week 6	End of Week 9	End of Week 12
Neck					
Chest					
Upper Arm/L					
Upper Arm/R					
Waist					
Hips					
Thigh/L					
Thigh/R					
Calf/L					
Calf/R					

Of course, you will still want to keep track of your scale weight. Below I have included a chart for body weight and composition. Remember to (1) only weigh yourself once a week, (2) always weigh yourself at the same time of day, (3) always weigh with either no clothes or the same clothes. I have included a space for your percentage of body fat to lean muscle if you want to keep track of that as well. See chapter 2, page 44 for instructions on calculating body composition.

■ Getting Started

Below I have chosen three different basic workout routines for each of the three metabolic types. If you are unfamiliar with the format of

	Date	Body Weight	Body Composition
Week 1			
Week 2			
Week 3			
Week 4			
Week 5			
Week 6			
Week 7			
Week 8			
Week 9			
Week 10			
Week 11			
Week 12			

any of these exercises, there are great illustrated exercise books that I can refer you to that will help you with posture and alignment. These include Bill Pearl's revised edition of *Getting Stronger: Weight Training for Men and Women,* and Arnold Schwarzenegger and Bill Dobbins's *The New Encyclopedia of Modern Bodybuilding.* Another great source for pictures and directions for doing weight exercises correctly are the many fine interactive Internet websites. These include www.plantetkc.com/exrx, www.nuticise.com, www.fitnesslink.com, www.globalfitness.com, http://en.fitness.com, www.efit.com, www.indiadiets.com, www.acefitness.com. As your strength and endurance increase, these websites can even fill the role of a personal trainer, providing you with more challenging workouts. For additional exercise information, you can access my website, www.pfcnutrition.com.

As for the length of your workout, I suggest an hour to an hour and a half. If you have never exercised before, or are deconditioned, start with half an hour and gradually increase your time weekly. If you are working out three days per week, combine your weight training with your cardiovascular exercises in the proper proportions. But also keep in mind that you can lift weights three days a week and perform your cardio exercises on a different day of the week if it is more convenient for you, based on your lifestyle.

How can you tell when you are using too much weight? If you are new to weights and resistance exercises, I suggest you start with the lowest setting on the machine or the lightest free weights and slowly add weight in 5-to-10-pound increments. Begin with 1 set of repetitions (the number of reps per set per exercise is suggested in each workout chart below) and slowly build up to 3, 4, or 5 sets, depending on the exercise and workout format.

An appropriate amount of weight is the amount that is comfortable for you to maintain proper joint stability and alignment. Warning signs that you are using too much weight include not being able to control the weight during the exercise, arching your back when lifting, excessively squeezing your neck and jaw, tremors and shaking during the movement, and not being able to catch your breath. If you find yourself using muscle groups, body parts, or movements that are not meant for that particular exercise, you should reduce your weight. For example, you shouldn't be pushing with your hands if you are using a machine designed to work your abdominal muscles—your abdominals are supposed to do all the work. If you are doing the exercise correctly, you will feel slight muscular burning caused by the repetitions of muscular contraction and extension. However, don't confuse joint pain or muscular pain with this healthy burning and tingling sensation. There is a distinct difference between the two.

Recovery time. Be sure to allow yourself some recovery time in between each set to allow your muscles to recuperate. I suggest 45 seconds to a minute for the upper body and back, and slightly longer than that if needed when training the lower body—the legs and buttocks.

A common question I hear is whether or not you can exercise on two consecutive days, or whether it is necessary to always rest a day between workouts. The answer depends upon what kind of workout you are performing. There are a variety of different exercise patterns. In one you would train your entire body three days a week, with a day of rest in between. Exercise programs that *can* be done on consecutive days are four-, five-, or six-day workouts that break your body into either individual body parts or groups of body parts trained on specific days with adequate rest periods in between each *muscle group*. For example, a five-day workout is designed to train one body part a day. Day one is chest, day two is legs, day three is shoulders, day four is back, day five is arms. Days six and seven are off.

■ A Basic Workout Program for the Fat-and-Protein-Efficient Metabolism

If you are a fat-and-protein-efficient individual, your primary mode of exercise will be weight training because your body gets strong quickly and experiences its greatest physique changes by pushing against resistance or lifting something heavy. This type of physique, which is heavily muscled and designed for strength rather than long-term endurance, will find cardiovascular training more challenging. Therefore, your workout should ideally consist of 1 hour of weight lifting or resistance exercises and a minimum of 30 minutes of cardiovascular work. How many times a week depends upon the exercise program you have chosen.

The physique of a fat-and-protein-efficient individual can handle heavier weights and lower repetitions within each set—between 8 and 15 reps per exercise set. With this type of regimen, your body will respond rapidly, developing greater strength and shape. After you complete your weight training, finish with 30 minutes to 1 hour of cardiovascular training (how much is dependent on lifestyle, time constraints, and individual needs). If you have only an hour a day to work out, then I suggest that you do your cardiovascular exercise on the days you are not training with weights. You won't feel as comfortable with the cardio aspect of your fitness program as you do with your weight training, but it is still an important part of your overall fitness program.

Below is a basic workout program for a fat-and-protein-efficient individual. This program is the same whether you are male or female. Your basic three-day exercise program will consist of two alternating parts, A and B. Your seven-day schedule will be structured in the following way:

3-Day Total-Body Workout for a Fat-and-Protein-Efficient Metabolism

Day 1: Workout A

Day 2: Off (or cardio day)

Day 3: Workout B

Day 4: Off (or cardio day)

Day 5: Workout A

Day 6: Off (or cardio day)

Day 7: Off

Start your second week with Workout B and continue to alternate.

List of Exercises for the Fat-and-Protein-Efficient Metabolism 3-Day Workout

Workout A: Chest, Back, Biceps, Triceps

Warm-up: 5 to 10 minutes

CHEST

Barbell bench press, incline

Low-incline dumbbell bench press

Seated horizontal bench press machine

Flat-bench flys

Pec deck (optional)

BACK

Seated flex torso support cable row

Seated cable rows

Wide-grip pulldowns, front

Close-grip pulldowns, front

BICEPS

Standing straight-bar curls

Horizontal cable curl machine

Seated cable preacher curls (optional)

TRICEPS

Standing tricep pushdowns

Overhead seated cable extension superset (optional)

Standing reverse tricep pushdowns superset

Workout B: Legs and Shoulders

Warm-up: 10 minutes

LEGS

Leg extensions

Hack squat machine (low incline) or horizontal squat press machine

Leg press machine

Leg extensions

Leg curl superset with hamtractor

SHOULDERS

Seated machine shoulder press

Standing dumbbell lateral raises

Reverse pec deck deltoid pulls

Standing dumbbell shrugs

Abdominals and Calves: Do at the End of Both Workouts A and B

ABDOMINALS

High-incline bent-knee sit-ups

Hanging leg raises

Crunches

CALVES

Standing calf raises

Cooldown: 3 to 5 minutes

Here is an exercise log for the three-day workout program for the fat-and-protein-efficient metabolism. I have suggested the ideal number of sets and reps for a foundation workout program, but you will probably start with only one or two sets and work your way up. I have left the amount of weight blank so that you can fill in whatever pounds are comfortable for you at the time. Don't forget to always warm up and cool down. Do all exercises in the order in which they are listed for correct postural stability and strength. If you perform the exercises out of order, this could result in poor posture and possible injury. I prefer Cybex, Flex, and Icarian machines for some of the following exercises, but any reliable equipment line used by your gym, such as Nautilus, is perfectly acceptable.

3-Day Workout Program for the Fat-and-Protein-Efficient Metabolism

Workout A: Chest, Back, Biceps, Triceps, Abdominals, Calves

CHEST

Barbell bench press, incline

Wt.											
Rep.	10	8	8	10	15						
Set	1	2	3	4	5						

Low-incline dumbbell bench press

Wt.											
Rep.	10	10	10	15							
Set	1	2	3	4							

Seated horizontal bench press machine

Wt.											
Rep.	12	12	15	15							
Set	1	2	3	4							

Flat-bench flys

Wt.											
Rep.	12	12	12								
Set	1	2	3								

Pec deck (optional)

Wt.											
Rep.	12	12	12								
Set	1	2	3								

BACK

Seated torso support cable row

Wt.											
Rep.	10	10	12	15							
Set	1	2	3	4							

Seated cable rows

Wt.											
Rep.	10	10	10	10							
Set	1	2	3	4							

Wide-grip pulldowns, front

Wt.											
Rep.	10	8	8	12	15						
Set	1	2	3	4	5						

Close-grip pulldowns, front

Wt.										
Rep.	15	15								
Set	1	2								

BICEPS

Standing straight-bar curls

Wt.										
Rep.	10	8	8	12	15					
Set	1	2	3	4	5					

Horizontal cable curl machine

Wt.										
Rep.	12	12	12							
Set	1	2	3							

Seated cable preacher curls (optional)

Wt.										
Rep.	12	12	12							
Set	1	2	3							

TRICEPS

Standing tricep pushdowns

Wt.										
Rep.	10	8	8	12	15					
Set	1	2	3	4	5					

Overhead seated cable extension superset (optional)

Wt.										
Rep.	12	12	12							
Set	1	2	3							

Standing reverse tricep pushdowns superset

Wt.										
Rep.	12	12	12							
Set	1	2	3							

Cardiovascular Workout

Date							
Mode							
Duration							
Intensity							

Workout B: Legs and Shoulders

LEGS

Leg extensions

Wt.												
Rep.	20	20	20									
Set	1	2	3									

Hack squat machine (low incline) or horizontal squat press machine

Wt.												
Rep.	15	15	15	15								
Set	1	2	3	4								

Leg press flex machine

Wt.												
Rep.	15	15	15	15								
Set	1	2	3	4								

Leg extensions

Wt.												
Rep.	30	30										
Set	1	2										

Leg curl superset with hamtractor

Wt.												
Rep.	15	15	15	20								
Set	1	2	3	4								

SHOULDERS

Seated machine shoulder press

Wt.												
Rep.	10	10	10	10								
Set	1	2	3	4								

Standing dumbbell lateral raises

Wt.												
Rep.	12	12	12	12								
Set	1	2	3	4								

Reverse pec deck deltoid pulls

Wt.												
Rep.	15	15	15									
Set	1	2	3									

Standing dumbbell shrugs										
Wt.										
Rep.	10	10	10							
Set	1	2	3							

Cardiovascular Workout										
Date										
Mode										
Duration										
Intensity										

The following exercises for the abdominal muscles and the calves are to be done at the end of *both* Workouts A and B.

Workouts A and B: Abdominals, Calves

ABDOMINALS

High-incline bent-knee sit-ups										
Wt.										
Rep.	15	15	15	15						
Set										

Hanging leg raises										
Wt.										
Rep.	20	20	20	20						
Set										

Crunches										
Wt.										
Rep.	20	20	20	20						
Set										

CALVES

Standing calf raises										
Wt.										
Rep.	20	20	20	20						
Set										

■ A Basic Workout Program for the Carbohydrate-Efficient Metabolism

If you are a carbohydrate-efficient individual, your primary mode of exercise will be cardiovascular because you excel at all forms of endurance exercise. You should begin your workout with an hour of aerobic exercise, such as stair stepping, riding a stationary bike, running on the treadmill, or using a rower or climber. Finish off with half an hour of weights. If you feel that you don't have enough time to exercise for an hour and a half, you can spread your workout throughout the week, doing weight training on some days and cardiovascular training on others, as long as you do these activities in the proper proportions.

Your tall and lanky physique type doesn't carry a lot of muscle tissue but has great muscular endurance. Therefore, your weight workout will be most effective if you perform it as a circuit program, moving rapidly from one exercise or machine to another, maintaining a high repetition scheme of 12 to 20 reps per set per body part. To enable this high amount of repetition, you will use slightly less weight than a fat-and-protein-efficient individual would. This will enable you to maintain constant muscular expansion and contraction in your movements over an extended period of time.

Since you are an expert at cardiovascular work, you have considerable capacity to sustain long, extended exercise programs. The three-day total-body workout below will support your inborn cardiovascular efficiency. Do all exercises in the order in which they are listed for correct postural stability and strength. If you perform the exercises out of order, this could result in poor posture and possible injury.

3-Day Total-Body Workout for a Carbohydrate-Efficient Metabolism
Day 1: Workout
Day 2: Off (or cardio day)
Day 3: Workout
Day 4: Off (or cardio day)
Day 5: Workout
Day 6: Off (or cardio day)
Day 7: Off

List of Exercises for the
Carbohydrate-Efficient Metabolism 3-Day Workout

Chest, Shoulders, Back, Legs, Arms, Abdominals

Warm-up: 5 to 10 minutes

CHEST

Machine bench press

Low-incline dumbbell flys

Pec dec flys

SHOULDERS

Seated machine shoulder press

Seated dumbbell lateral raises

BACK

Wide-grip pulldowns, front

Seated row machine torso support

LEGS

Leg extensions

Inner/outer thigh machine

Leg curl

TRICEPS AND BICEPS

Standing tricep pushdowns

Standing bicep curl or machine curl

ABDOMINALS

Seated incline abdominal crunches

CALVES

Calf raises, seated or standing

Cooldown: 3 to 5 minutes

Here is an exercise log to help you keep track of your progress. Don't forget to take the time to warm up and cool down.

Cardiovascular Exercise Log

DATE	MODE	DURATION	INTENSITY

3-Day Workout for the Carbohydrate-Efficient Metabolism

Chest, Shoulders, Back, Legs, Triceps, Biceps, Abdominals

CHEST

Machine bench press

Wt.											
Rep.	12	12	12								
Set	1	2	3								

Low-incline dumbbell flys

Wt.											
Rep.	12	12	12								
Set	1	2	3								

Pec dec flys

Wt.											
Rep.	15	15									
Set	1	2									

SHOULDERS

Seated machine shoulder press

Wt.											
Rep.	12	12	12								
Set	1	2	3								

Seated dumbbell lateral raises

Wt.											
Rep	12	12	12								
Set	1	2	3								

BACK

Wide-grip pulldowns, front

Wt.											
Rep.	12	12	12	12							
Set	1	2	3	4							

Seated row machine torso support

Wt.											
Rep.	12	12	12								
Set	1	2	3								

LEGS

Leg extensions

Wt.											
Rep.	20	20	20								
Set	1	2	3								

Inner/outer thigh machine

Wt.											
Rep.	20	20	20								
Set	1	2	3								

Leg curl

Wt.											
Rep.	20	20	20								
Set	1	2	3								

TRICEPS AND BICEPS

Standing tricep pushdowns

Wt.											
Rep.	12	12	12								
Set	1	2	3								

Machine bicep curl or machine curl

Wt.											
Rep.	12	12	12								
Set	1	2	3								

ABDOMINALS

Seat incline abdominal crunches

Wt.											
Rep.	15	15	15								
Set	1	2	3								

CALVES

Calf raises, seated or standing

Wt.											
Rep.	15	15	15								
Set	1	2	3								

■ A Basic Workout Program for the Dual Metabolism

Since the dual metabolism combines both strength and endurance, these individuals should divide their workout program equally between both types of exercises, ideally doing 45 minutes of weight training and 45 minutes of cardiovascular. If you have this type of metabolism, you will find that you improve evenly at both. If you do not have time for an hour and a half of exercise a day, then simply do the cardio and strength-training components of your program on different days, keeping them in proper proportion. Below is a basic workout program for the dual metabolism.

3-Day Total-Body Workout for the Dual Metabolism

Day 1: Workout

Day 2: Off (or cardio day)

Day 3: Workout

Day 4: Off (or cardio day)

Day 5: Workout

Day 6: Off (or cardio day)

Day 7: Off

List of Exercises for the Dual Metabolism 3-Day Workout

Chest, Shoulders, Back, Legs, Arms, Abdominals

Warm-up: 5 to 10 minutes

CHEST

Machine bench press

Pec dec flys

SHOULDERS

Seated machine shoulder press

Seated machine lateral raises

BACK

Wide-grip pulldowns, front

Seated cable rows

LEGS

Leg extensions

Inner/outer thigh machine

Leg curl

TRICEPS AND BICEPS

Standing tricep pushdowns

Machine bicep curl

Machine triceps extensions, seated

ABDOMINALS

Bent-knee sit-ups or abdominal crunch machine

Leg raises (knees bent) (optional—do not perform if lower-back or hip problems exist)

Cooldown: 3 to 5 minutes

Here is an exercise log to help you keep track of your progress. The dual metabolism can perform both cardiovascular exercises and resistance exercises with equal ability. Therefore, you should begin your workout with cardio one day, then with weights the next, alternating between the two. Remember, always make sure that you warm up and cool down. Do all exercises in the order in which they are listed for correct postural stability and strength. If you perform the exercises out of order, this could result in poor posture and possible injury.

Cardiovascular Exercise Log

DATE	MODE	DURATION	INTENSITY

3-Day Workout Program for the Dual Metabolism

Chest, Shoulders, Back, Legs, Triceps, Biceps, Abdominals

CHEST

Machine bench press

Wt.										
Rep.	10	10	10	15						
Set	1	2	3	4						

Pec dec flys

Wt.										
Rep.	15	15	15	15						
Set	1	2	3	4						

SHOULDERS

Seated machine shoulder press

Wt.										
Rep.	10	10	10	12						
Set	1	2	3	4						

Seated machine lateral raises

Wt.										
Rep.	12	12	12							
Set	1	2	3							

BACK

Wide-grip pulldowns, front

Wt.										
Rep.	10	10	10	12						
Set	1	2	3	4						

Seated cable rows

Wt.										
Rep.	10	10	10	12						
Set	1	2	3	4						

LEGS

Leg extensions

Wt.										
Rep.	20	20	20	20						
Set	1	2	3	4						

Inner/outer thigh machine

Wt.										
Rep.	20	20	20	20						
Set	1	2	3	4						

Leg curl

Wt.										
Rep.	20	20	20	20						
Set	1	2	3	4						

TRICEPS AND BICEPS

Standing tricep pushdowns

Wt.										
Rep.	12	12	12							
Set	1	2	3							

Machine bicep curl										
Wt.										
Rep.	12	12	12							
Set	1	2	3							

Machine tricep extensions, seated										
Wt.										
Rep.	12	12	12							
Set	1	2	3							

ABDOMINALS

Bent-knee sit-ups or abdominal crunch machine										
Wt.										
Rep.	20	20	20	20						
Set	1	2	3	4						

Leg raises (knees bent) (optional—do not perform if lower-back or hip problems exist										
Wt.										
Rep.	20	20	20	20						
Set	1	2	3	4						

■ What If You Do Not Belong to a Gym?

If you don't want to take the time or expense to join a gym, most exercises listed above can be performed using stretch straps. You can purchase these either at your local sporting goods store or through my website, www.pfcnutrition.com. When you purchase these products, you will receive an instruction booklet that teaches you exercises to tone and condition each part of the body. These exercises will resemble those found in this book.

Whatever you decide to do, know that your metabolically appropriate nutritional program will help you to achieve fitness results that have always seemed beyond your reach. This combination of nutrition and exercise tailored to your unique metabolic needs will increase your performance levels, health, endurance, and self-confidence, keeping your body young, your mind sharp and clear, and your outlook on life joyous.

Part II

The Food **Programs**

The Fat-and-Protein-Efficient Food Program

12-Week Instructions and Meal Plans for Caloric Levels 1–11

Determine your level by choosing the caloric range closest to the caloric number determined by your metabolic scenario:

Level	Caloric Range of Level
1	Under 1,200
2	1,201–1,365
3	1,366–1,480
4	1,481–1,685
5	1,686–1,805
6	1,806–2,180
7	2,181–2,330
8	2,331–2,450
9	2,451–2,765
10	2,766–3,065
11	3,066 and up

Do not forget the option of adding items from the Free Foods List in appendix C to these meal plans. For example, when you are having oatmeal or cereal, you may add ½ cup nonfat milk; when you are having salad, you can add up to 2 tablespoons low-fat dressing per day; when you have steamed vegetables, you are allowed 1 tablespoon of nondairy butter per day. Also, beverages such as tea, coffee, and diet soda can be added to your meal plans, but they *do not* count toward your daily water intake.

During certain weeks Meal 1 is listed as a Fruit 1 and a two-scoop whey protein shake. The whey shake is not mandatory for the program, but we have chosen to use the shake during some weeks because whey protein offers the highest, most biologically efficient form of protein. To make this shake you need to buy a zero carbohydrate whey shake either at your health food store or from my website, www.pfcnutrition.com. Make sure that one scoop equals between 70 and 85 calories. To make the shake, blend one serving of fruit, two scoops of whey protein powder, some ice, and water according to your desired consistency and drink this as your first meal. If you choose not to do the shake, then the whey portion of Meal 1 becomes a Meat 2, for example, two eggs.

■ Weekly Instructions for the Fat-and-Protein-Efficient Metabolism (for All Levels)

Below are just a few things to keep in mind as you begin each week of your program, no matter what level you are using.

Week 1. In this first week, also known as your Foundation Food Program, you'll be laying groundwork for the coming weeks of the program. This week we want you to get used to eating more times during the day, drinking more water, and getting to know your list of foods. If this week seems like a drastic change from your normal eating habits, do the best you can.

Week 2. You'll notice that the meal pattern this week is the same as last week. Your challenge this week, and from now on, is to eliminate from your diet the foods in the Bread subcategory from the larger Bread category. There are lots of great foods in the Bread category that are not what most people think of as "bread," so get to know and love these choices. For optimum results, eliminate, as best you can, all regular rising breads, including bagels, cakes, muffins, and bread. I know this may be a huge challenge, just do the best you can.

Week 3. Congratulations on your success last week! I hope you're getting used to cutting out those breads. This week, you'll be bumping up your percentage of protein and cutting back on carbohydrates just a little. You'll probably notice only one or two changes in the menu. Keep up the good work and don't forget to drink that water.

Week 4—Reassessment Week. Great job last week! This week, you'll notice fewer or no carbohydrates in the evening. Remember, your body needs those carbs during the day when you're active—not at night when you're sleeping. The other challenge is to go the whole week without eating *any* red meat. All your Meat category foods should consist of fish, poultry, eggs, and maybe a little soy.

Week 5. Fantastic! You've made it to Week 5, also known as "fish week." Eat fish for dinner every night this week. Any fish you like is fine, but try to enjoy as much fresh fish as you can. Experiment with a type of fish that you've never tried before. Try a new fish recipe you've been meaning to make. If you are allergic to seafood, have skinless chicken breast every night.

Week 6. Congratulations! You've made it to Week 6. You'll notice that you are slowly cutting back on carbohydrate and increasing protein. Don't let yourself get bored—this week, try a new vegetable you've never tried before. You're doing great. How's the water intake?

Week 7. You've made it to lucky Week 7! You must be feeling fantastic by now. You're now at the point where the Bread category has been completely cut out of your nighttime meals. You'll be continuing this way through Week 12, so you'd better get used to it. Remember, you need protein at night to rebuild your muscle, not carbohydrate. And be sure to keep eating all your meals in order.

Week 8—Reassessment Week. Week 8 is great! You're getting really good at this, keep up the good work. No special instructions for you this week. Just enjoy your success. And we hope you are getting used to avoiding the bread "breads."

Week 9. Week 9! You're really cooking—just don't cook any red meat this week. If you liked Week 4, then you'll love Week 9, because it's another no-red-meat week. Stick with fish, poultry, and eggs in your Meat category. By choosing only low-fat protein sources, you will utilize your own fat stores for energy.

Week 10. Congratulations! You've made it through nine weeks of the Turn Up the Heat program. Since you're doing so well, get ready for Week 10, which is fondly referred to as "Hell Week." Are you ready for one week of nutritional hell? You'll be eating very few carbs this week since your body is becoming more adept at utilizing fat instead of sugars for energy. You can do it! (Don't worry, you'll get them back, I promise.) And here's something to look forward to—a treat day is only six days away!

Week 11. Fantastic job! How do you feel? Can you gear up for another week of nutritional hell? You're getting ready for some big changes, so follow Week 11's menu and you'll soon be allowed some of the things you've been missing.

Week 12. Congratulations—you did it! Eleven weeks, wow! Week 12 is the last menu before you start again. Do a good job this week and enjoy your treat day. After this week, you have a choice—you can either reassess your caloric level and continue your weight loss, or you can start your maintenance program. If you choose to continue your weight loss, you will reassess your caloric level and begin again with Week 1 (remember—you were even allowed to have bread back then), moving down a level, maintaining your current level, or moving up a level, depending on your answers to the reassessment evaluation on page 76. Or, you may be happy with your weight loss and choose to stabilize your current weight and begin your maintenance program, at which point you would maintain the menu pattern for Week 12. Keep up the great work.

Fat-and-Protein-Efficient Food Program

Level 1

Week 1	Category	Exchanges	Sample food	Quantity
Meal 1	Bread	2	bagel	⅔ large
	Fruit	1	cantaloupe	½ item

Meal 2	Fruit	1	apple	1 item
Meal 3	Bread	3	pita	1½ item
	Meat	2	turkey	2 ounces
	Vegetable	1	romaine lettuce	3 cups
Meal 4	Fruit	1	plum	2 items
Meal 5	Bread	1½	baked potato	½ item
	Meat	4	salmon	4 ounces
	Vegetable	2	spinach	4 cups
Meal 6	Fruit	1	pear	1 item

Week 2	Category	Exchanges	Sample food	Quantity
Meal 1	Bread	2	oatmeal	1 cup
	Fruit	1	banana	½ item
Meal 2	Fruit	1	peach	2 small items
Meal 3	Bread	3	white rice	1 cup
	Meat	2	tuna	4 ounces
	Vegetable	1	tomato	1 item
Meal 4	Fruit	1	grapes	1 cup
Meal 5	Bread	1½	corn	¾ cup
	Meat	4	chicken	4 ounces
	Vegetable	2	green beans	2 cups
Meal 6	Fruit	1	strawberries	½ cup

Week 3	Category	Exchanges	Sample food	Quantity
Meal 1	Bread	2	bran flakes	1 cup
	Fruit	1	raspberries	1 cup
Meal 2	Fruit	1	watermelon	1 cup
Meal 3	Bread	3	white rice	1 cup
	Meat	2	shrimp	4 ounces
	Vegetable	1	zucchini	1 cup
Meal 4	Fruit	1	apple	1 item
	Meat (Nut)	1	peanut butter	1 tablespoon
Meal 5	Meat	4	flank steak	4 ounces
	Vegetable	3	asparagus	3 cups
Meal 6	Fruit	1	orange	1 item

Week 4	Category	Exchanges	Sample food	Quantity
Meal 1	Bread	2	cream of wheat	1 cup
	Fruit	1	grapefruit	1 item

Meal 2	Fruit	1	grapes	1 cup
Meal 3	Bread	3	kidney beans	1 cup
	Meat	4	tuna	8 ounces
	Vegetable	1	romaine lettuce	3 cups
Meal 4	Fruit	1	banana	½ item
	Meat (Nut)	1	almond butter	1 tablespoon
Meal 5	Meat	4	chicken	4 ounces
	Vegetable	3	peppers	3 cups
Meal 6	Fruit	1	papaya	½ item

Week 5

	Category	Exchanges	Sample food	Quantity
Meal 1	Bread	2	oatmeal	1 cup
	Fruit	1	blueberries	1 cup
Meal 2	Fruit	1	apple	1 item
	Meat (Nut)	1	peanut butter	1 tablespoon
Meal 3	Bread	1½	corn tortilla	1½ items
	Meat	4	chicken	4 ounces
	Vegetable	1	peppers	1 cup
Meal 4	Fruit	1	apricot	3 items
	Meat (Nut)	1	cashews	⅛ cup
Meal 5	Meat	4	whitefish	8 ounces
	Vegetable	3	spinach	6 cups
Meal 6	Fruit	1	figs	1 large item

Week 6

	Category	Exchanges	Sample food	Quantity
Meal 1	Bread	2	shredded wheat	2 large biscuits
	Fruit	1	strawberries	1½ cups
	Meat	1	egg	1 item
Meal 2	Meat (Nut)	1	Brazil nuts	⅛ cup
Meal 3	Bread	1½	artichoke	1½ items
	Meat	4	salmon	4 ounces
	Vegetable	1	asparagus	1 cup
Meal 4	Fruit	1	banana	½ item
	Meat (Nut)	1	peanut butter	1 tablespoon
Meal 5	Fruit	1	orange	1 item
Meal 6	Meat	4	chicken	4 ounces
	Vegetable	3	broccoli	3 cups

Week 7

	Category	Exchanges	Sample food	Quantity
Meal 1	Bread	2	bran flakes	1 cup
	Fruit	1	blueberries	1 cup
	Meat	1	egg	1 item
Meal 2	Meat (Nut)	1	pecans	⅛ cup
Meal 3	Bread	1½	yams	½ cup
	Meat	4	catfish	4 ounces
	Vegetable	1	collards	2 cups
Meal 4	Meat (Nut)	1	cashew butter	1 tablespoon
	Vegetable	1	celery	2 cups
Meal 5	Meat	2	turkey	2 ounces
Meal 6	Meat	4	chicken	4 ounces
	Vegetable	3	romaine lettuce	9 cups

Week 8

	Category	Exchanges	Sample food	Quantity
Meal 1	Bread	2	oatmeal	1 cup
	Fruit	1	banana	½ item
Meal 2	Meat	1	egg	1 item
Meal 3	Bread	1½	garbanzo beans	⅜ cup
	Meat	4	chicken	4 ounces
	Vegetable	1	romaine lettuce	3 cups
Meal 4	Meat (Nut)	1	peanut butter	1 tablespoon
	Vegetable	1	jicama	½ cup
Meal 5	Meat	2	tuna	4 ounces
Meal 6	Meat	4	sirloin	4 ounces
	Vegetable	3	tomato	3 items

Week 9

	Category	Exchanges	Sample food	Quantity
Meal 1	Fruit	1	melon, honeydew	⅙ item
	Meat	2	egg white	6 items
Meal 2	Vegetable	1	carrots	½ cup
Meal 3	Bread	1½	potato	¾ cup
	Meat	4	tuna	8 ounces
	Vegetable	3	romaine lettuce	9 cups
Meal 4	Meat (Nut)	1	soynut butter	1 tablespoon
	Vegetable	1	celery	2 cups
Meal 5	Meat	6	turkey	6 ounces
	Vegetable	3	mushrooms	6 cups

Week 10

	Category	Exchanges	Sample food	Quantity
Meal 1	Fruit	1	mango	½ item
	Shake	2	whey protein shake	2 scoops
Meal 2	Meat	1	egg	1 item
Meal 3	Meat	4	flank steak	4 ounces
	Vegetable	3	peppers	3 cups
Meal 4	Meat (Nut)	1	olives	20 items
	Vegetable	1	cucumber	2 cups
Meal 5	Meat	2	turkey	2 ounces
Meal 6	Meat	4	snapper	8 ounces
	Vegetable	3	Brussels sprouts	3 cups

Week 11

	Category	Exchanges	Sample food	Quantity
Meal 1	Fruit	1	grapefruit	1 item
	Meat	2	egg	2 items
Meal 2	Vegetable	1	celery	2 cups
Meal 3	Meat	4	halibut	8 ounces
	Vegetable	3	cabbage	6 cups
Meal 4	Fruit	1	apple	1 item
	Meat (Nut)	1	peanut butter	1 tablespoon
Meal 5	Meat	2	tuna	4 ounces
Meal 6	Meat	4	chicken	4 ounces
	Vegetable	3	green beans	3 cups

Week 12

	Category	Exchanges	Sample food	Quantity
Meal 1	Fruit	1	banana	½ item
	Shake	2	whey protein shake	2 scoops
Meal 2	Meat	1	egg white	3 items
Meal 3	Bread	1½	lentils	½ cup
	Meat	4	chicken	4 ounces
	Vegetable	2	carrot	1 cup
Meal 4	Meat (Nut)	1	almond butter	1 tablespoon
	Vegetable	1	celery	2 cups
Meal 5	Meat	2	turkey	2 ounces
Meal 6	Meat	4	salmon	4 ounces
	Vegetable	3	spinach	6 cups

Level 2

Week 1

Category	Exchanges	Sample food	Quantity
Meal 1			
Bread	2	bagel	⅔ item
Fruit	1	cantaloupe	½ item
Meal 2			
Fruit	1	apple	1 item
Meal 3			
Bread	3	pita	1½ items
Meat	4	turkey	4 ounces
Vegetable	1	romaine lettuce	3 cups
Meal 4			
Fruit	1	plum	2 items
Meal 5			
Bread	1½	baked potato	½ item
Meat	4	salmon	4 ounces
Vegetable	2	spinach	4 cups
Meal 6			
Fruit	1	pear	1 item

Week 2

Category	Exchanges	Sample food	Quantity
Meal 1			
Bread	2	oatmeal	1 cup
Fruit	1	banana	½ item
Meal 2			
Fruit	1	peach	2 small items
Meal 3			
Bread	3	white rice	1 cup
Meat	4	tuna	8 ounces
Vegetable	1	tomato	1 item
Meal 4			
Fruit	1	grapes	1 cup
Meal 5			
Bread	1½	corn	¾ cup
Meat	4	chicken breast	4 ounces
Vegetable	2	green beans	2 cups
Meal 6			
Fruit	1	strawberries	1½ cups

Week 3

Category	Exchanges	Sample food	Quantity
Meal 1			
Bread	2	bran flakes	1 cup
Fruit	1	raspberries	1 cup
Meat	1	egg	1 item
Meal 2			
Fruit	1	watermelon	1 cup
Meal 3			
Bread	3	white rice	1 cup
Meat	4	shrimp	8 ounces
Vegetable	1	zucchini	1 cup
Meal 4			
Fruit	1	apple	1 item

Meal 5	Bread	1½	tortilla	1½ items
	Meat	4	flank steak	4 ounces
	Vegetable	2	peppers	2 cups
Meal 6	Fruit	1	orange	1 item

Week 4

	Category	Exchanges	Sample food	Quantity
Meal 1	Bread	2	cream of wheat	1 cup
	Fruit	1	grapefruit	1 item
	Meat	1	egg white	3 items
Meal 2	Fruit	1	grapes	1 cup
Meal 3	Bread	3	kidney beans	1 cup
	Meat	4	tuna	8 ounces
	Vegetable	1	romaine lettuce	3 cups
Meal 4	Fruit	1	apricot	3 items
Meal 5	Bread	1½	couscous	¾ cup
	Meat	4	chicken	4 ounces
	Vegetable	2	tomato	2 items

Week 5

	Category	Exchanges	Sample food	Quantity
Meal 1	Bread	2	oatmeal	1 cup
	Fruit	1	blueberries	1 cup
	Meat	1	egg	1 item
Meal 2	Fruit	1	pear	1 item
Meal 3	Bread	3	corn tortilla	3 items
	Meat	4	chicken	4 ounces
	Vegetable	1	peppers	1 cup
Meal 4	Fruit	1	apple	1 item
	Meat (Nut)	1	peanut butter	1 tablespoon
Meal 5	Meat	4	whitefish	8 ounces
	Vegetable	3	spinach	6 cups

Week 6

	Category	Exchanges	Sample food	Quantity
Meal 1	Bread	2	shredded wheat	2 large biscuits
	Fruit	1	strawberries	1½ cups
	Meat	1	egg white	3 items
Meal 2	Fruit	1	pineapple	1 cup
Meal 3	Bread	3	artichoke	3 items
	Meat	4	salmon	4 ounces
	Vegetable	1	asparagus	1 cup

Meal 4	Fruit	I	orange	I item
	Meat (Nut)	I	Brazil nuts	⅛ cup
Meal 5	Meat	6	chicken	6 ounces
	Vegetable	3	broccoli	3 cups

Week 7

	Category	Exchanges	Sample food	Quantity
Meal I	Bread	2	bran flakes	I cup
	Fruit	I	blueberries	I cup
	Meat	I	egg	I item
Meal 2	Fruit	I	mango	½ item
Meal 3	Bread	I ½	yams	½ cup
	Meat	4	catfish	4 ounces
	Vegetable	I	collards	2 cups
Meal 4	Fruit	I	banana	½ item
	Meat (Nut)	I	almond butter	I tablespoon
Meal 5	Meat	6	chicken	6 ounces
	Vegetable	3	romaine lettuce	9 cups

Week 8

	Category	Exchanges	Sample food	Quantity
Meal I	Bread	2	oatmeal	I cup
	Meat	I	egg	I item
Meal 2	Fruit	I	banana	½ item
Meal 3	Bread	I ½	garbanzo beans	⅜ cup
	Meat	4	chicken	4 ounces
	Vegetable	I	romaine lettuce	3 cups
Meal 4	Fruit	I	apple	I item
	Meat (Nut)	I	peanut butter	I tablespoon
Meal 5	Meat	6	sirloin	6 ounces
	Vegetable	3	tomato	3 items

Week 9

	Category	Exchanges	Sample food	Quantity
Meal I	Bread	2	cream of rice	I cup
	Meat	I	egg	I item
Meal 2	Fruit	I	melon, honeydew	⅛ item
Meal 3	Bread	I ½	split peas	½ cup
	Meat	4	tuna	8 ounces
	Vegetable	I	romaine lettuce	3 cups
Meal 4	Fruit	I	grapes	I cup
	Meat (Nut)	I	pecans	⅛ cup

Meal 5	Meat	2	turkey	2 ounces
Meal 6	Meat	4	turkey	4 ounces
	Vegetable	3	mushrooms	6 cups

Week 10

	Category	Exchanges	Sample food	Quantity
Meal 1	Fruit	1	banana	½ item
	Shake	2	whey protein shake	2 scoops
Meal 2	Fruit	1	nectarine	1 item
Meal 3	Meat	4	flank steak	4 ounces
	Vegetable	1	peppers	1 cup
Meal 4	Meat (Nut)	1	peanut butter	1 tablespoon
	Vegetable	1	celery	2 cups
Meal 5	Meat	2	turkey	2 ounces
Meal 6	Meat	4	snapper	8 ounces
	Vegetable	3	Brussels sprouts	3 cups

Week 11

	Category	Exchanges	Sample food	Quantity
Meal 1	Fruit	1	mango	½ item
	Shake	2	whey protein shake	2 scoops
Meal 2	Vegetable	1	carrots	½ cup
Meal 3	Meat	4	halibut	8 ounces
	Vegetable	2	cabbage	4 cups
Meal 4	Meat (Nut)	1	soynut butter	1 tablespoon
	Vegetable	1	celery	2 cups
Meal 5	Meat	2	tuna	4 ounces
Meal 6	Meat	4	chicken	4 ounces
	Vegetable	3	green beans	3 cups

Week 12

	Category	Exchanges	Sample food	Quantity
Meal 1	Fruit	1	blueberries	1 cup
	Shake	2	whey protein shake	2 scoops
Meal 2	Fruit	1	pear	1 item
Meal 3	Bread	1½	lentils	½ cup
	Meat	4	chicken	4 ounces
	Vegetable	2	spinach	4 cups
Meal 4	Meat (Nut)	1	avocado	⅓ item
	Vegetable	1	jicama	½ cup
Meal 5	Meat	6	salmon	6 ounces
	Vegetable	3	spinach	6 cups

Level 3

Week 1

Meal	Category	Exchanges	Sample food	Quantity
Meal 1	Bread	2	bagel	⅔ item
	Fruit	1	cantaloupe	½ item
Meal 2	Fruit	1	apple	1 item
Meal 3	Bread	3	pita	1 ½ items
	Meat	4	turkey	4 ounces
	Vegetable	1	romaine lettuce	3 cups
Meal 4	Fruit	1	plum	2 items
Meal 5	Bread	3	baked potato	1 item
	Meat	4	salmon	4 ounces
	Vegetable	2	spinach	4 cups
Meal 6	Fruit	1	pear	1 item

Week 2

Meal	Category	Exchanges	Sample food	Quantity
Meal 1	Bread	2	oatmeal	1 cup
	Fruit	1	banana	½ item
Meal 2	Fruit	1	peach	2 small items
Meal 3	Bread	3	white rice	1 cup
	Meat	4	tuna	8 ounces
	Vegetable	1	tomato	1 item
Meal 4	Fruit	1	grapes	1 cup
Meal 5	Bread	3	corn	1 ½ cups
	Meat	4	chicken breast	4 ounces
	Vegetable	2	green beans	2 cups
Meal 6	Fruit	1	strawberries	1 ½ cups

Week 3

Meal	Category	Exchanges	Sample food	Quantity
Meal 1	Bread	2	bran flakes	1 cup
	Fruit	1	raspberries	1 cup
Meal 2	Fruit	1	watermelon	1 cup
Meal 3	Bread	3	white rice	1 cup
	Meat	4	shrimp	8 ounces
	Vegetable	2	zucchini	2 cups
Meal 4	Fruit	1	apple	1 item
Meal 5	Bread	1 ½	tortilla	1 ½ items
	Meat	4	flank steak	4 ounces
	Vegetable	2	peppers	2 cups
Meal 6	Fruit	1	orange	1 item

Week 4

	Category	Exchanges	Sample food	Quantity
Meal 1	Bread	2	cream of wheat	1 cup
	Fruit	1	grapefruit	1 item
Meal 2	Fruit	1	grapes	1 cup
Meal 3	Bread	3	kidney beans	1 cup
	Meat	4	tuna	8 ounces
	Vegetable	2	romaine lettuce	6 cups
Meal 4	Fruit	1	apricot	3 items
Meal 5	Meat	4	chicken	4 ounces
	Vegetable	3	tomato	3 items
Meal 6	Bread	1	popcorn	1 cup
	Fruit	1	pear	1 item

Week 5

	Category	Exchanges	Sample food	Quantity
Meal 1	Bread	2	oatmeal	1 cup
	Fruit	1	blueberries	1 cup
	Meat	1	egg	1 item
Meal 2	Fruit	1	pear	1 item
Meal 3	Bread	3	corn tortilla	3 items
	Meat	4	chicken	4 ounces
	Vegetable	2	peppers	2 cups
Meal 4	Fruit	1	apple	1 item
	Meat (Nut)	1	peanut butter	1 tablespoon
Meal 5	Meat	4	whitefish	8 ounces
	Vegetable	3	spinach	6 cups
Meal 6	Fruit	1	peach	2 small items

Week 6

	Category	Exchanges	Sample food	Quantity
Meal 1	Bread	2	shredded wheat	2 large biscuits
	Fruit	1	strawberries	1½ cups
	Meat	1	egg white	3 items
Meal 2	Fruit	1	pineapple	1 cup
Meal 3	Bread	1½	artichoke	1½ items
	Meat	4	salmon	4 ounces
	Vegetable	2	asparagus	2 cups
Meal 4	Fruit	1	orange	1 item
	Meat (Nut)	1	Brazil nuts	⅛ cup

Meal 5	Meat	6	chicken	6 ounces
	Vegetable	3	broccoli	3 cups
Meal 6	Fruit	1	papaya	½ item

Week 7

	Category	Exchanges	Sample food	Quantity
Meal 1	Fruit	1	blueberries	1 cup
	Meat	2	egg	2 items
Meal 2	Fruit	1	apple	1 item
	Meat (Nut)	1	peanut butter	1 tablespoon
Meal 3	Bread	1½	yams	½ cup
	Meat	4	catfish	4 ounces
	Vegetable	2	collards	4 cups
Meal 4	Meat (Nut)	1	almond butter	1 tablespoon
	Vegetable	1	celery	2 cups
Meal 5	Meat	6	chicken	6 ounces
	Vegetable	3	romaine lettuce	9 cups
Meal 6	Fruit	1	strawberries	1½ cups

Week 8

	Category	Exchanges	Sample food	Quantity
Meal 1	Fruit	1	orange	1 item
	Meat	2	egg white	6 items
Meal 2	Fruit	1	banana	½ item
	Meat (Nut)	1	peanut butter	1 tablespoon
Meal 3	Bread	1½	split peas	½ cup
	Meat	4	salmon	4 ounces
	Vegetable	2	spinach	4 cups
Meal 4	Meat (Nut)	1	avocado	⅓ item
	Vegetable	1	jicama	½ cup
Meal 5	Meat	2	tuna	4 ounces
Meal 6	Meat	4	sirloin	4 ounces
	Vegetable	3	tomato	3 items

Week 9

	Category	Exchanges	Sample food	Quantity
Meal 1	Fruit	1	mango	½ item
	Shake	2	whey protein shake	2 scoops
Meal 2	Vegetable	1	carrots	½ cup

Meal 3	Bread	1½	garbanzo beans	⅜ cup
	Meat	4	chicken	4 ounces
	Vegetable	2	romaine lettuce	6 cups
Meal 4	Meat (Nut)	1	pecans	⅛ cup
	Vegetable	1	celery	2 cups
Meal 5	Meat	2	turkey	2 ounces
Meal 6	Meat	4	turkey	4 ounces
	Vegetable	3	mushrooms	6 cups

Week 10

	Category	Exchanges	Sample food	Quantity
Meal 1	Fruit	1	banana	½ item
	Shake	2	whey protein shake	2 scoops
Meal 2	Vegetable	1	carrots	½ cup
Meal 3	Meat	4	tuna	8 ounces
	Vegetable	3	romaine lettuce	9 cups
Meal 4	Meat (Nut)	1	peanut butter	1 tablespoon
	Vegetable	1	celery	2 cups
Meal 5	Meat	2	turkey	2 ounces
Meal 6	Meat	4	snapper	8 ounces
	Vegetable	3	Brussels sprouts	3 cups

Week 11

	Category	Exchanges	Sample food	Quantity
Meal 1	Fruit	1	grapefruit	1 item
	Meat	2	egg	2 items
Meal 2	Fruit	1	nectarine	1 item
Meal 3	Bread	1½	tortilla	1½ items
	Meat	4	flank steak	4 ounces
	Vegetable	2	peppers	2 cups
Meal 4	Meat (Nut)	1	almonds	⅛ cup
	Vegetable	1	broccoli	1 cup
Meal 5	Meat	2	tuna	4 ounces
Meal 6	Meat	4	chicken	4 ounces
	Vegetable	3	green beans	3 cups

Week 12

	Category	Exchanges	Sample food	Quantity
Meal 1	Fruit	1	apricot	3 items
	Meat	2	egg white	6 items
Meal 2	Fruit	1	pear	1 item

Meal 3	Bread	1½	lentils	½ cup
	Meat	4	chicken	4 ounces
	Vegetable	2	carrots	I cup
Meal 4	Meat (Nut)	I	olives	20 items
	Vegetable	I	cucumbers	2 cups
Meal 5	Meat	2	turkey	2 ounces
Meal 6	Meat	4	halibut	8 ounces
	Vegetable	3	spinach	6 cups

Level 4

Week 1

	Category	Exchanges	Sample food	Quantity
Meal I	Bread	3	bagel	I item
	Fruit	I	cantaloupe	½ item
Meal 2	Fruit	I	apple	I item
Meal 3	Bread	3	pita	1½ items
	Meat	4	turkey	4 ounces
	Vegetable	I	romaine lettuce	3 cups
Meal 4	Fruit	I	plum	2 items
	Meat (Nut)	I	almonds	⅛ cup
Meal 5	Bread	3	baked potato	I item
	Meat	4	salmon	4 ounces
	Vegetable	2	spinach	4 cups
Meal 6	Bread	I	popcorn	I cup
	Fruit	I	pear	I item

Week 2

	Category	Exchanges	Sample food	Quantity
Meal I	Bread	3	oatmeal	1½ cups
	Fruit	I	banana	½ item
Meal 2	Fruit	I	peach	2 small items
Meal 3	Bread	3	white rice	I cup
	Meat	4	tuna	8 ounces
	Vegetable	I	tomato	I item
Meal 4	Fruit	I	apple	I item
	Meat (Nut)	I	peanut butter	I tablespoon
Meal 5	Bread	3	corn	1½ cups
	Meat	4	chicken breast	4 ounces
	Vegetable	2	green beans	2 cups
Meal 6	Bread	I	whole wheat crackers	I ounce
	Fruit	I	strawberries	1½ cups

Week 3

Meal	Category	Exchanges	Sample food	Quantity
Meal 1	Bread	3	bran flakes	1½ cups
	Fruit	1	raspberries	1 cup
Meal 2	Fruit	1	watermelon	1 cup
Meal 3	Bread	3	white rice	1 cup
	Meat	4	shrimp	8 ounces
	Vegetable	1	zucchini	1 cup
Meal 4	Fruit	1	apple	1 item
	Meat (Nut)	1	almond butter	1 tablespoon
Meal 5	Bread	1½	tortilla	1½ items
	Meat	4	flank steak	4 ounces
	Vegetable	2	peppers	2 cups
Meal 6	Bread	1	popcorn	1 cup
	Fruit	1	orange	1 item

Week 4

Meal	Category	Exchanges	Sample food	Quantity
Meal 1	Bread	3	cream of wheat	1½ cups
	Fruit	1	grapefruit	1 item
Meal 2	Fruit	1	grapes	1 cup
Meal 3	Bread	3	kidney beans	1 cup
	Meat	4	tuna	8 ounces
	Vegetable	1	romaine lettuce	3 cups
Meal 4	Fruit	1	apricot	3 items
	Meat (Nut)	1	Brazil nuts	⅛ cup
Meal 5	Bread	1½	couscous	¾ cup
	Meat	6	chicken	6 ounces
	Vegetable	2	tomato	2 items
Meal 6	Bread	1	rice cakes	2 items
	Fruit	1	pear	1 item

Week 5

Meal	Category	Exchanges	Sample food	Quantity
Meal 1	Bread	3	oatmeal	1½ cups
	Fruit	1	blueberries	1 cup
	Meat	1	egg	1 item
Meal 2	Fruit	1	pear	1 item
Meal 3	Bread	3	corn tortilla	3 items
	Meat	4	chicken	4 ounces
	Vegetable	1	peppers	1 cup

Meal 4	Fruit	1	apple	1 item
	Meat (Nut)	1	peanut butter	1 tablespoon
Meal 5	Bread	1½	wild rice	½ cup
	Meat	6	whitefish	12 ounces
	Vegetable	2	spinach	4 cups
Meal 6	Bread	1	popcorn	1 cup
	Fruit	1	peach	2 small items

Week 6

	Category	Exchanges	Sample food	Quantity
Meal 1	Bread	3	shredded wheat	3 large biscuits
	Fruit	1	strawberries	1½ cups
	Meat	1	egg white	3 items
Meal 2	Fruit	1	pineapple	1 cup
Meal 3	Bread	3	artichoke	3 items
	Meat	4	salmon	4 ounces
	Vegetable	1	asparagus	1 cup
Meal 4	Fruit	1	orange	1 item
	Meat (Nut)	1	Brazil nuts	⅛ cup
Meal 5	Meat	8	chicken	8 ounces
	Vegetable	3	broccoli	3 cups
Meal 6	Fruit	1	papaya	½ item

Week 7

	Category	Exchanges	Sample food	Quantity
Meal 1	Bread	3	cream of rice	1½ cups
	Fruit	1	banana	½ item
	Meat	1	egg	1 item
Meal 2	Fruit	1	apple	1 item
	Meat (Nut)	1	peanut butter	1 tablespoon
Meal 3	Bread	1½	yams	½ cup
	Meat	4	catfish	4 ounces
	Vegetable	2	collards	4 cups
Meal 4	Fruit	1	apple	1 item
	Meat (Nut)	1	almond butter	1 tablespoon
Meal 5	Meat	8	chicken	8 ounces
	Vegetable	3	romaine lettuce	9 cups
Meal 6	Fruit	1	strawberries	1½ cups

Week 8

Meal	Category	Exchanges	Sample food	Quantity
Meal 1	Bread	2	potato	1 cup
	Fruit	1	orange	1 item
	Meat	2	egg white	6 items
Meal 2	Fruit	1	banana	½ item
	Meat (Nut)	1	sesame butter	1 tablespoon
Meal 3	Bread	1½	garbanzo beans	⅜ cup
	Meat	4	chicken	4 ounces
	Vegetable	2	romaine lettuce	6 cups
Meal 4	Fruit	1	jicama	½ cup
	Meat (Nut)	1	avocado	⅓ item
Meal 5	Meat	8	sirloin	8 ounces
	Vegetable	3	tomato	3 items

Week 9

Meal	Category	Exchanges	Sample food	Quantity
Meal 1	Fruit	1	mango	½ item
	Shake	2	whey protein shake	2 scoops
Meal 2	Fruit	1	nectarine	1 item
	Meat (Nut)	1	cashews	⅛ cup
Meal 3	Bread	1½	lentils	½ cup
	Meat	4	chicken	4 ounces
	Vegetable	2	carrots	1 cup
Meal 4	Meat (Nut)	1	pecans	⅛ cup
	Vegetable	1	celery	2 cups
Meal 5	Meat	2	turkey	2 ounces
Meal 6	Meat	8	turkey	8 ounces
	Vegetable	3	mushrooms	6 cups
Meal 7	Fruit	1	pear	1 item

Week 10

Meal	Category	Exchanges	Sample food	Quantity
Meal 1	Fruit	1	banana	½ item
	Shake	2	whey protein shake	2 scoops
Meal 2	Meat	1	egg	1 item
Meal 3	Meat	4	salmon	4 ounces
	Vegetable	2	spinach	4 cups
Meal 4	Meat (Nut)	1	peanut butter	1 tablespoon
	Vegetable	1	celery	2 cups
Meal 5	Meat	2	turkey	2 ounces

Meal 6	Meat	8	snapper	16 ounces
	Vegetable	3	Brussels sprouts	3 cups
Meal 7	Fruit	I	figs	I large item

Week 11	Category	Exchanges	Sample food	Quantity
Meal 1	Fruit	2	grapefruit	2 items
	Meat	2	egg	2 items
Meal 2	Meat (Nut)	I	almonds	⅛ cup
	Vegetable	I	jicama	½ cup
Meal 3	Bread	1½	tortilla	1½ items
	Meat	4	flank steak	4 ounces
	Vegetable	2	peppers	2 cups
Meal 4	Meat (Nut)	I	almonds	⅛ cup
	Vegetable	I	peppers	I cup
Meal 5	Meat	2	tuna	4 ounces
Meal 6	Meat	8	chicken	8 ounces
	Vegetable	3	green beans	3 cups

Week 12	Category	Exchanges	Sample food	Quantity
Meal 1	Fruit	2	apricot	6 items
	Meat	2	egg white	6 items
Meal 2	Fruit	I	pear	I item
Meal 3	Bread	1½	split peas	½ cup
	Meat	4	salmon	4 ounces
	Vegetable	2	spinach	4 cups
Meal 4	Meat (Nut)	I	olives	20 items
	Vegetable	I	cucumbers	2 cups
Meal 5	Meat	2	turkey	2 ounces
Meal 6	Meat	8	halibut	16 ounces
	Vegetable	3	asparagus	3 cups
Meal 7	Fruit	I	papaya	½ item

Level 5

Week 1	Category	Exchanges	Sample food	Quantity
Meal 1	Bread	3	bagel	I item
	Fruit	I	cantaloupe	½ item
	Meat	I	egg	I item
Meal 2	Fruit	I	apple	I item
	Meat (Nut)	I	peanut butter	I tablespoon

Meal 3	Bread	3	pita	1½ items
	Meat	4	turkey	4 ounces
	Vegetable	1	romaine lettuce	3 cups
Meal 4	Fruit	1	plum	2 items
	Meat (Nut)	1	almonds	⅛ cup
Meal 5	Bread	3	baked potato	1 item
	Meat	4	salmon	4 ounces
	Vegetable	2	spinach	4 cups
Meal 6	Bread	1	popcorn	1 cup
	Fruit	1	pear	1 item

Week 2

	Category	**Exchanges**	**Sample food**	**Quantity**
Meal 1	Bread	3	oatmeal	1½ cups
	Fruit	1	banana	½ item
	Meat	1	egg white	3 items
Meal 2	Fruit	1	peach	2 small items
	Meat (Nut)	1	cashews	⅛ cup
Meal 3	Bread	3	white rice	1 cup
	Meat	4	tuna	8 ounces
	Vegetable	1	tomato	1 item
Meal 4	Fruit	1	apple	1 item
	Meat (Nut)	1	peanut butter	1 tablespoon
Meal 5	Bread	3	corn	1½ cups
	Meat	4	chicken breast	4 ounces
	Vegetable	2	green beans	2 cups
Meal 6	Bread	1	whole wheat crackers	1 ounce
	Fruit	1	strawberries	1½ cups

Week 3

	Category	**Exchanges**	**Sample food**	**Quantity**
Meal 1	Bread	3	bran flakes	1½ cups
	Fruit	1	raspberries	1 cup
	Meat	1	egg	1 item
Meal 2	Fruit	1	watermelon	1 cup
	Meat (Nut)	1	cashews	⅛ cup
Meal 3	Bread	3	white rice	1 cup
	Meat	4	shrimp	8 ounces
	Vegetable	1	zucchini	1 cup
Meal 4	Fruit	1	apple	1 item
	Meat (Nut)	1	almond butter	1 tablespoon

Meal 5	Bread	3	tortilla	3 items
	Meat	6	flank steak	6 ounces
	Vegetable	2	peppers	2 cups
Meal 6	Bread	I	popcorn	I cup
	Fruit	I	orange	I item

Week 4

	Category	Exchanges	Sample food	Quantity
Meal 1	Bread	3	cream of wheat	1½ cups
	Fruit	I	grapefruit	I item
	Meat	I	egg white	3 items
Meal 2	Fruit	I	grapes	I cup
	Meat (Nut)	I	walnuts	⅛ cup
Meal 3	Bread	3	kidney beans	I cup
	Meat	4	tuna	8 ounces
	Vegetable	I	romaine lettuce	3 cups
Meal 4	Fruit	I	apricot	3 items
	Meat (Nut)	I	Brazil nuts	⅛ cup
Meal 5	Bread	3	couscous	1½ cups
	Meat	8	chicken	8 ounces
	Vegetable	2	tomato	2 items
Meal 6	Bread	I	rice cakes	2 items
	Fruit	I	papaya	½ item

Week 5

	Category	Exchanges	Sample food	Quantity
Meal 1	Bread	3	oatmeal	1½ cups
	Fruit	I	blueberries	I cup
	Meat	I	egg	I item
Meal 2	Fruit	I	pear	I item
	Meat (Nut)	I	almonds	⅛ cup
Meal 3	Bread	3	corn tortilla	3 items
	Meat	4	chicken	4 ounces
	Vegetable	I	peppers	I cup
Meal 4	Fruit	I	apple	I item
	Meat (Nut)	I	peanut butter	I tablespoon
Meal 5	Meat	2	turkey	2 ounces
Meal 6	Bread	1½	wild rice	½ cup
	Meat	8	whitefish	16 ounces
	Vegetable	2	spinach	4 cups

Week 6

	Category	Exchanges	Sample food	Quantity
Meal 1	Bread	3	shredded wheat	3 large biscuits
	Fruit	1	strawberries	1½ cups
	Meat	1	egg white	3 items
Meal 2	Fruit	1	papaya	½ item
	Meat (Nut)	1	avocado	⅓ item
Meal 3	Bread	3	artichoke	3 items
	Meat	4	salmon	4 ounces
	Vegetable	1	asparagus	1 cup
Meal 4	Fruit	1	orange	1 item
	Meat (Nut)	1	Brazil nuts	⅛ cup
Meal 5	Meat	2	tuna	4 ounces
Meal 6	Meat	8	chicken	8 ounces
	Vegetable	3	broccoli	3 cups

Week 7

	Category	Exchanges	Sample food	Quantity
Meal 1	Bread	2	cream of rice	1 cup
	Fruit	1	banana	½ item
	Meat	2	egg	2 items
Meal 2	Fruit	1	apple	1 item
	Meat (Nut)	1	peanut butter	1 tablespoon
Meal 3	Bread	3	yams	1 cup
	Meat	4	catfish	4 ounces
	Vegetable	1	collards	2 cups
Meal 4	Fruit	1	pineapple	1 cup
	Meat (Nut)	1	almonds	⅛ cup
Meal 5	Meat	2	turkey	2 ounces
Meal 6	Meat	8	chicken	8 ounces
	Vegetable	3	romaine lettuce	9 cups

Week 8

	Category	Exchanges	Sample food	Quantity
Meal 1	Bread	2	potato	1 cup
	Fruit	1	orange	1 item
	Meat	2	egg white	6 items
Meal 2	Fruit	1	banana	½ item
	Meat (Nut)	1	sesame butter	1 tablespoon
Meal 3	Bread	3	garbanzo beans	¾ cup
	Meat	4	chicken	4 ounces
	Vegetable	1	romaine lettuce	3 cups

	Category	Exchanges	Sample food	Quantity
Meal 4	Meat (Nut)	1	avocado	⅓ item
	Vegetable	1	jicama	½ cup
Meal 5	Meat	2	tuna	4 ounces
Meal 6	Meat	8	sirloin	8 ounces
	Vegetable	3	tomato	3 items

Week 9

	Category	Exchanges	Sample food	Quantity
Meal 1	Bread	2	bran flakes	1 cup
	Fruit	1	blueberries	1 cup
	Meat	2	egg	2 items
Meal 2	Fruit	1	nectarine	1 item
	Meat (Nut)	1	cashews	⅛ cup
Meal 3	Bread	1½	lentils	½ cup
	Meat	4	chicken	4 ounces
	Vegetable	2	carrots	1 cup
Meal 4	Meat (Nut)	1	pecans	⅛ cup
	Vegetable	1	celery	2 cups
Meal 5	Meat	2	turkey	2 ounces
Meal 6	Meat	8	turkey	8 ounces
	Vegetable	3	mushrooms	6 cups
Meal 7	Fruit	1	pear	1 item

Week 10

	Category	Exchanges	Sample food	Quantity
Meal 1	Fruit	2	orange	2 items
	Meat	2	egg	2 items
Meal 2	Meat (Nut)	1	almond butter	1 tablespoon
	Vegetable	1	jicama	½ cup
Meal 3	Meat	4	flank steak	4 ounces
	Vegetable	3	peppers	3 cups
Meal 4	Meat (Nut)	1	peanut butter	1 tablespoon
	Vegetable	1	celery	2 cups
Meal 5	Meat	4	turkey	4 ounces
Meal 6	Meat	8	snapper	16 ounces
	Vegetable	3	Brussels sprouts	3 cups

Week 11

	Category	Exchanges	Sample food	Quantity
Meal 1	Fruit	2	mango	1 item
	Shake	2	whey protein shake	2 scoops

Meal 2	Meat (Nut)	1	pumpkin seeds	⅛ cup
	Vegetable	1	celery	2 cups
Meal 3	Meat	4	salmon	4 ounces
	Vegetable	3	spinach	6 cups
Meal 4	Meat (Nut)	1	almonds	⅛ cup
	Vegetable	1	peppers	1 cup
Meal 5	Meat	4	tuna	8 ounces
Meal 6	Meat	8	chicken	8 ounces
	Vegetable	3	green beans	3 cups

Week 12

	Category	Exchanges	Sample food	Quantity
Meal 1	Fruit	2	grapefruit	2 items
	Meat	2	egg	2 items
Meal 2	Meat (Nut)	1	olives	20 items
	Vegetable	1	cucumbers	2 cups
Meal 3	Bread	1½	split peas	½ cup
	Meat	4	salmon	4 ounces
	Vegetable	2	spinach	4 cups
Meal 4	Fruit	1	apple	1 item
	Meat (Nut)	1	peanut butter	1 tablespoon
Meal 5	Meat	2	turkey	2 ounces
Meal 6	Meat	8	halibut	16 ounces
	Vegetable	3	asparagus	3 cups
Meal 7	Fruit	1	figs	1 large item

Level 6

Week 1

	Category	Exchanges	Sample food	Quantity
Meal 1	Bread	3	bagel	1 item
	Fruit	1	cantaloupe	½ item
	Meat	2	egg	2 items
Meal 2	Fruit	1	apple	1 item
	Meat (Nut)	1	peanut butter	1 tablespoon
Meal 3	Bread	3	pita	1½ items
	Meat	4	turkey	4 ounces
	Vegetable	1	romaine lettuce	3 cups
Meal 4	Fruit	1	plum	2 items
	Meat (Nut)	1	almonds	⅛ cup

Meal 5	Bread	3	baked potato	1 item
	Meat	8	salmon	8 ounces
	Vegetable	2	spinach	4 cups
Meal 6	Bread	1	popcorn	1 cup
	Fruit	2	pear	2 items

Week 2

	Category	**Exchanges**	**Sample food**	**Quantity**
Meal 1	Bread	3	oatmeal	1½ cups
	Fruit	1	banana	½ item
	Meat	2	egg white	6 items
Meal 2	Fruit	1	peach	2 small items
	Meat (Nut)	1	cashews	⅛ cup
Meal 3	Bread	3	white rice	1 cup
	Meat	4	tuna	8 ounces
	Vegetable	1	tomato	1 item
Meal 4	Fruit	1	apple	1 item
	Meat (Nut)	1	peanut butter	1 tablespoon
Meal 5	Bread	3	corn	1½ cups
	Meat	8	chicken breast	8 ounces
	Vegetable	2	green beans	2 cups
Meal 6	Bread	1	whole wheat crackers	1 ounce
	Fruit	2	strawberries	3 cups

Week 3

	Category	**Exchanges**	**Sample food**	**Quantity**
Meal 1	Bread	3	bran flakes	1½ cups
	Fruit	1	raspberries	1 cup
	Meat	2	egg	2 items
Meal 2	Fruit	1	watermelon	1 cup
	Meat (Nut)	1	cashews	⅛ cup
Meal 3	Bread	3	white rice	1 cup
	Meat	4	shrimp	8 ounces
	Vegetable	1	zucchini	1 cup
Meal 4	Fruit	1	apple	1 item
	Meat (Nut)	1	almond butter	1 tablespoon
Meal 5	Bread	3	tortilla	3 items
	Meat	8	flank steak	8 ounces
	Vegetable	2	peppers	2 cups

Meal 6	Bread	I	popcorn	I cup
	Fruit	I	orange	I item

Week 4

	Category	Exchanges	Sample food	Quantity
Meal I	Bread	3	cream of wheat	1½ cups
	Fruit	I	grapefruit	I item
	Meat	2	egg white	6 items
Meal 2	Fruit	I	grapes	I cup
	Meat (Nut)	I	walnuts	⅛ cup
Meal 3	Bread	3	kidney beans	I cup
	Meat	6	tuna	12 ounces
	Vegetable	2	romaine lettuce	6 cups
Meal 4	Fruit	I	apricot	3 items
	Meat (Nut)	I	Brazil nuts	⅛ cup
Meal 5	Bread	1½	couscous	¾ cup
	Meat	8	chicken	8 ounces
	Vegetable	3	tomato	3 items
Meal 6	Fruit	I	papaya	½ item

Week 5

	Category	Exchanges	Sample food	Quantity
Meal I	Bread	3	oatmeal	1½ cups
	Fruit	I	blueberries	I cup
	Meat	2	egg	2 items
Meal 2	Fruit	I	pear	I item
	Meat (Nut)	I	almonds	⅛ cup
Meal 3	Bread	3	corn tortilla	3 items
	Meat	6	chicken	6 ounces
	Vegetable	2	peppers	2 cups
Meal 4	Meat (Nut)	I	peanut butter	I tablespoon
	Vegetable	I	celery	2 cups
Meal 5	Bread	1½	wild rice	½ cup
	Meat	8	whitefish	16 ounces
	Vegetable	3	spinach	6 cups

Week 6

	Category	Exchanges	Sample food	Quantity
Meal I	Bread	3	shredded wheat	3 large biscuits
	Fruit	I	strawberries	1½ cups
	Meat	2	egg white	6 items

Meal 2	Fruit	I	papaya	½ item
	Meat (Nut)	I	avocado	⅓ item
Meal 3	Bread	3	artichoke	3 items
	Meat	6	salmon	6 ounces
	Vegetable	2	asparagus	2 cups
Meal 4	Meat (Nut)	I	Brazil nuts	⅛ cup
	Vegetable	I	carrots	½ cup
Meal 5	Meat	2	tuna	4 ounces
Meal 6	Meat	8	chicken	8 ounces
	Vegetable	3	broccoli	3 cups
Meal 7	Fruit	I	orange	I item

Week 7

	Category	Exchanges	Sample food	Quantity
Meal I	Bread	3	cream of rice	I½ cups
	Fruit	I	banana	½ item
	Meat	2	egg	2 items
Meal 2	Fruit	I	apple	I item
	Meat (Nut)	I	peanut butter	I tablespoon
Meal 3	Bread	I½	yams	½ cup
	Meat	6	catfish	6 ounces
	Vegetable	2	collards	4 cups
Meal 4	Meat (Nut)	I	almonds	⅛ cup
	Vegetable	I	cucumber	2 cups
Meal 5	Meat	2	turkey	2 ounces
Meal 6	Meat	8	chicken	8 ounces
	Vegetable	3	romaine lettuce	9 cups
Meal 7	Fruit	I	strawberries	I½ cups

Week 8

	Category	Exchanges	Sample food	Quantity
Meal I	Fruit	2	orange	2 items
	Meat	2	egg white	6 items
Meal 2	Fruit	I	banana	½ item
	Meat (Nut)	I	sesame butter	I tablespoon
Meal 3	Bread	I½	garbanzo beans	⅜ cup
	Meat	8	chicken	8 ounces
	Vegetable	3	romaine lettuce	9 cups
Meal 4	Meat (Nut)	I	avocado	⅓ item
	Vegetable	I	jicama	½ cup

Meal 5	Meat	2	tuna	4 ounces
Meal 6	Meat	8	sirloin	8 ounces
	Vegetable	3	tomato	3 items
Meal 7	Fruit	I	pear	I item

Week 9

	Category	Exchanges	Sample food	Quantity
Meal I	Fruit	2	blueberries	2 cups
	Meat	2	egg	2 items
Meal 2	Meat (Nut)	I	cashews	⅛ cup
	Vegetable	I	carrots	½ cup
Meal 3	Meat	8	chicken	8 ounces
	Vegetable	3	summer squash	3 cups
Meal 4	Meat (Nut)	I	peanut butter	I tablespoon
	Vegetable	I	celery	2 cups
Meal 5	Meat	4	turkey	4 ounces
Meal 6	Meat	8	turkey	8 ounces
	Vegetable	3	mushrooms	6 cups
Meal 7	Fruit	I	nectarine	I item

Week 10

	Category	Exchanges	Sample food	Quantity
Meal I	Fruit	I	mango	½ item
	Shake	2	whey protein shake	2 scoops
Meal 2	Meat (Nut)	I	almond butter	I tablespoon
	Vegetable	I	jicama	½ cup
Meal 3	Meat	8	flank steak	8 ounces
	Vegetable	3	peppers	3 cups
Meal 4	Meat (Nut)	I	peanut butter	I tablespoon
	Vegetable	I	celery	2 cups
Meal 5	Meat	4	turkey	4 ounces
Meal 6	Meat	8	snapper	16 ounces
	Vegetable	3	Brussels sprouts	3 cups

Week 11

	Category	Exchanges	Sample food	Quantity
Meal I	Fruit	I	banana	½ item
	Shake	2	whey protein shake	2 scoops
Meal 2	Meat (Nut)	I	pumpkin seeds	⅛ cup
	Vegetable	I	celery	2 cups

Meal 3	Bread	1½	lentils	½ cup
	Meat	8	chicken	8 ounces
	Vegetable	3	carrots	1½ cups
Meal 4	Meat (Nut)	1	almonds	⅛ cup
	Vegetable	1	peppers	1 cup
Meal 5	Meat	4	tuna	8 ounces
Meal 6	Meat	8	salmon	8 ounces
	Vegetable	3	green beans	3 cups

Week 12

	Category	Exchanges	Sample food	Quantity
Meal 1	Fruit	2	grapefruit	2 items
	Meat	3	egg	3 items
Meal 2	Meat (Nut)	1	olives	20 items
	Vegetable	1	cucumbers	2 cups
Meal 3	Bread	1½	split peas	½ cup
	Meat	8	chicken	8 ounces
	Vegetable	3	spinach	6 cups
Meal 4	Meat (Nut)	1	peanut butter	1 tablespoon
	Vegetable	1	celery	2 cups
Meal 5	Meat	4	turkey	4 ounces
Meal 6	Meat	12	halibut	24 ounces
	Vegetable	3	asparagus	3 cups
Meal 7	Fruit	1	figs	1 large item

Level 7

Week 1

	Category	Exchanges	Sample food	Quantity
Meal 1	Bread	3	bagel	1 item
	Fruit	1	cantaloupe	½ item
	Meat	2	egg	2 items
Meal 2	Fruit	1	apple	1 item
	Meat (Nut)	1	peanut butter	1 tablespoon
Meal 3	Bread	3	pita	1½ items
	Meat	4	turkey	4 ounces
	Vegetable	1	romaine lettuce	3 cups
Meal 4	Fruit	1	plum	2 items
	Meat (Nut)	1	almonds	⅛ cup

Meal 5	Fruit	I	watermelon	I cup
Meal 6	Bread	3	baked potato	I item
	Meat	8	salmon	8 ounces
	Vegetable	2	spinach	4 cups
Meal 7	Bread	2	popcorn	2 cups
	Fruit	2	pear	2 items

Week 2

	Category	Exchanges	Sample food	Quantity
Meal I	Bread	3	oatmeal	I ½ cups
	Fruit	I	banana	½ item
	Meat	2	egg white	6 items
Meal 2	Fruit	I	peach	2 small items
	Meat (Nut)	I	cashews	⅛ cup
Meal 3	Bread	3	white rice	I cup
	Meat	4	tuna	8 ounces
	Vegetable	I	tomato	I item
Meal 4	Fruit	I	apple	I item
	Meat (Nut)	I	peanut butter	I tablespoon
Meal 5	Fruit	I	nectarine	I item
Meal 6	Bread	3	corn	I ½ cups
	Meat	8	chicken breast	8 ounces
	Vegetable	2	green beans	2 cups
Meal 7	Bread	2	whole wheat crackers	2 ounces
	Fruit	2	strawberries	3 cups

Week 3

	Category	Exchanges	Sample food	Quantity
Meal I	Bread	3	bran flakes	I ½ cups
	Fruit	I	raspberries	I cup
	Meat	2	egg	2 items
Meal 2	Fruit	I	watermelon	I cup
	Meat (Nut)	I	cashews	⅛ cup
Meal 3	Bread	3	white rice	I cup
	Meat	4	shrimp	8 ounces
	Vegetable	I	zucchini	I cup
Meal 4	Fruit	I	apple	I item
	Meat (Nut)	I	almond butter	I tablespoon
Meal 5	Fruit	I	grapes	I cup
	Meat	2	turkey	2 ounces

Meal 6	Bread	3	tortilla	3 items
	Meat	8	flank steak	8 ounces
	Vegetable	2	peppers	2 cups
Meal 7	Fruit	I	orange	I item

Week 4

	Category	Exchanges	Sample food	Quantity
Meal I	Bread	3	cream of wheat	1½ cups
	Fruit	I	grapefruit	I item
	Meat	2	egg white	6 items
Meal 2	Fruit	I	grapes	I cup
	Meat (Nut)	I	walnuts	⅛ cup
Meal 3	Bread	3	kidney beans	I cup
	Meat	4	tuna	8 ounces
	Vegetable	I	romaine lettuce	3 cups
Meal 4	Fruit	I	apricot	3 items
	Meat (Nut)	I	Brazil nuts	⅛ cup
Meal 5	Fruit	I	melon, cantaloupe	½ item
	Meat	2	tuna	4 ounces
Meal 6	Bread	1½	couscous	¾ cup
	Meat	10	chicken	10 ounces
	Vegetable	2	tomato	2 items
Meal 7	Fruit	I	papaya	½ item

Week 5

	Category	Exchanges	Sample food	Quantity
Meal I	Bread	3	oatmeal	1½ cups
	Fruit	I	blueberries	I cup
	Meat	4	egg	4 items
Meal 2	Fruit	I	pear	I item
	Meat (Nut)	I	almonds	⅛ cup
Meal 3	Bread	3	corn tortilla	3 items
	Meat	4	chicken	4 ounces
	Vegetable	I	peppers	I cup
Meal 4	Fruit	I	banana	½ item
	Meat (Nut)	I	peanut butter	I tablespoon
Meal 5	Fruit	I	cranberries	I cup
	Meat	2	turkey	2 ounces
Meal 6	Bread	1½	wild rice	½ cup
	Meat	10	whitefish	20 ounces
	Vegetable	3	spinach	6 cups

Week 6

Category	Exchanges	Sample food	Quantity
Meal 1			
Bread	3	shredded wheat	3 large biscuits
Fruit	1	strawberries	1½ cups
Meat	4	egg white	12 items
Meal 2			
Fruit	1	papaya	½ item
Meat (Nut)	1	avocado	⅓ item
Meal 3			
Bread	3	artichoke	3 items
Meat	4	salmon	4 ounces
Vegetable	1	asparagus	1 cup
Meal 4			
Fruit	1	peach	2 small items
Meat (Nut)	1	Brazil nuts	⅛ cup
Meal 5			
Fruit	1	apple	1 item
Meat	4	tuna	8 ounces
Meal 6			
Meat	10	chicken	10 ounces
Vegetable	3	broccoli	3 cups

Week 7

Category	Exchanges	Sample food	Quantity
Meal 1			
Bread	3	cream of rice	1½ cups
Fruit	1	banana	½ item
Meat	4	egg	4 items
Meal 2			
Fruit	1	apple	1 item
Meat (Nut)	1	peanut butter	1 tablespoon
Meal 3			
Bread	1½	yams	½ cup
Meat	8	catfish	8 ounces
Vegetable	2	collards	4 cups
Meal 4			
Meat (Nut)	1	almonds	⅛ cup
Vegetable	1	cucumber	2 cups
Meal 5			
Meat	4	turkey	4 ounces
Vegetable	1	beets	½ cup
Meal 6			
Meat	10	chicken	10 ounces
Vegetable	3	romaine lettuce	9 cups

Week 8

Category	Exchanges	Sample food	Quantity
Meal 1			
Bread	3	potato	1½ cups
Fruit	1	orange	1 item
Meat	4	egg white	12 items
Meal 2			
Meat (Nut)	1	sesame butter	1 tablespoon
Vegetable	1	celery	2 cups

Meal 3	Bread	1½	garbanzo beans	⅜ cup
	Meat	8	chicken	8 ounces
	Vegetable	2	romaine lettuce	6 cups
Meal 4	Meat (Nut)	1	avocado	⅓ item
	Vegetable	1	jicama	½ cup
Meal 5	Meat	4	tuna	8 ounces
	Vegetable	1	onions	½ cup
Meal 6	Meat	10	sirloin	10 ounces
	Vegetable	3	tomato	3 items
Meal 7	Fruit	1	pear	1 item

Week 9

	Category	Exchanges	Sample food	Quantity
Meal 1	Fruit	1	mango	½ item
	Shake	2	whey protein shake	2 scoops
Meal 2	Meat (Nut)	1	cashews	⅛ cup
	Vegetable	1	carrots	½ cup
Meal 3	Bread	1½	corn	¾ cup
	Meat	8	chicken	8 ounces
	Vegetable	2	summer squash	2 cups
Meal 4	Meat (Nut)	1	peanut butter	1 tablespoon
	Vegetable	1	celery	2 cups
Meal 5	Meat	4	turkey	4 ounces
	Vegetable	1	tomato	1 item
Meal 6	Meat	10	turkey	10 ounces
	Vegetable	3	mushrooms	6 cups

Week 10

	Category	Exchanges	Sample food	Quantity
Meal 1	Fruit	1	banana	½ item
	Shake	2	whey protein shake	2 scoops
Meal 2	Meat (Nut)	1	almond butter	1 tablespoon
	Vegetable	1	jicama	½ cup
Meal 3	Meat	8	flank steak	8 ounces
	Vegetable	2	peppers	2 cups
Meal 4	Meat (Nut)	1	olives	20 items
	Vegetable	1	cucumbers	2 cups
Meal 5	Meat	4	turkey	4 ounces
	Vegetable	1	green beans	1 cup

Meal 6	Meat	10	snapper	20 ounces
	Vegetable	3	Brussels sprouts	3 cups
Meal 7	Fruit	1	pear	1 item

Week 11

	Category	Exchanges	Sample food	Quantity
Meal 1	Fruit	2	blueberries	2 cups
	Shake	2	whey protein shake	2 scoops
Meal 2	Meat (Nut)	1	pumpkin seeds	1/8 cup
	Vegetable	1	celery	2 cups
Meal 3	Bread	1½	lentils	½ cup
	Meat	8	chicken	8 ounces
	Vegetable	2	carrots	1 cup
Meal 4	Meat (Nut)	1	almonds	1/8 cup
	Vegetable	1	peppers	1 cup
Meal 5	Meat	4	tuna	8 ounces
	Vegetable	1	jicama	½ cup
Meal 6	Meat	10	salmon	10 ounces
	Vegetable	3	cauliflower	3 cups

Week 12

	Category	Exchanges	Sample food	Quantity
Meal 1	Fruit	2	grapefruit	2 items
	Meat	3	egg	3 items
Meal 2	Fruit	1	apple	1 item
	Meat (Nut)	1	peanut butter	1 tablespoon
Meal 3	Bread	1½	split peas	½ cup
	Meat	8	chicken	8 ounces
	Vegetable	2	spinach	4 cups
Meal 4	Meat (Nut)	1	soynut butter	1 tablespoon
	Vegetable	1	celery	2 cups
Meal 5	Meat	4	turkey	4 ounces
	Vegetable	1	broccoli	1 cup
Meal 6	Meat	10	halibut	20 ounces
	Vegetable	3	asparagus	3 cups
Meal 7	Fruit	1	figs	1 large item

Level 8

Week 1

	Category	Exchanges	Sample food	Quantity
Meal 1	Bread	3	bagel	1 item
	Fruit	1	cantaloupe	½ item
	Meat	2	egg	2 items
Meal 2	Fruit	1	apple	1 item
	Meat (Nut)	1	peanut butter	1 tablespoon
Meal 3	Bread	3	pita	1½ items
	Meat	4	turkey	4 ounces
	Vegetable	1	romaine lettuce	3 cups
Meal 4	Fruit	1	plum	2 items
	Meat (Nut)	1	almonds	⅛ cup
Meal 5	Fruit	1	watermelon	1 cup
	Meat	2	turkey	2 ounces
Meal 6	Bread	3	baked potato	1 item
	Meat	8	salmon	8 ounces
	Vegetable	2	spinach	4 cups
Meal 7	Bread	2	popcorn	2 cups
	Fruit	2	pear	2 items

Week 2

	Category	Exchanges	Sample food	Quantity
Meal 1	Bread	3	oatmeal	1½ cups
	Fruit	1	banana	½ item
	Meat	2	egg white	6 items
Meal 2	Fruit	1	peach	2 small items
	Meat (Nut)	1	cashews	⅛ cup
Meal 3	Bread	3	white rice	1 cup
	Meat	4	tuna	8 ounces
	Vegetable	1	tomato	1 item
Meal 4	Fruit	1	apple	1 item
	Meat (Nut)	1	peanut butter	1 tablespoon
Meal 5	Fruit	1	nectarine	1 item
	Meat	2	turkey	2 ounces
Meal 6	Bread	3	corn	1½ cups
	Meat	8	chicken breast	8 ounces
	Vegetable	2	green beans	2 cups
Meal 7	Bread	2	whole wheat crackers	2 ounces
	Fruit	2	strawberries	3 cups

Week 3

Category	Exchanges	Sample food	Quantity
Meal 1			
Bread	3	bran flakes	1½ cups
Fruit	1	raspberries	1 cup
Meat	2	egg	2 items
Meal 2			
Fruit	1	watermelon	1 cup
Meat (Nut)	1	cashews	⅛ cup
Meal 3			
Bread	3	white rice	1 cup
Meat	4	shrimp	8 ounces
Vegetable	1	zucchini	1 cup
Meal 4			
Fruit	1	apple	1 item
Meat (Nut)	1	almond butter	1 tablespoon
Meal 5			
Fruit	1	grapes	1 cup
Meat	2	turkey	2 ounces
Meat (Nut)	1	walnuts	⅛ cup
Meal 6			
Bread	1½	tortilla	1½ items
Meat	8	flank steak	8 ounces
Vegetable	2	peppers	2 cups
Meal 7			
Bread	2	popcorn	2 cups
Fruit	2	orange	2 item

Week 4

Category	Exchanges	Sample food	Quantity
Meal 1			
Bread	3	cream of wheat	1½ cups
Fruit	1	grapefruit	1 item
Meat	2	egg white	6 items
Meal 2			
Fruit	1	grapes	1 cup
Meat (Nut)	1	walnuts	⅛ cup
Meal 3			
Bread	3	kidney beans	1 cup
Meat	4	tuna	8 ounces
Vegetable	1	romaine lettuce	3 cups
Meal 4			
Fruit	1	apricot	3 items
Meat (Nut)	1	Brazil nuts	⅛ cup
Meal 5			
Fruit	1	melon, cantaloupe	½ item
Meat	2	tuna	4 ounces
Meat (Nut)	1	cashews	⅛ cup
Meal 6			
Bread	1½	couscous	¾ cup
Meat	10	chicken	10 ounces
Vegetable	3	tomato	3 items
Meal 7			
Fruit	2	papaya	1 item

Week 5

	Category	Exchanges	Sample food	Quantity
Meal 1	Bread	3	oatmeal	1½ cups
	Fruit	1	blueberries	1 cup
	Meat	2	egg	2 items
Meal 2	Fruit	1	pear	1 item
	Meat (Nut)	1	almonds	⅛ cup
Meal 3	Bread	1½	corn tortilla	1½ items
	Meat	6	chicken	6 ounces
	Vegetable	2	peppers	2 cups
Meal 4	Fruit	1	banana	½ item
	Meat (Nut)	1	peanut butter	1 tablespoon
Meal 5	Fruit	1	cranberries	1 cup
	Meat	2	turkey	2 ounces
	Meat (Nut)	1	avocado	⅓ item
Meal 6	Bread	1½	wild rice	½ cup
	Meat	10	whitefish	20 ounces
	Vegetable	3	spinach	6 cups
Meal 7	Fruit	2	strawberries	3 cups

Week 6

	Category	Exchanges	Sample food	Quantity
Meal 1	Bread	3	shredded wheat	3 large biscuits
	Fruit	1	strawberries	1½ cups
	Meat	2	egg white	6 items
Meal 2	Fruit	1	papaya	½ item
	Meat (Nut)	1	avocado	⅓ item
Meal 3	Bread	1½	artichoke	1½ items
	Meat	6	salmon	6 ounces
	Vegetable	2	asparagus	2 cups
Meal 4	Fruit	1	peach	2 small items
	Meat (Nut)	1	Brazil nuts	⅛ cup
Meal 5	Meat	4	tuna	8 ounces
Meal 6	Bread	1½	winter squash	¾ cup
	Meat	10	chicken	10 ounces
	Vegetable	3	broccoli	3 cups
Meal 7	Fruit	2	nectarine	2 items

Week 7

	Category	Exchanges	Sample food	Quantity
Meal 1	Bread	3	cream of rice	1½ cups
	Fruit	1	banana	½ item
	Meat	2	egg	2 items
Meal 2	Fruit	1	apple	1 item
	Meat (Nut)	1	peanut butter	1 tablespoon
Meal 3	Bread	1½	yams	½ cup
	Meat	8	catfish	8 ounces
	Vegetable	2	collards	4 cups
Meal 4	Meat (Nut)	1	almonds	⅛ cup
	Vegetable	1	cucumber	2 cups
Meal 5	Meat	4	turkey	4 ounces
Meal 6	Meat	12	chicken	12 ounces
	Vegetable	3	romaine lettuce	9 cups
Meal 7	Fruit	2	plum	4 items

Week 8

	Category	Exchanges	Sample food	Quantity
Meal 1	Bread	3	potato	1½ cups
	Fruit	1	orange	1 item
	Meat	3	egg white	9 items
Meal 2	Fruit	1	banana	½ item
	Meat (Nut)	1	sesame butter	1 tablespoon
Meal 3	Bread	1½	garbanzo beans	⅜ cup
	Meat	8	chicken	8 ounces
	Vegetable	2	romaine lettuce	6 cups
Meal 4	Meat (Nut)	1	avocado	⅓ item
	Vegetable	1	jicama	½ cup
Meal 5	Meat	4	tuna	8 ounces
Meal 6	Meat	12	sirloin	12 ounces
	Vegetable	3	spinach	6 cups

Week 9

	Category	Exchanges	Sample food	Quantity
Meal 1	Fruit	2	mango	1 item
	Shake	2	whey protein shake	2 scoops
Meal 2	Meat (Nut)	1	cashews	⅛ cup
	Vegetable	1	carrots	½ cup
Meal 3	Bread	1½	corn	¾ cup
	Meat	8	chicken	8 ounces
	Vegetable	2	summer squash	2 cups

Meal 4	Meat (Nut)	I	peanut butter	I tablespoon
	Vegetable	I	celery	2 cups
Meal 5	Meat	4	turkey	4 ounces
Meal 6	Meat	12	turkey	12 ounces
	Vegetable	3	mushrooms	6 cups
Meal 7	Fruit	I	orange	I item

Week 10

	Category	Exchanges	Sample food	Quantity
Meal I	Fruit	2	banana	I item
	shake	2	whey protein shake	2 scoops
Meal 2	Meat (Nut)	I	almond butter	I tablespoon
	Vegetable	I	jicama	½ cup
Meal 3	Meat	8	flank steak	8 ounces
	Vegetable	3	peppers	3 cups
Meal 4	Meat (Nut)	I	olives	20 items
	Vegetable	I	cucumbers	2 cups
Meal 5	Meat	4	tuna	8 ounces
Meal 6	Meat	12	turkey	12 ounces
	Vegetable	3	green beans	3 cups

Week 11

	Category	Exchanges	Sample food	Quantity
Meal I	Bread	3	bran flakes	1½ cups
	Fruit	I	blueberries	I cup
	Meat	3	egg white	9 items
Meal 2	Meat (Nut)	I	pumpkin seeds	⅛ cup
	Vegetable	I	celery	2 cups
Meal 3	Bread	1½	lentils	½ cup
	Meat	8	chicken	8 ounces
	Vegetable	2	carrots	I cup
Meal 4	Fruit	I	pear	I item
	Meat (Nut)	I	almonds	⅛ cup
Meal 5	Meat	4	tuna	8 ounces
Meal 6	Meat	12	salmon	12 ounces
	Vegetable	3	asparagus	3 cups

Week 12

	Category	Exchanges	Sample food	Quantity
Meal I	Bread	3	corn grits	1½ cups
	Fruit	I	grapefruit	I item
	Meat	3	egg	3 items

Meal 2	Meat (Nut)	1	peanut butter	1 tablespoon
	Vegetable	1	celery	2 cups
Meal 3	Bread	1½	split peas	½ cup
	Meat	8	chicken	8 ounces
	Vegetable	2	spinach	4 cups
Meal 4	Fruit	1	apple	1 item
	Meat (Nut)	1	soynut butter	1 tablespoon
Meal 5	Meat	4	turkey	4 ounces
Meal 6	Fruit	1	figs	1 large item
Meal 7	Meat	12	halibut	24 ounces
	Vegetable	3	broccoli	3 cups

Level 9

Week 1	Category	Exchanges	Sample food	Quantity
Meal 1	Bread	4	bagel	1⅓ items
	Fruit	1	cantaloupe	½ item
	Meat	2	egg	2 items
Meal 2	Fruit	1	apple	1 item
	Meat (Nut)	1	peanut butter	1 tablespoon
Meal 3	Bread	3	pita	1½ items
	Meat	8	turkey	8 ounces
	Vegetable	1	romaine lettuce	3 cups
Meal 4	Fruit	1	plum	2 items
	Meat (Nut)	1	almonds	⅛ cup
Meal 5	Fruit	1	watermelon	1 cup
	Meat	2	turkey	2 ounces
Meal 6	Bread	3	baked potato	1 item
	Meat	8	salmon	8 ounces
	Vegetable	2	spinach	4 cups
Meal 7	Bread	2	popcorn	2 cups
	Fruit	2	pear	2 items

Week 2	Category	Exchanges	Sample food	Quantity
Meal 1	Bread	4	oatmeal	2 cups
	Fruit	1	banana	½ item
	Meat	2	egg white	6 items
Meal 2	Fruit	1	peach	2 small items
	Meat (Nut)	1	cashews	⅛ cup

Meal 3	Bread	3	white rice	I cup
	Meat	8	tuna	I6 ounces
	Vegetable	I	tomato	I item
Meal 4	Fruit	I	apple	I item
	Meat (Nut)	I	peanut butter	I tablespoon
Meal 5	Fruit	I	nectarine	I item
	Meat	2	turkey	2 ounces
Meal 6	Bread	3	corn	I½ cups
	Meat	8	chicken breast	8 ounces
	Vegetable	2	green beans	2 cups
Meal 7	Bread	2	whole wheat crackers	2 ounces
	Fruit	2	strawberries	3 cups

Week 3

	Category	Exchanges	Sample food	Quantity
Meal I	Bread	4	bran flakes	2 cups
	Fruit	I	raspberries	I cup
	Meat	2	egg	2 items
Meal 2	Fruit	I	watermelon	I cup
	Meat (Nut)	I	cashews	⅛ cup
Meal 3	Bread	3	white rice	I cup
	Meat	8	shrimp	I6 ounces
	Vegetable	I	zucchini	I cup
Meal 4	Fruit	I	apple	I item
	Meat (Nut)	I	almond butter	I tablespoon
Meal 5	Meat	4	turkey	4 ounces
	Vegetable	I	tomato	I item
Meal 6	Bread	I½	tortilla	I½ items
	Meat	8	flank steak	8 ounces
	Vegetable	3	peppers	3 cups
Meal 7	Bread	I	popcorn	I cup
	Fruit	2	orange	2 items

Week 4

	Category	Exchanges	Sample food	Quantity
Meal I	Bread	4	cream of wheat	2 cups
	Fruit	I	grapefruit	I item
	Meat	2	egg white	6 items
Meal 2	Fruit	I	grapes	I cup
	Meat (Nut)	I	walnuts	⅛ cup

Meal 3	Bread	3	kidney beans	1 cup
	Meat	8	tuna	16 ounces
	Vegetable	1	romaine lettuce	3 cups
Meal 4	Fruit	1	apricot	3 items
	Meat (Nut)	1	Brazil nuts	⅛ cup
Meal 5	Meat	4	tuna	8 ounces
	Vegetable	1	celery	2 cups
Meal 6	Bread	1½	couscous	¾ cup
	Meat	10	chicken	10 ounces
	Vegetable	3	tomato	3 items
Meal 7	Fruit	2	papaya	1 item

Week 5	Category	Exchanges	Sample food	Quantity
Meal 1	Bread	3	oatmeal	1½ cups
	Fruit	1	blueberries	1 cup
	Meat	3	egg	3 items
Meal 2	Fruit	1	pear	1 item
	Meat (Nut)	1	almonds	⅛ cup
Meal 3	Bread	3	corn tortilla	3 items
	Meat	8	chicken	8 ounces
	Vegetable	1	peppers	1 cup
Meal 4	Fruit	1	banana	½ item
	Meat (Nut)	1	peanut butter	1 tablespoon
Meal 5	Meat	4	turkey	4 ounces
	Vegetable	1	eggplant	1 cup
Meal 6	Bread	1½	wild rice	½ cup
	Meat	10	whitefish	20 ounces
	Vegetable	3	spinach	6 cups

Week 6	Category	Exchanges	Sample food	Quantity
Meal 1	Bread	3	shredded wheat	3 large biscuits
	Fruit	1	strawberries	1½ cups
	Meat	4	egg white	12 items
Meal 2	Fruit	1	papaya	½ item
	Meat (Nut)	1	avocado	⅓ item
Meal 3	Bread	3	artichoke	3 items
	Meat	8	salmon	8 ounces
	Vegetable	1	asparagus	1 cup

Meal 4	Fruit	I	peach	2 small items
	Meat (Nut)	I	Brazil nuts	⅛ cup
Meal 5	Meat	4	tuna	8 ounces
	Vegetable	I	celery	2 cups
Meal 6	Meat	12	chicken	12 ounces
	Vegetable	3	broccoli	3 cups

Week 7

	Category	Exchanges	Sample food	Quantity
Meal I	Bread	3	cream of rice	1½ cups
	Fruit	I	banana	½ item
	Meat	4	egg	4 items
Meal 2	Fruit	I	apple	I items
	Meat (Nut)	I	peanut butter	I tablespoon
Meal 3	Bread	1½	yams	½ cup
	Meat	8	catfish	8 ounces
	Vegetable	2	collards	4 cups
Meal 4	Fruit	I	apricot	3 items
	Meat (Nut)	I	almonds	⅛ cup
Meal 5	Meat	4	turkey	4 ounces
	Vegetable	I	beets	½ cup
Meal 6	Meat	12	chicken	12 ounces
	Vegetable	3	romaine lettuce	9 cups
Meal 7	Fruit	I	plum	2 items

Week 8

	Category	Exchanges	Sample food	Quantity
Meal I	Fruit	2	orange	2 items
	Meat	4	egg white	12 items
Meal 2	Fruit	I	banana	½ item
	Meat (Nut)	I	sesame butter	I tablespoon
Meal 3	Bread	1½	garbanzo beans	⅜ cup
	Meat	8	chicken	8 ounces
	Vegetable	2	romaine lettuce	6 cups
Meal 4	Meat (Nut)	I	avocado	⅓ item
	Vegetable	I	jicama	½ cup
Meal 5	Meat	4	tuna	8 ounces
	Vegetable	I	celery	2 cups
Meal 6	Meat	16	sirloin	16 ounces
	Vegetable	3	tomato	3 items

Week 9

	Category	Exchanges	Sample food	Quantity
Meal 1	Fruit	2	melon, honeydew	⅓ item
	Meat	4	egg	4 items
Meal 2	Meat (Nut)	1	cashews	⅛ cup
	Vegetable	1	carrots	½ cup
Meal 3	Meat	8	chicken	8 ounces
	Vegetable	2	summer squash	2 cups
Meal 4	Meat (Nut)	1	peanut butter	1 tablespoon
	Vegetable	1	celery	2 cups
Meal 5	Meat	4	tuna	8 ounces
	Vegetable	1	romaine lettuce	3 cups
Meal 6	Meat	16	turkey	16 ounces
	Vegetable	3	mushrooms	6 cups

Week 10

	Category	Exchanges	Sample food	Quantity
Meal 1	Fruit	2	mango	1 item
	Shake	2	whey protein shake	2 scoops
Meal 2	Meat (Nut)	1	almond butter	1 tablespoon
	Vegetable	1	jicama	½ cup
Meal 3	Meat	8	flank steak	8 ounces
	Vegetable	2	peppers	2 cups
Meal 4	Meat (Nut)	1	olives	20 items
	Vegetable	1	cucumbers	2 cups
Meal 5	Meat	4	tuna	8 ounces
	Vegetable	1	tomato	1 item
Meal 6	Meat	16	turkey	16 ounces
	Vegetable	3	green beans	3 cups
Meal 7	Fruit	1	papaya	½ item

Week 11

	Category	Exchanges	Sample food	Quantity
Meal 1	Fruit	2	banana	1 item
	Shake	2	whey protein shake	2 scoops
Meal 2	Meat (Nut)	1	pumpkin seeds	⅛ cup
	Vegetable	1	celery	2 cups
Meal 3	Bread	1½	lentils	½ cup
	Meat	8	chicken	8 ounces
	Vegetable	2	carrots	1 cup
Meal 4	Meat (Nut)	1	almonds	⅛ cup
	Vegetable	1	broccoli	1 cup

Meal 5	Meat	4	tuna	8 ounces
	Vegetable	1	peppers	1 cup
Meal 6	Meat	16	salmon	16 ounces
	Vegetable	3	asparagus	3 cups
Meal 7	Fruit	1	pear	1 item

Week 12

	Category	Exchanges	Sample food	Quantity
Meal 1	Bread	3	bran flakes	1½ cups
	Fruit	1	blueberries	1 cup
	Meat	4	egg white	12 items
Meal 2	Fruit	1	apple	1 item
	Meat (Nut)	1	peanut butter	1 tablespoon
Meal 3	Bread	1½	split peas	½ cup
	Meat	8	chicken	8 ounces
	Vegetable	2	spinach	4 cups
Meal 4	Meat (Nut)	1	soynut butter	1 tablespoon
	Vegetable	1	jicama	½ cup
Meal 5	Meat	4	turkey	4 ounces
	Vegetable	1	Brussels sprouts	1 cup
Meal 6	Meat	16	halibut	32 ounces
	Vegetable	3	tomato	3 items
Meal 7	Fruit	1	figs	1 large item

Level 10

Week 1

	Category	Exchanges	Sample food	Quantity
Meal 1	Bread	4	bagel	1⅓ items
	Fruit	1	cantaloupe	½ item
	Meat	3	egg	3 items
Meal 2	Fruit	1	apple	1 item
	Meat (Nut)	1	peanut butter	1 tablespoon
Meal 3	Bread	3	pita	1½ items
	Meat	8	turkey	8 ounces
	Vegetable	1	romaine lettuce	3 cups
Meal 4	Fruit	1	plum	2 items
	Meat (Nut)	1	almonds	⅛ cup
Meal 5	Fruit	1	mango	½ item
	Meat	2	turkey	2 ounces

Meal 6	Bread	3	baked potato	I item
	Meat	12	salmon	12 ounces
	Vegetable	2	spinach	4 cups
Meal 7	Bread	2	popcorn	2 cups
	Fruit	2	pear	2 items

Week 2

	Category	Exchanges	Sample food	Quantity
Meal I	Bread	4	oatmeal	2 cups
	Fruit	I	banana	½ item
	Meat	3	egg white	9 items
Meal 2	Fruit	I	peach	2 small items
	Meat (Nut)	I	cashews	⅛ cup
Meal 3	Bread	3	white rice	I cup
	Meat	8	tuna	16 ounces
	Vegetable	I	tomato	I item
Meal 4	Fruit	I	apple	I item
	Meat (Nut)	I	peanut butter	I tablespoon
Meal 5	Fruit	I	nectarine	I item
	Meat	2	turkey	2 ounces
Meal 6	Bread	3	corn	I½ cups
	Meat	12	chicken breast	12 ounces
	Vegetable	2	green beans	2 cups
Meal 7	Bread	2	whole wheat crackers	2 ounces
	Fruit	2	strawberries	3 cups

Week 3

	Category	Exchanges	Sample food	Quantity
Meal I	Bread	4	bran flakes	2 cups
	Fruit	I	raspberries	I cup
	Meat	3	egg	3 items
Meal 2	Fruit	I	watermelon	I cup
	Meat (Nut)	I	Brazil nuts	⅛ cup
Meal 3	Bread	3	white rice	I cup
	Meat	8	shrimp	16 ounces
	Vegetable	I	zucchini	I cup
Meal 4	Fruit	I	apple	I item
	Meat (Nut)	I	almond butter	I tablespoon
Meal 5	Fruit	I	pear	I item
	Meat	4	tuna	8 ounces

Meal 6	Bread	1½	tortilla	1½ items
	Meat	12	flank steak	12 ounces
	Vegetable	2	peppers	2 cups
Meal 7	Bread	1	popcorn	1 cup
	Fruit	1	orange	1 item

Week 4

	Category	Exchanges	Sample food	Quantity
Meal 1	Bread	4	cream of wheat	2 cups
	Fruit	1	grapefruit	1 item
	Meat	3	egg white	9 items
Meal 2	Fruit	1	grapes	1 cup
	Meat (Nut)	1	walnuts	⅛ cup
Meal 3	Bread	3	couscous	1½ cups
	Meat	8	chicken	8 ounces
	Vegetable	1	tomato	1 item
Meal 4	Fruit	1	apricot	3 items
	Meat (Nut)	1	Brazil nuts	⅛ cup
Meal 5	Fruit	1	melon, cantaloupe	½ item
	Meat	4	tuna	8 ounces
Meal 6	Meat	16	salmon	16 ounces
	Vegetable	2	asparagus	2 cups
Meal 7	Fruit	1	papaya	½ item

Week 5

	Category	Exchanges	Sample food	Quantity
Meal 1	Bread	3	oatmeal	1½ cups
	Fruit	1	blueberries	1 cup
	Meat	4	egg	4 items
Meal 2	Fruit	1	pear	1 item
	Meat (Nut)	1	almonds	⅛ cup
Meal 3	Bread	3	corn tortilla	3 items
	Meat	8	chicken	8 ounces
	Vegetable	1	peppers	1 cup
Meal 4	Meat (Nut)	1	peanut butter	1 tablespoon
	Vegetable	1	celery	2 cups
Meal 5	Meat	4	turkey	4 ounces
	Vegetable	1	eggplant	1 cup
Meal 6	Meat	16	whitefish	32 ounces
	Vegetable	2	spinach	4 cups
Meal 7	Fruit	1	pear	1 item

Week 6

Category	Exchanges	Sample food	Quantity
Meal 1			
Bread	3	shredded wheat	3 large biscuits
Fruit	1	strawberries	1½ cups
Meat	4	egg white	12 items
Meal 2			
Fruit	1	papaya	½ item
Meat (Nut)	1	avocado	⅓ item
Meal 3			
Bread	1½	artichoke	1½ items
Meat	8	salmon	8 ounces
Vegetable	1	spinach	2 cups
Meal 4			
Meat	8	tuna	16 ounces
Vegetable	1	onions, green	1 cup
Meal 5			
Meat (Nut)	1	Brazil nuts	⅛ cup
Vegetable	1	carrots	½ cup
Meal 6			
Meat	16	chicken	16 ounces
Vegetable	2	broccoli	2 cups
Meal 7			
Fruit	1	plum	2 items

Week 7

Category	Exchanges	Sample food	Quantity
Meal 1			
Bread	3	cream of rice	1½ cups
Fruit	1	banana	½ item
Meat	4	egg	4 items
Meal 2			
Meat (Nut)	1	peanut butter	1 tablespoon
Vegetable	1	celery	2 cups
Meal 3			
Bread	1½	yams	½ cup
Meat	8	catfish	8 ounces
Vegetable	1	collards	2 cups
Meal 4			
Meat	8	turkey	8 ounces
Vegetable	1	tomato	1 item
Meal 5			
Meat (Nut)	1	almonds	⅛ cup
Vegetable	1	cucumber	2 cups
Meal 6			
Meat	16	chicken	16 ounces
Vegetable	2	romaine lettuce	6 cups

Week 8

Category	Exchanges	Sample food	Quantity
Meal 1			
Fruit	2	orange	2 items
Meat	4	egg white	12 items
Meal 2			
Meat (Nut)	1	sesame butter	1 tablespoon
Vegetable	1	celery	2 cups

Meal 3	Bread	1½	garbanzo beans	⅜ cup
	Meat	8	chicken	8 ounces
	Vegetable	1	romaine lettuce	3 cups
Meal 4	Meat	8	tuna	16 ounces
	Vegetable	1	peppers	1 cup
Meal 5	Meat (Nut)	1	avocado	⅓ item
	Vegetable	1	jicama	½ cup
Meal 6	Meat	16	sirloin	16 ounces
	Vegetable	2	tomato	2 items

Week 9

	Category	Exchanges	Sample food	Quantity
Meal 1	Fruit	2	mango	1 item
	Shake	2	whey protein shake	2 scoops
Meal 2	Meat (Nut)	1	cashews	⅛ cup
	Vegetable	1	carrots	½ cup
Meal 3	Bread	1½	pasta	1½ ounces
	Meat	8	chicken	8 ounces
	Vegetable	1	tomato	1 item
Meal 4	Meat	8	tuna	16 ounces
	Vegetable	1	romaine lettuce	3 cups
Meal 5	Meat (Nut)	1	peanut butter	1 tablespoon
	Vegetable	1	celery	2 cups
Meal 6	Meat	16	turkey	16 ounces
	Vegetable	2	mushrooms	4 cups

Week 10

	Category	Exchanges	Sample food	Quantity
Meal 1	Fruit	2	banana	1 item
	Shake	2	whey protein shake	2 scoops
Meal 2	Meat (Nut)	1	almond butter	1 tablespoon
	Vegetable	1	jicama	½ cup
Meal 3	Meat	8	flank steak	8 ounces
	Vegetable	3	peppers	3 cups
Meal 4	Meat	8	tuna	16 ounces
	Vegetable	2	tomato	2 items
Meal 5	Meat (Nut)	1	olives	20 items
	Vegetable	1	cucumbers	2 cups
Meal 6	Meat	16	snapper	32 ounces
	Vegetable	2	green beans	2 cups

Week 11

Meal	Category	Exchanges	Sample food	Quantity
Meal 1	Bread	3	corn grits	1½ cups
	Fruit	1	grapefruit	1 item
	Meat	4	egg	4 items
Meal 2	Meat (Nut)	1	pumpkin seeds	⅛ cup
	Vegetable	1	celery	2 cups
Meal 3	Bread	1½	lentils	½ cup
	Meat	8	chicken	8 ounces
	Vegetable	2	carrots	1 cup
Meal 4	Meat	8	tuna	16 ounces
	Vegetable	2	peppers	2 cups
Meal 5	Meat (Nut)	1	almonds	⅛ cup
	Vegetable	1	broccoli	1 cup
Meal 6	Meat	16	salmon	16 ounces
	Vegetable	2	asparagus	2 cups

Week 12

Meal	Category	Exchanges	Sample food	Quantity
Meal 1	Bread	3	bran flakes	1½ cups
	Fruit	1	melon, honeydew	⅙ item
	Meat	4	egg white	12 items
Meal 2	Meat (Nut)	1	peanut butter	1 tablespoon
	Vegetable	1	celery	2 cups
Meal 3	Bread	1½	split peas	½ cup
	Meat	8	chicken	8 ounces
	Vegetable	2	spinach	4 cups
Meal 4	Meat	8	turkey	8 ounces
	Vegetable	2	tomato	2 items
Meal 5	Meat (Nut)	1	soynut butter	1 tablespoon
	Vegetable	1	jicama	½ cup
Meal 6	Meat	16	halibut	32 ounces
	Vegetable	2	Brussels sprouts	2 cups
Meal 7	Fruit	1	figs	1 large item

Level 11

Week 1

Meal	Category	Exchanges	Sample food	Quantity
Meal 1	Bread	4	bagel	1⅓ items
	Fruit	2	cantaloupe	1 item
	Meat	3	egg	3 items

Meal 2	Fruit	I	apple	I item
	Meat (Nut)	I	peanut butter	I tablespoon
Meal 3	Bread	3	pita	1½ items
	Meat	8	turkey	8 ounces
	Vegetable	I	romaine lettuce	3 cups
Meal 4	Fruit	I	plum	2 items
	Meat (Nut)	I	almonds	⅛ cup
Meal 5	Fruit	I	watermelon	I cup
	Meat	4	turkey	4 ounces
Meal 6	Bread	3	baked potato	I item
	Meat	12	salmon	12 ounces
	Vegetable	2	spinach	4 cups
Meal 7	Bread	2	popcorn	2 cups
	Fruit	2	pear	2 items

Week 2

	Category	Exchanges	Sample food	Quantity
Meal I	Bread	4	oatmeal	2 cups
	Fruit	2	banana	I item
	Meat	3	egg white	9 items
Meal 2	Fruit	I	peach	2 small items
	Meat (Nut)	I	cashews	⅛ cup
Meal 3	Bread	3	white rice	I cup
	Meat	8	tuna	16 ounces
	Vegetable	I	tomato	I item
Meal 4	Fruit	I	apple	I item
	Meat (Nut)	I	peanut butter	I tablespoon
Meal 5	Fruit	I	nectarine	I item
	Meat	4	turkey	4 ounces
Meal 6	Bread	3	corn	1½ cups
	Meat	12	chicken breast	12 ounces
	Vegetable	2	green beans	2 cups
Meal 7	Bread	2	whole wheat crackers	2 ounces
	Fruit	2	strawberries	3 cups

Week 3

	Category	Exchanges	Sample food	Quantity
Meal I	Bread	4	bran flakes	2 cups
	Fruit	2	raspberries	2 cups
	Meat	3	egg	3 items

Meal 2	Fruit	I	watermelon	I cup
	Meat (Nut)	I	cashews	⅛ cup
Meal 3	Bread	3	white rice	I cup
	Meat	8	shrimp	I6 ounces
	Vegetable	I	zucchini	I cup
Meal 4	Fruit	I	apple	I item
	Meat (Nut)	I	almond butter	I tablespoon
Meal 5	Fruit	I	pear	I item
	Meat	4	tuna	8 ounces
Meal 6	Bread	I½	tortilla	I½ items
	Meat	I6	flank steak	I6 ounces
	Vegetable	2	peppers	2 cups
Meal 7	Bread	2	popcorn	2 cups
	Fruit	2	orange	2 items

Week 4

	Category	Exchanges	Sample food	Quantity
Meal I	Bread	4	cream of wheat	2 cups
	Fruit	2	grapefruit	2 items
	Meat	4	egg white	I2 items
Meal 2	Fruit	I	grapes	I cup
	Meat (Nut)	I	walnuts	⅛ cup
Meal 3	Bread	3	couscous	I½ cups
	Meat	8	chicken	8 ounces
	Vegetable	I	tomato	I item
Meal 4	Fruit	I	apricot	3 items
	Meat (Nut)	I	Brazil nuts	⅛ cup
Meal 5	Fruit	I	melon, cantaloupe	½ item
	Meat	4	tuna	8 ounces
Meal 6	Meat	I6	salmon	I6 ounces
	Vegetable	2	asparagus	2 cups
Meal 7	Bread	2	papaya	I item
	Fruit	2	rice cakes	4 items

Week 5

	Category	Exchanges	Sample food	Quantity
Meal I	Bread	4	oatmeal	2 cups
	Fruit	2	blueberries	2 cups
	Meat	4	egg	4 items
Meal 2	Fruit	I	pear	I item
	Meat (Nut)	I	almonds	⅛ cup

	Category	Exchanges	Sample food	Quantity
Meal 3	Bread	3	corn tortilla	3 items
	Meat	8	chicken	8 ounces
	Vegetable	I	peppers	I cup
Meal 4	Fruit	I	banana	½ item
	Meat (Nut)	I	peanut butter	I tablespoon
Meal 5	Meat	8	turkey	8 ounces
	Vegetable	I	eggplant	I cup
Meal 6	Meat	16	whitefish	32 ounces
	Vegetable	3	spinach	6 cups
Meal 7	Bread	I	granola	⅛ cup
	Fruit	I	pear	I item

Week 6

	Category	Exchanges	Sample food	Quantity
Meal I	Bread	4	shredded wheat	4 large biscuits
	Fruit	2	strawberries	3 cups
	Meat	4	egg white	12 items
Meal 2	Fruit	I	papaya	½ item
	Meat (Nut)	I	avocado	⅓ item
Meal 3	Bread	1½	artichoke	1½ items
	Meat	8	salmon	8 ounces
	Vegetable	2	spinach	4 cups
Meal 4	Fruit	I	carrots	½ cup
	Meat (Nut)	I	Brazil nuts	⅛ cup
Meal 5	Meat	8	tuna	16 ounces
	Vegetable	I	onions, green	I cup
Meal 6	Meat	16	chicken	16 ounces
	Vegetable	3	broccoli	3 cups
Meal 7	Bread	I	popcorn	I cup
	Fruit	I	plum	2 items

Week 7

	Category	Exchanges	Sample food	Quantity
Meal I	Bread	4	cream of rice	2 cups
	Fruit	2	banana	I item
	Meat	6	egg	6 items
Meal 2	Fruit	I	apple	I item
	Meat (Nut)	I	peanut butter	I tablespoon
Meal 3	Bread	1½	yams	½ cup
	Meat	8	catfish	8 ounces
	Vegetable	2	collards	4 cups

Meal 4	Meat (Nut)	2	almonds	¼ cup
	Vegetable	I	cucumber	2 cups
Meal 5	Meat	8	turkey	8 ounces
	Vegetable	I	tomato	I item
Meal 6	Meat	16	chicken	16 ounces
	Vegetable	3	romaine lettuce	9 cups

Week 8

	Category	Exchanges	Sample food	Quantity
Meal I	Bread	4	bran flakes	2 cups
	Fruit	2	orange	2 items
	Meat	6	egg white	18 items
Meal 2	Fruit	I	papaya	½ item
	Meat	2	chicken	2 ounces
	Meat (Nut)	I	avocado	⅓ item
Meal 3	Bread	1½	garbanzo beans	⅜ cup
	Meat	8	chicken	8 ounces
	Vegetable	2	romaine lettuce	6 cups
Meal 4	Meat (Nut)	2	cashew butter	2 tablespoons
	Vegetable	I	jicama	½ cup
Meal 5	Meat	8	tuna	16 ounces
	Vegetable	I	peppers	I cup
Meal 6	Meat	16	sirloin	16 ounces
	Vegetable	3	tomato	3 items

Week 9

	Category	Exchanges	Sample food	Quantity
Meal I	Fruit	2	melon, cantaloupe	I item
	Meat	8	egg	8 items
Meal 2	Meat	2	turkey	2 ounces
	Meat (Nut)	I	avocado	⅓ item
Meal 3	Meat	12	chicken	12 ounces
	Vegetable	3	tomato	3 items
Meal 4	Meat (Nut)	2	peanut butter	2 tablespoons
	Vegetable	I	celery	2 cups
Meal 5	Meat	8	tuna	16 ounces
	Vegetable	I	romaine lettuce	3 cups
Meal 6	Meat	16	turkey	16 ounces
	Vegetable	3	mushrooms	6 cups
Meal 7	Fruit	I	strawberries	1½ cups

Week 10

	Category	Exchanges	Sample food	Quantity
Meal 1	Fruit	2	mango	1 item
	Shake	2	whey protein shake	2 scoops
Meal 2	Meat	4	turkey	4 ounces
	Meat (Nut)	1	almonds	⅛ cup
Meal 3	Meat	12	flank steak	12 ounces
	Vegetable	3	peppers	3 cups
Meal 4	Meat (Nut)	2	olives	40 items
	Vegetable	1	cucumbers	2 cups
Meal 5	Meat	8	tuna	16 ounces
	Vegetable	1	tomato	1 item
Meal 6	Meat	16	turkey	16 ounces
	Vegetable	3	green beans	3 cups
Meal 7	Fruit	1	peach	2 small items

Week 11

	Category	Exchanges	Sample food	Quantity
Meal 1	Bread	4	corn grits	2 cups
	Fruit	2	grapefruit	2 items
	Meat	6	egg	6 items
Meal 2	Meat	4	turkey	4 ounces
	Meat (Nut)	1	pumpkin seeds	⅛ cup
Meal 3	Meat	12	sea bass	24 ounces
	Vegetable	3	asparagus	3 cups
Meal 4	Fruit	1	banana	½ item
	Meat (Nut)	1	sesame butter	1 tablespoon
Meal 5	Meat	8	chicken	8 ounces
	Vegetable	1	spinach	2 cups
Meal 6	Meat	16	halibut	32 ounces
	Vegetable	3	Brussels sprouts	3 cups

Week 12

	Category	Exchanges	Sample food	Quantity
Meal 1	Fruit	2	banana	1 item
	Shake	2	whey protein shake	2 scoops
Meal 2	Meat	4	tuna	8 ounces
	Meat (Nut)	1	sunflower seeds	⅛ cup
Meal 3	Bread	1½	lentils	½ cup
	Meat	12	chicken	12 ounces
	Vegetable	2	carrots	1 cup

Meal 4	Fruit	1	soynut butter	1 tablespoon
	Meat (Nut)	1	apple	1 item
Meal 5	Meat	8	ground beef	8 ounces
	Vegetable	1	tomato	1 item
Meal 6	Meat	16	turkey	16 ounces
	Vegetable	3	cabbage	6 cups
Meal 7	Fruit	1	figs	1 large item

The Carbohydrate-Efficient Food Program

12-Week Instructions and Meal Plans for Caloric Levels 1–11

Determine your level by choosing the caloric range closest to the caloric number determined by your metabolic scenario:

Level	Caloric Range of Level
1	Under 1,200
2	1,201–1,365
3	1,366–1,480
4	1,481–1,685
5	1,686–1,805
6	1,806–2,180
7	2,181–2,330
8	2,331–2,450
9	2,451–2,765
10	2,766–3,065
11	3,066 and up

Do not forget the option of adding items from the Free Foods List in appendix C to these meal plans. For example, when you are having oatmeal or cereal, you may add ½ cup nonfat milk; when you are having salad, you can add up to 2 tablespoons of low-fat dressing per day; when you have steamed vegetables, you are allowed 1 tablespoon of nondairy butter per day. Also, beverages such as tea, coffee, and diet soda may be added to your meal plans, but they *do not* count toward your daily water intake.

During certain weeks Meal 1 is listed as a Fruit 1 and a two-scoop whey protein shake. The whey shake is not mandatory for the program, but we have chosen to use the shake during some weeks because whey protein offers the highest, most biologically efficient form of protein. To make this shake you need to buy a zero carbohydrate whey shake either at your health food store or from my website, www.pfcnutrition.com. Make sure that one scoop equals between 70 to 85 calories. To make the shake, blend one serving of fruit, two scoops of whey protein powder, some ice, and water according to your desired consistency and drink this as your first meal. If you choose not to do the shake, then the whey portion of Meal 1 becomes a Meat 2, for example, two eggs.

■ Weekly Instructions for the Carbohydrate-Efficient Metabolism (for All Levels)

Below are just a few things to keep in mind as you begin each week of your program, no matter what level you are using.

Week 1. In this first week, also known as your Foundation Food Program, you'll be laying the groundwork for the coming weeks of the program. This week we want you to get used to eating more times during the day, drinking more water, and getting to know your list of foods. If this week seems like a drastic change from your normal eating habits, do the best you can.

Week 2. You'll notice that the meal pattern this week is the same as last week. Your challenge this week, and from now on, is to eliminate from your diet the foods in the Bread subcategory from the larger Bread category. There are lots of great foods in the Bread category that are not what most people think of as "bread," so get to know and love these choices. For optimum results, eliminate, as best you can, all regular rising breads, including bagels, cakes, muffins, and bread. I know this may be a huge challenge, just do the best you can.

Week 3. Congratulations on your success last week! I hope you're getting used to cutting out those breads. This week, you'll be adjusting your protein, fat, and carbohydrate intakes just a little. You'll probably notice only one or two changes in the menu. Keep up the good work and don't forget to drink that water.

Week 4—Reassessment Week. Great job last week! This week comes with a challenge: Go the whole week without eating *any* red meat. All your Meat category foods should consist of fish, poultry, eggs, and maybe a little soy.

Week 5. Fantastic! You've made it to Week 5, also known as "fish week." Eat fish for dinner every night this week. Any fish you like is fine, but try to enjoy as much fresh fish as you can. Experiment with a type of fish that you've never tried before. Try a new fish recipe you've been meaning to make. If you are allergic to seafood, have skinless chicken breast every night.

Week 6. Congratulations! You've made it to Week 6. You'll notice that we keep adjusting your number of meals and ratio of protein, fat, and carbohydrate intake. By spacing out the carbohydrates this way, you'll utilize them as an energy source more effectively. Don't let yourself get bored—this week, try a new vegetable you've never tried before. You're doing great. How's the water intake?

Week 7. You've made it to lucky Week 7! You must be feeling fantastic by now. You're now at the point where you will be reducing the amount of carbohydrate that you eat at night, while increasing its amount in the daytime meals. You'll be continuing this through Week 12, so you'd better get used to it. Remember, you need protein at night to rebuild your muscle, not carbohydrate. And be sure to keep eating all your meals in order.

Week 8—Reassessment Week. Week 8 is great! You should be getting really good at this by now, keep up the good work. No special instructions for you this week. Just enjoy your success. And we hope you are getting used to avoiding the bread "breads."

Week 9. Week Nine! You're really cooking—just don't cook any red meat this week. If you liked Week 4, then you'll love Week 9, because it's another no-red-meat week. Stick with fish, poultry, and eggs in your Meat category. By choosing only low-fat protein sources, you will utilize your own fat stores for energy.

Week 10. Congratulations! You've made it through nine weeks of the Turn Up the Heat program. Since you're doing so well, get ready for Week 10, which is fondly referred to as "Hell Week." Are you ready for one week of nutritional hell? You'll be eating fewer calories than normal this week. You can do it. (Don't worry, you'll get them back, I promise.) And here's something to look forward to—a treat day is only six days away.

Week 11. Fantastic job! How do you feel? Can you gear up for another week of nutritional hell? You're getting ready for some big changes, so follow Week 11's menu and you'll soon be allowed some of the things you've been missing.

Week 12. Congratulations—you did it! Eleven weeks, wow! Week 12 is the last menu before you start again. Do a good job this week and enjoy your treat day. After this week, you have a choice—you can either reassess your caloric level and continue your weight loss, or you can start your maintenance program. If you choose to continue your weight loss, you will reassess your caloric level and begin again with Week 1 (remember—you were even allowed to have bread back then!), moving down a level, maintaining your current level, or moving up a level, depending on your answers to the reassessment evaluation on page 76. Or, you may be happy with your weight loss and choose to stabilize your current weight and begin your maintenance program, at which point you would maintain the menu pattern for Week 12. Keep up the great work.

Carbohydrate-Efficient Food Program

Level I

Week 1

	Category	Exchanges	Sample food	Quantity
Meal 1	Bread	2	bagel	⅔ large item
	Fruit	1	cantaloupe	½ item
Meal 2	Fruit	1	apple	1 item
Meal 3	Bread	3	pita	1½ items
	Meat	2	turkey	2 ounces
	Vegetable	1	romaine lettuce	3 cups
Meal 4	Fruit	1	plum	2 items
Meal 5	Bread	1½	baked potato	½ item
	Meat	4	salmon	4 ounces
	Vegetable	2	spinach	4 cups
Meal 6	Fruit	1	pear	1 item

Week 2

	Category	Exchanges	Sample food	Quantity
Meal 1	Bread	2	oatmeal	1 cup
	Fruit	1	banana	½ item
Meal 2	Fruit	1	peach	2 small items
Meal 3	Bread	3	white rice	1 cup
	Meat	2	tuna	4 ounces
	Vegetable	1	tomato	1 item
Meal 4	Fruit	1	grapes	1 cup
Meal 5	Bread	1½	corn	¾ cup
	Meat	4	chicken breast	4 ounces
	Vegetable	2	green beans	2 cups
Meal 6	Fruit	1	strawberries	1½ cups

Week 3

	Category	Exchanges	Sample food	Quantity
Meal 1	Bread	2	bran flakes	1 cup
	Fruit	1	raspberries	1 cup
Meal 2	Fruit	1	watermelon	1 cup
Meal 3	Bread	3	white rice	1 cup
	Meat	4	shrimp	8 ounces
	Vegetable	1	zucchini	1 cup
Meal 4	Fruit	1	apple	1 item

Meal 5	Bread	1½	tortilla, flour	1½ items
	Meat	4	flank steak	4 ounces
	Vegetable	2	asparagus	2 cups
Meal 6	Fruit	1	orange	1 item

Week 4

	Category	Exchanges	Sample food	Quantity
Meal 1	Bread	2	cream of wheat	1 cup
	Fruit	1	grapefruit	1 item
Meal 2	Fruit	1	grapes	1 cup
Meal 3	Bread	1½	kidney beans	1½ cups
	Meat	4	tuna	8 ounces
	Vegetable	1	romaine lettuce	3 cups
Meal 4	Bread	1½	popcorn	1½ cups
Meal 5	Fruit	1	banana	½ item
Meal 6	Bread	1½	pasta	1½ ounces
	Meat	4	chicken	4 ounces
	Vegetable	2	peppers	2 cups
Meal 7	Fruit	1	papaya	½ item

Week 5

	Category	Exchanges	Sample food	Quantity
Meal 1	Bread	2	oatmeal	1 cup
	Fruit	1	blueberries	1 cup
Meal 2	Fruit	1	apple	1 item
Meal 3	Bread	1½	corn tortilla	1½ items
	Meat	2	chicken	2 ounces
	Vegetable	1	peppers	1 cup
Meal 4	Bread	1½	potato	¾ cup
	Meat	2	tuna	4 ounces
	Vegetable	1	romaine lettuce	3 cups
Meal 5	Fruit	1	apricot	3 items
Meal 6	Bread	1½	brown rice	½ cup
	Meat	4	whitefish	8 ounces
	Vegetable	2	spinach	4 cups
Meal 7	Fruit	1	figs	1 large item

Week 6

	Category	Exchanges	Sample food	Quantity
Meal 1	Bread	2	shredded wheat	2 large biscuits
	Fruit	1	strawberries	1½ cups
Meal 2	Fruit	1	banana	½ item

Meal 3	Bread	1½	artichoke	1½ items
	Meat	2	salmon	2 ounces
	Vegetable	1	asparagus	1 cup
Meal 4	Bread	1½	winter squash	¾ cup
	Meat	2	turkey	2 ounces
	Vegetable	1	tomato	1 item
Meal 5	Fruit	1	orange	1 item
Meal 6	Meat	4	chicken	4 ounces
	Vegetable	2	broccoli	2 cups
Meal 7	Bread	1	popcorn	1 cup
	Fruit	1	apple sauce	½ cup

Week 7

	Category	Exchanges	Sample food	Quantity
Meal 1	Fruit	1	banana	½ item
	Meat (Nut)	1	peanut butter	1 tablespoon
Meal 2	Bread	2	bran flakes	1 cup
	Fruit	1	blueberries	1 cup
Meal 3	Bread	1½	yams	½ cup
	Meat	2	catfish	2 ounces
	Vegetable	1	collards	2 cups
Meal 4	Meat	2	tuna	4 ounces
	Vegetable	1	celery	2 cups
Meal 5	Fruit	1	apple	1 item
	Meat (Nut)	1	cashew butter	1 tablespoon
Meal 6	Meat	4	chicken	4 ounces
	Vegetable	2	romaine lettuce	6 cups
Meal 7	Fruit	1	apricot	3 items

Week 8

	Category	Exchanges	Sample food	Quantity
Meal 1	Fruit	1	strawberries	1½ cups
	Shake	2	whey protein shake	2 scoops
Meal 2	Fruit	1	apple	1 item
Meal 3	Bread	1½	garbanzo beans	⅜ cup
	Meat	2	chicken	2 ounces
	Vegetable	1	romaine lettuce	3 cups
Meal 4	Meat	2	tuna	4 ounces
	Vegetable	1	jicama	½ cup
Meal 5	Fruit	1	banana	½ item
	Meat (Nut)	1	peanut butter	1 tablespoon

Meal 6	Bread	1½	potato, baked	½ item
	Meat	4	sirloin	4 ounces
	Vegetable	2	tomato	2 items

Week 9

	Category	Exchanges	Sample food	Quantity
Meal 1	Fruit	1	banana	½ item
	Shake	2	whey protein shake	2 scoops
Meal 2	Fruit	1	tangerine	2 items
Meal 3	Bread	1½	potato	¾ cup
	Meat	2	tuna	4 ounces
	Vegetable	1	romaine lettuce	3 cups
Meal 4	Bread	1½	lentils	½ cup
	Vegetable	1	tomato	1 item
Meal 5	Fruit	1	apple	1 item
	Meat (Nut)	1	soynut butter	1 tablespoon
Meal 6	Bread	1½	corn	¾ cup
	Meat	4	turkey	4 ounces
	Vegetable	2	mushrooms	4 cups

Week 10

	Category	Exchanges	Sample food	Quantity
Meal 1	Fruit	1	mango	½ item
	Shake	2	whey protein shake	2 scoops
Meal 2	Fruit	1	cherries	½ cup
Meal 3	Bread	1½	tortilla, corn	1½ items
	Meat	2	flank steak	2 ounces
	Vegetable	1	peppers	1 cup
Meal 4	Bread	1½	garbanzo beans	⅜ cup
	Vegetable	1	cucumber	2 cups
Meal 5	Fruit	1	cranberries	1 cup
	Meat	2	turkey	2 ounces
Meal 6	Bread	1½	white rice	½ cup
	Meat	2	snapper	4 ounces
	Vegetable	2	Brussels sprouts	2 cups

Week 11

	Category	Exchanges	Sample food	Quantity
Meal 1	Bread	2	granola	¼ cup
	Fruit	1½	grapes	1½ cups
Meal 2	Fruit	1	grapefruit	1 item

Meal 3	Bread	1½	tortilla, corn	1½ items
	Meat	2	halibut	4 ounces
	Vegetable	1	cabbage	2 cups
Meal 4	Bread	1½	pasta	1½ ounces
	Vegetable	1	tomato	1 item
Meal 5	Fruit	1	apple	1 item
Meal 6	Bread	1½	corn	¾ cup
	Meat	4	chicken	4 ounces
	Vegetable	2	green beans	2 cups

Week 12

	Category	Exchanges	Sample food	Quantity
Meal 1	Bread	2	oatmeal	1 cup
	Fruit	1	banana	½ item
Meal 2	Fruit	1	peach	2 small items
Meal 3	Bread	1½	lentils	½ cup
	Meat	4	chicken	4 ounces
	Vegetable	1	carrots	½ cup
Meal 4	Bread	1½	popcorn	1½ cups
	Vegetable	1	green beans	1 cup
Meal 5	Fruit	1	pineapple	1 cup
Meal 6	Bread	1½	brown rice	½ cup
	Meat	4	salmon	4 ounces
	Vegetable	2	spinach	4 cups

Level 2

Week 1

	Category	Exchanges	Sample food	Quantity
Meal 1	Bread	2	bagel	⅔ large item
	Fruit	1	cantaloupe	½ item
Meal 2	Fruit	1	apple	1 item
Meal 3	Bread	3	pita	1½ items
	Meat	4	turkey	4 ounces
	Vegetable	1	romaine lettuce	3 cups
Meal 4	Fruit	1	plum	2 items
Meal 5	Bread	1½	baked potato	½ item
	Meat	4	salmon	4 ounces
	Vegetable	2	spinach	4 cups
Meal 6	Fruit	1	pear	1 item

Week 2

Category	Exchanges	Sample food	Quantity
Meal 1			
Bread	2	oatmeal	1 cup
Fruit	1	banana	½ item
Meal 2			
Fruit	1	peach	2 small items
Meal 3			
Bread	3	white rice	1 cup
Meat	4	tuna	8 ounces
Vegetable	1	tomato	1 item
Meal 4			
Fruit	1	grapes	1 cup
Meal 5			
Bread	1½	corn	¾ cup
Meat	4	chicken breast	4 ounces
Vegetable	2	green beans	2 cups
Meal 6			
Fruit	1	strawberries	1½ cups

Week 3

Category	Exchanges	Sample food	Quantity
Meal 1			
Bread	2	bran flakes	1 cup
Fruit	1	raspberries	1 cup
Meal 2			
Fruit	1	watermelon	1 cup
Meal 3			
Bread	3	white rice	1 cup
Meat	4	shrimp	8 ounces
Vegetable	1	zucchini	1 cup
Meal 4			
Fruit	1	banana	½ item
Meal 5			
Fruit	1	apple	1 item
Meal 6			
Bread	1½	tortilla	1½ items
Meat	4	flank steak	4 ounces
Vegetable	2	peppers	2 cups

Week 4

Category	Exchanges	Sample food	Quantity
Meal 1			
Bread	2	cream of wheat	1 cup
Fruit	1	grapefruit	1 item
Meal 2			
Fruit	1	grapes	1 cup
Meal 3			
Bread	1½	kidney beans	½ cup
Meat	4	tuna	8 ounces
Vegetable	2	romaine lettuce	6 cups
Meal 4			
Bread	1½	popcorn	1½ cups
Vegetable	1	jicama	½ cup
Meal 5			
Fruit	1	apricot	3 items
Meal 6			
Bread	1½	couscous	¾ cup
Meat	4	chicken	4 ounces
Vegetable	2	tomato	2 items

Week 5

	Category	Exchanges	Sample food	Quantity
Meal 1	Bread	2	oatmeal	1 cup
	Fruit	1	blueberries	1 cup
Meal 2	Fruit	1	pear	1 item
Meal 3	Bread	1½	corn tortilla	1½ items
	Meat	4	chicken	4 ounces
	Vegetable	2	peppers	2 cups
Meal 4	Bread	1½	pasta	1½ ounces
	Vegetable	1	broccoli	1 cup
Meal 5	Fruit	1	apple	1 item
Meal 6	Meat	4	whitefish	8 ounces
	Vegetable	2	spinach	4 cups
Meal 7	Bread	1	rice cakes	2 items
	Fruit	1	kiwi	2 items

Week 6

	Category	Exchanges	Sample food	Quantity
Meal 1	Bread	2	shredded wheat	2 large biscuits
	Fruit	1	strawberries	1½ cups
Meal 2	Fruit	1	pineapple	1 cup
Meal 3	Bread	1½	artichoke	1½ items
	Meat	2	salmon	2 ounces
	Vegetable	2	asparagus	2 cups
Meal 4	Bread	1½	winter squash	¾ cup
	Meat	2	turkey	2 ounces
	Vegetable	1	tomato	1 item
Meal 5	Fruit	1	orange	1 item
Meal 6	Meat	4	chicken	4 ounces
	Vegetable	2	broccoli	2 cups
Meal 7	Bread	1	popcorn	1 cup
	Fruit	1	applesauce	½ cup

Week 7

	Category	Exchanges	Sample food	Quantity
Meal 1	Bread	2	bran flakes	1 cup
	Fruit	1½	blueberries	1½ cups
Meal 2	Fruit	1	mango	½ item
Meal 3	Bread	1½	yams	½ cup
	Meat	2	catfish	2 ounces
	Vegetable	2	collards	4 cups

Meal 4	Bread	1½	garbanzo beans	⅜ cup
	Vegetable	1	celery	2 cups
Meal 5	Fruit	1	banana	½ item
	Meat (Nut)	1	almond butter	1 tablespoon
Meal 6	Meat	6	chicken	6 ounces
	Vegetable	2	romaine lettuce	6 cups
Meal 7	Fruit	1	apricot	3 items

Week 8

	Category	Exchanges	Sample food	Quantity
Meal 1	Fruit	1	banana	½ item
	Meat (Nut)	1	peanut butter	1 tablespoon
Meal 2	Bread	2	oatmeal	1 cup
	Fruit	1	blueberries	1 cup
Meal 3	Bread	1½	kidney beans	½ cup
	Meat	2	chicken	2 ounces
	Vegetable	1	romaine lettuce	3 cups
Meal 4	Bread	1½	tortilla, flour	1½ items
	Meat	2	chicken	2 ounces
	Vegetable	1	tomato	1 item
Meal 5	Fruit	1	apple	1 item
	Meat (Nut)	1	almond butter	1 tablespoon
Meal 6	Meat	4	sirloin	4 ounces
	Vegetable	2	asparagus	2 cups
Meal 7	Fruit	1	grapes	1 cup

Week 9

	Category	Exchanges	Sample food	Quantity
Meal 1	Fruit	1	apple	1 item
	Meat (Nut)	1	peanut butter	1 tablespoon
Meal 2	Bread	2	cream of rice	1 cup
	Fruit	1	melon, honeydew	⅛ item
Meal 3	Bread	1½	split peas	½ cup
	Meat	2	tuna	4 ounces
	Vegetable	1	romaine lettuce	3 cups
Meal 4	Bread	1½	tortilla	1½ items
	Meat	1	egg	1 item
Meal 5	Fruit	1	grapes	1 cup
	Meat (Nut)	1	pecans	⅛ cup
Meal 6	Meat	4	turkey	4 ounces
	Vegetable	2	mushrooms	4 cups

| **Meal 7** | Bread | I | cream of wheat | ½ cup |
| | Fruit | I | papaya | ½ item |

Week 10

	Category	Exchanges	Sample food	Quantity
Meal 1	Fruit	I	banana	½ item
	Shake	2	whey protein shake	2 scoops
Meal 2	Fruit	I	nectarine	I item
	Meat (Nut)	I	almonds	⅛ cup
Meal 3	Bread	I½	potato, baked	½ item
	Meat	2	flank steak	2 ounces
	Vegetable	I	peppers	I cup
Meal 4	Bread	I½	rice cakes	3 items
	Meat	I	turkey	I ounce
Meal 5	Fruit	I	cherries	½ cup
Meal 6	Bread	I½	corn	¾ cup
	Meat	4	snapper	8 ounces
	Vegetable	2	Brussels sprouts	2 cups

Week 11

	Category	Exchanges	Sample food	Quantity
Meal 1	Fruit	I	mango	½ item
	Shake	2	whey protein shake	2 scoops
Meal 2	Fruit	I	apple	I item
	Meat (Nut)	I	peanut butter	I tablespoon
Meal 3	Bread	I½	tortilla, corn	I½ items
	Meat	2	halibut	4 ounces
	Vegetable	I	cabbage	2 cups
Meal 4	Bread	I½	pasta	I½ ounces
	Meat	I	chicken	I ounce
Meal 5	Fruit	I	grapes	I cup
Meal 6	Bread	I½	brown rice	½ cup
	Meat	4	chicken	4 ounces
	Vegetable	2	green beans	2 cups

Week 12

	Category	Exchanges	Sample food	Quantity
Meal 1	Bread	2	granola	¼ cup
	Fruit	I	blueberries	I cup
Meal 2	Fruit	I	pear	I item

Meal 3	Bread	1½	lentils	½ cup
	Meat	2	chicken	2 ounces
	Vegetable	1	spinach	2 cups
Meal 4	Bread	1½	spaghetti	¾ cup
	Meat	2	ground beef	2 ounces
	Vegetable	1	tomato	1 item
Meal 5	Fruit	1	banana	½ item
	Meat (Nut)	1	sesame butter	1 tablespoon
Meal 6	Fruit	1	orange	1 item
Meal 7	Bread	1½	couscous	¾ cup
	Meat	4	salmon	4 ounces
	Vegetable	2	spinach	4 cups

Level 3

Week 1

	Category	Exchanges	Sample food	Quantity
Meal 1	Bread	2	bagel	⅔ large item
	Fruit	1	cantaloupe	½ item
Meal 2	Fruit	1	apple	1 item
Meal 3	Bread	3	pita	1½ items
	Meat	4	turkey	4 ounces
	Vegetable	1	romaine lettuce	3 cups
Meal 4	Fruit	1	plum	2 items
Meal 5	Bread	3	baked potato	1 item
	Meat	4	salmon	4 ounces
	Vegetable	2	spinach	4 cups
Meal 6	Fruit	1	pear	1 item

Week 2

	Category	Exchanges	Sample food	Quantity
Meal 1	Bread	2	oatmeal	1 cup
	Fruit	1	banana	½ item
Meal 2	Fruit	1	peach	2 small items
Meal 3	Bread	3	white rice	1 cup
	Meat	4	tuna	8 ounces
	Vegetable	1	tomato	1 item
Meal 4	Fruit	1	grapes	1 cup
Meal 5	Bread	3	corn	1½ cups
	Meat	4	chicken breast	4 ounces
	Vegetable	2	green beans	2 cups
Meal 6	Fruit	1	strawberries	1½ cups

Week 3

	Category	Exchanges	Sample food	Quantity
Meal 1	Bread	2	bran flakes	1 cup
	Fruit	1	raspberries	1 cup
Meal 2	Fruit	1	watermelon	1 cup
Meal 3	Bread	3	white rice	1 cup
	Meat	4	shrimp	8 ounces
	Vegetable	2	zucchini	2 cups
Meal 4	Fruit	1	apple	1 item
Meal 5	Bread	1½	tortilla	1½ items
	Meat	4	flank steak	4 ounces
	Vegetable	2	peppers	2 cups
Meal 6	Bread	1	popcorn	1 cup
	Fruit	1	orange	1 item

Week 4

	Category	Exchanges	Sample food	Quantity
Meal 1	Bread	2	cream of wheat	1 cup
	Fruit	1	grapefruit	1 item
Meal 2	Fruit	1	grapes	1 cup
Meal 3	Bread	1½	kidney beans	½ cup
	Meat	4	tuna	4 ounces
	Vegetable	2	romaine lettuce	6 cups
Meal 4	Bread	1½	popcorn	1½ cups
	Vegetable	1	jicama	½ cup
Meal 5	Fruit	1	apricot	3 items
Meal 6	Bread	1½	pasta	1½ ounces
	Meat	4	chicken	4 ounces
	Vegetable	2	tomato	2 items

Week 5

	Category	Exchanges	Sample food	Quantity
Meal 1	Fruit	2	pear	2 items
Meal 2	Bread	2	oatmeal	1 cup
Meal 3	Bread	1½	corn tortilla	1½ items
	Meat	4	chicken	4 ounces
	Vegetable	2	peppers	2 cups
Meal 4	Bread	1½	green peas	¾ cup
	Vegetable	1	romaine lettuce	3 cups
Meal 5	Fruit	1	apple	1 item

Meal 6	Bread	1½	brown rice	½ cup
	Meat	4	whitefish	8 ounces
	Vegetable	2	spinach	4 cups

Week 6

	Category	Exchanges	Sample food	Quantity
Meal 1	Fruit	2	strawberries	3 cups
Meal 2	Bread	2	shredded wheat	2 large biscuits
Meal 3	Bread	1½	artichoke	1½ items
	Meat	4	salmon	4 ounces
	Vegetable	1	asparagus	1 cup
Meal 4	Fruit	1	Brazil nuts	⅛ cup
	Meat (Nut)	1	orange	1 item
Meal 5	Bread	1½	winter squash	¾ cup
	Meat	4	chicken	4 ounces
	Vegetable	2	broccoli	2 cups
Meal 6	Fruit	1	papaya	½ item

Week 7

	Category	Exchanges	Sample food	Quantity
Meal 1	Bread	2	wheat flakes	1 cup
	Fruit	1	blueberries	1 cup
Meal 2	Meat	1	egg	1 item
Meal 3	Bread	1½	yams	½ cup
	Meat	4	catfish	4 ounces
	Vegetable	2	collards	4 cups
Meal 4	Fruit	1	apple	1 item
	Meat (Nut)	1	peanut butter	1 tablespoon
Meal 5	Bread	1½	black beans	½ cup
	Meat	4	chicken	4 ounces
	Vegetable	3	romaine lettuce	9 cups
Meal 6	Fruit	1	strawberries	1½ cups

Week 8

	Category	Exchanges	Sample food	Quantity
Meal 1	Bread	2	potato	1 cup
	Fruit	1	orange	1 item
Meal 2	Meat	1	egg white	3 items
Meal 3	Bread	3	split peas	1 cup
	Meat	2	salmon	2 ounces
	Vegetable	3	spinach	6 cups

	Category	Exchanges	Sample food	Quantity
Meal 4	Fruit	I	banana	½ item
	Meat (Nut)	I	peanut butter	I tablespoon
Meal 5	Meat	4	sirloin	4 ounces
	Vegetable	3	tomato	3 items
Meal 6	Bread	I	rice cakes	2 items
	Fruit	I	mango	½ item

Week 9

	Category	Exchanges	Sample food	Quantity
Meal I	Bread	2	Grapenuts	½ cup
	Fruit	I	raspberries	I cup
Meal 2	Meat	I	egg	I item
Meal 3	Bread	3	garbanzo beans	¾ cup
	Vegetable	3	romaine lettuce	9 cups
Meal 4	Bread	I ½	lentils	½ cup
	Vegetable	I	tomato	I item
Meal 5	Fruit	I	apple	I item
	Meat (Nut)	I	peanut butter	I tablespoon
Meal 6	Meat	4	turkey	4 ounces
	Vegetable	3	mushrooms	6 cups
Meal 7	Fruit	I	figs	I large item

Week 10

	Category	Exchanges	Sample food	Quantity
Meal I	Fruit	I	banana	½ item
	Shake	2	whey protein shake	2 scoops
Meal 2	Fruit	I	cherries	½ cup
Meal 3	Bread	I ½	garbanzo beans	⅜ cup
	Meat	2	tuna	4 ounces
	Vegetable	I	romaine lettuce	3 cups
Meal 4	Bread	I ½	potato	¾ cup
	Vegetable	I	tomato	I item
Meal 5	Fruit	I	tangerine	2 items
Meal 6	Meat	4	snapper	8 ounces
	Vegetable	3	Brussels sprouts	3 cups
Meal 7	Fruit	I	grapes	I cup

Week 11

	Category	Exchanges	Sample food	Quantity
Meal I	Fruit	I	mango	½ item
	Shake	2	whey protein shake	2 scoops

Meal 2	Fruit	1	nectarine	1 item
Meal 3	Bread	1½	tortilla	1½ items
	Meat	2	flank steak	2 ounces
	Vegetable	1	peppers	1 cup
Meal 4	Bread	1½	split peas	½ cup
	Vegetable	1	carrots	½ cup
Meal 5	Fruit	1	applesauce	½ cup
Meal 6	Bread	1½	pasta	1½ ounces
	Meat	4	chicken	4 ounces
	Vegetable	2	green beans	2 cups

Week 12

	Category	Exchanges	Sample food	Quantity
Meal 1	Bread	2	oatmeal	1 cup
	Fruit	1	apricot	3 items
Meal 2	Fruit	1	pear	1 item
Meal 3	Bread	1½	lentils	½ cup
	Meat	2	chicken	2 ounces
	Vegetable	1	carrots	½ cup
Meal 4	Bread	1½	rice	½ cup
	Vegetable	1	onions	½ cup
Meal 5	Fruit	1	apple	1 item
	Meat (Nut)	1	almond butter	1 tablespoon
Meal 6	Bread	1½	sweet potato	½ item
	Meat	4	halibut	8 ounces
	Vegetable	2	spinach	4 cups

Level 4

Week 1

	Category	Exchanges	Sample food	Quantity
Meal 1	Bread	3	bagel	1 large item
	Fruit	1	cantaloupe	½ item
Meal 2	Fruit	1	apple	1 item
Meal 3	Bread	3	pita	1½ items
	Meat	4	turkey	4 ounces
	Vegetable	1	romaine lettuce	3 cups
Meal 4	Fruit	1	plum	2 items
	Meat (Nut)	1	almonds	⅛ cup
Meal 5	Bread	3	baked potato	1 item
	Meat	4	salmon	4 ounces
	Vegetable	2	spinach	4 cups

| Meal 6 | Bread | I | popcorn | I cup |
| | Fruit | I | pear | I item |

Week 2

	Category	Exchanges	Sample food	Quantity
Meal 1	Bread	3	oatmeal	1½ cups
	Fruit	I	banana	½ item
Meal 2	Fruit	I	peach	2 small items
Meal 3	Bread	3	white rice	I cup
	Meat	4	tuna	8 ounces
	Vegetable	I	tomato	I item
Meal 4	Fruit	I	apple	I item
	Meat (Nut)	I	peanut butter	I tablespoon
Meal 5	Bread	3	corn	1½ cups
	Meat	4	chicken breast	4 ounces
	Vegetable	2	green beans	2 cups
Meal 6	Bread	I	whole wheat crackers	I ounce
	Fruit	I	strawberries	1½ cups

Week 3

	Category	Exchanges	Sample food	Quantity
Meal 1	Bread	3	bran flakes	1½ cups
	Fruit	I	raspberries	I cup
Meal 2	Fruit	I	watermelon	I cup
Meal 3	Bread	3	white rice	I cup
	Meat	4	shrimp	8 ounces
	Vegetable	I	zucchini	I cup
Meal 4	Fruit	I	apple	I item
	Meat (Nut)	I	almond butter	I tablespoon
Meal 5	Bread	3	tortilla	3 items
	Meat	4	flank steak	4 ounces
	Vegetable	2	peppers	2 cups
Meal 6	Bread	I	popcorn	I cup
	Fruit	I	orange	I item

Week 4

	Category	Exchanges	Sample food	Quantity
Meal 1	Bread	3	cream of wheat	1½ cups
	Fruit	I	grapefruit	I item
Meal 2	Fruit	I	grapes	I cup
	Meat (Nut)	I	almonds	⅛ cup

Meal 3	Bread	1½	kidney beans	½ cup
	Meat	4	tuna	8 ounces
	Vegetable	3	romaine lettuce	9 cups
Meal 4	Bread	1½	pasta	1½ ounces
	Vegetable	1	broccoli	1 cup
Meal 5	Fruit	1	apricot	3 items
	Meat (Nut)	1	Brazil nuts	⅛ cup
Meal 6	Bread	3	couscous	1½ cups
	Meat	4	chicken	4 ounces
	Vegetable	2	tomato	2 items
Meal 7	Fruit	1	pear	1 item

Week 5

	Category	Exchanges	Sample food	Quantity
Meal 1	Bread	3	oatmeal	1½ cups
	Fruit	1	blueberries	1 cup
	Meat	1	egg	1 item
Meal 2	Fruit	1	pear	1 item
Meal 3	Bread	1½	corn tortilla	1½ items
	Meat	4	chicken	4 ounces
	Vegetable	2	peppers	2 cups
Meal 4	Bread	1½	popcorn	1½ cups
	Vegetable	1	jicama	½ cup
Meal 5	Fruit	1	apple	1 item
	Meat (Nut)	1	peanut butter	1 tablespoon
Meal 6	Bread	1½	wild rice	½ cup
	Meat	4	whitefish	8 ounces
	Vegetable	3	spinach	6 cups
Meal 7	Fruit	1	peach	2 small items

Week 6

	Category	Exchanges	Sample food	Quantity
Meal 1	Bread	3	shredded wheat	3 large biscuits
	Fruit	1	strawberries	1½ cups
	Meat	1	egg white	3 items
Meal 2	Fruit	1	pineapple	1 cup
Meal 3	Bread	1½	artichoke	1½ items
	Meat	4	salmon	4 ounces
	Vegetable	2	asparagus	2 cups
Meal 4	Bread	1½	garbanzo beans	⅜ cup
	Vegetable	1	cucumber	2 cups

Meal 5	Fruit	I	orange	I item
	Meat (Nut)	I	Brazil nuts	⅛ cup
Meal 6	Bread	1½	winter squash	¾ cup
	Meat	4	chicken	4 ounces
	Vegetable	3	broccoli	3 cups
Meal 7	Bread	I	rice cakes	2 items
	Fruit	I	papaya	½ item

Week 7

	Category	Exchanges	Sample food	Quantity
Meal I	Bread	3	cream of rice	1½ cups
	Fruit	I	banana	½ item
	Meat	2	egg	2 items
Meal 2	Fruit	I	apple	I item
Meal 3	Bread	3	yams	I cup
	Meat	2	catfish	2 ounces
	Vegetable	3	collards	6 cups
Meal 4	Fruit	I	banana	½ item
	Meat (Nut)	I	peanut butter	I tablespoon
Meal 5	Bread	1½	brown rice	½ cup
	Meat	4	chicken	4 ounces
	Vegetable	2	romaine lettuce	6 cups
Meal 6	Bread	I	popcorn	I cup
	Fruit	I	strawberries	1½ cups

Week 8

	Category	Exchanges	Sample food	Quantity
Meal I	Bread	3	potato	I cup
	Fruit	I	orange	I item
	Meat	I	egg white	3 items
Meal 2	Fruit	I	banana	½ item
	Meat (Nut)	I	sesame butter	I tablespoon
Meal 3	Bread	1½	garbanzo beans	⅜ cup
	Meat	2	chicken	2 ounces
	Vegetable	2	romaine lettuce	6 cups
Meal 4	Fruit	I	apple	I item
	Meat (Nut)	I	almond butter	I tablespoon
Meal 5	Bread	1½	potato, baked	½ item
	Meat	4	sirloin	4 ounces
	Vegetable	3	tomato	3 items
Meal 6	Fruit	I	applesauce	½ cup

Week 9

	Category	Exchanges	Sample food	Quantity
Meal 1	Bread	3	Grapenuts	¾ cup
	Fruit	1	grapes	1 cup
	Meat	1	egg	1 item
Meal 2	Fruit	1	nectarine	1 item
	Meat (Nut)	1	cashews	⅛ cup
Meal 3	Bread	1½	lentils	½ cup
	Meat	2	chicken	2 ounces
	Vegetable	2	carrots	1 cup
Meal 4	Bread	1½	macaroni	¾ cup
	Vegetable	1	onions	½ cup
Meal 5	Fruit	1	banana	½ item
	Meat (Nut)	1	peanut butter	1 tablespoon
Meal 6	Bread	1½	artichoke	1½ items
	Meat	6	turkey	6 ounces
	Vegetable	3	mushrooms	6 cups
Meal 7	Fruit	1	pear	1 item

Week 10

	Category	Exchanges	Sample food	Quantity
Meal 1	Fruit	2	banana	1 item
	Shake	2	whey protein shake	2 scoops
Meal 2	Fruit	1	cherries	½ cup
Meal 3	Bread	1½	wild rice	½ cup
	Meat	4	salmon	4 ounces
	Vegetable	2	spinach	2 cups
Meal 4	Bread	1½	garbanzo beans	⅜ cup
	Vegetable	1	tomato	1 item
Meal 5	Fruit	1	tangerine	2 items
Meal 6	Meat	6	snapper	12 ounces
	Vegetable	2	Brussels sprouts	2 cups
Meal 7	Fruit	1	figs	1 large item

Week 11

	Category	Exchanges	Sample food	Quantity
Meal 1	Fruit	2	mango	1 item
	Shake	2	whey protein shake	2 scoops
Meal 2	Fruit	1	grapes	1 cup
Meal 3	Bread	1½	tortilla	1½ items
	Meat	4	flank steak	4 ounces
	Vegetable	2	peppers	2 cups

Meal 4	Bread	1½	pasta	1½ ounces
	Vegetable	1	tomato	1 item
Meal 5	Fruit	1	banana	½ item
	Meat (Nut)	1	peanut butter	1 tablespoon
Meal 6	Meat	6	chicken	6 ounces
	Vegetable	3	green beans	3 cups

Week 12

	Category	Exchanges	Sample food	Quantity
Meal 1	Bread	3	granola	⅜ cup
	Fruit	1	apricot	3 items
	Meat	1	egg white	3 items
Meal 2	Fruit	1	pear	1 item
Meal 3	Bread	1½	split peas	½ cup
	Meat	4	salmon	4 ounces
	Vegetable	2	spinach	4 cups
Meal 4	Bread	1½	corn	¾ cup
	Vegetable	1	green beans	1 cup
Meal 5	Fruit	1	pear	1 item
	Meat (Nut)	1	walnuts	⅛ cup
Meal 6	Bread	1½	white rice	½ cup
	Meat	6	halibut	12 ounces
	Vegetable	2	asparagus	2 cups

Level 5

Week 1

	Category	Exchanges	Sample food	Quantity
Meal 1	Bread	3	bagel	1 large item
	Fruit	1	cantaloupe	½ item
	Meat	1	egg	1 item
Meal 2	Fruit	1	apple	1 item
	Meat (Nut)	1	peanut butter	1 tablespoon
Meal 3	Bread	3	pita	1½ items
	Meat	4	turkey	4 ounces
	Vegetable	1	romaine lettuce	3 cups
Meal 4	Fruit	1	plum	2 items
	Meat (Nut)	1	almonds	⅛ cup
Meal 5	Bread	3	baked potato	1 item
	Meat	4	salmon	4 ounces
	Vegetable	2	spinach	4 cups

Meal 6	Bread	I	popcorn	I cup
	Fruit	I	pear	I item

Week 2

	Category	Exchanges	Sample food	Quantity
Meal I	Bread	3	oatmeal	1½ cups
	Fruit	I	banana	½ item
	Meat	I	egg white	3 items
Meal 2	Fruit	I	peach	2 small items
	Meat (Nut)	I	cashews	⅛ cup
Meal 3	Bread	3	white rice	I cup
	Meat	4	tuna	8 ounces
	Vegetable	I	tomato	I item
Meal 4	Fruit	I	apple	I item
	Meat (Nut)	I	peanut butter	I tablespoon
Meal 5	Bread	3	corn	1½ cups
	Meat	4	chicken breast	4 ounces
	Vegetable	2	green beans	2 cups
Meal 6	Bread	I	whole wheat crackers	I ounce
	Fruit	I	strawberries	1½ cups

Week 3

	Category	Exchanges	Sample food	Quantity
Meal I	Bread	3	bran flakes	1½ cups
	Fruit	I	raspberries	I cup
	Meat	I	egg	I item
Meal 2	Fruit	I	watermelon	I cup
	Meat (Nut)	I	cashews	⅛ cup
Meal 3	Bread	3	white rice	I cup
	Meat	4	shrimp	8 ounces
	Vegetable	I	zucchini	I cup
Meal 4	Fruit	I	apple	I item
	Meat (Nut)	I	almond butter	I tablespoon
Meal 5	Fruit	I	pear	I item
Meal 6	Bread	3	tortilla	3 items
	Meat	4	flank steak	4 ounces
	Vegetable	2	peppers	2 cups
Meal 7	Fruit	I	orange	I item

Week 4

	Category	Exchanges	Sample food	Quantity
Meal 1	Bread	3	cream of wheat	1½ cups
	Fruit	1	grapefruit	1 item
	Meat	1	egg white	3 items
Meal 2	Fruit	1	grapes	1 cup
	Meat (Nut)	1	walnuts	⅛ cup
Meal 3	Bread	1½	kidney beans	½ cup
	Meat	4	tuna	8 ounces
	Vegetable	1	romaine lettuce	3 cups
Meal 4	Bread	1½	pasta	1½ ounces
	Vegetable	1	broccoli	1 cup
Meal 5	Fruit	1	apricot	3 items
	Meat (Nut)	1	Brazil nuts	⅛ cup
Meal 6	Bread	1½	couscous	¾ cup
	Meat	4	chicken	4 ounces
	Vegetable	2	tomato	2 items
Meal 7	Bread	1	rice cakes	2 items
	Fruit	1	papaya	½ item

Week 5

	Category	Exchanges	Sample food	Quantity
Meal 1	Bread	3	oatmeal	1½ cups
	Fruit	1	blueberries	1 cup
	Meat	1	egg	1 item
Meal 2	Fruit	1	pear	1 item
	Meat (Nut)	1	almonds	⅛ cup
Meal 3	Bread	1½	corn tortilla	1½ items
	Meat	4	chicken	4 ounces
	Vegetable	1	peppers	1 cup
Meal 4	Bread	1½	popcorn	1½ cups
	Vegetable	1	jicama	½ cup
Meal 5	Fruit	1	apple	1 item
	Meat (Nut)	1	peanut butter	1 tablespoon
Meal 6	Meat	6	whitefish	12 ounces
	Vegetable	3	spinach	6 cups
Meal 7	Bread	1	rice cakes	2 items
	Fruit	1	kiwi	2 items

Week 6

Meal	Category	Exchanges	Sample food	Quantity
Meal 1	Bread	3	shredded wheat	3 large biscuits
	Fruit	1	strawberries	1½ cups
	Meat	1	egg white	3 items
Meal 2	Fruit	1	papaya	½ item
	Meat (Nut)	1	avocado	⅓ item
Meal 3	Bread	1½	artichoke	1½ items
	Meat	2	salmon	2 ounces
	Vegetable	2	asparagus	2 cups
Meal 4	Bread	1½	winter squash	¾ cup
	Meat	2	turkey	2 ounces
	Vegetable	1	tomato	1 item
Meal 5	Fruit	1	orange	1 item
	Meat (Nut)	1	Brazil nuts	⅛ cup
Meal 6	Bread	1½	brown rice	½ cup
	Meat	6	chicken	6 ounces
	Vegetable	3	broccoli	3 cups

Week 7

Meal	Category	Exchanges	Sample food	Quantity
Meal 1	Fruit	2	banana	1 item
	Meat (Nut)	1	peanut butter	1 tablespoon
Meal 2	Bread	3	potato	1½ cups
	Meat	1	egg	1 item
Meal 3	Bread	1½	yams	½ cup
	Meat	2	catfish	2 ounces
	Vegetable	2	collards	4 cups
Meal 4	Bread	1½	garbanzo beans	⅜ cup
	Meat	2	chicken	2 ounces
	Vegetable	1	celery	2 cups
Meal 5	Fruit	1	pineapple	1 cup
Meal 6	Meat	6	chicken	6 ounces
	Vegetable	3	romaine lettuce	9 cups
Meal 7	Fruit	1	orange	1 item

Week 8

Meal	Category	Exchanges	Sample food	Quantity
Meal 1	Fruit	1	mango	½ item
	Shake	2	whey protein shake	2 scoops
Meal 2	Fruit	1	banana	½ item
	Meat (Nut)	1	sesame butter	1 tablespoon

Meal 3	Bread	1½	garbanzo beans	⅜ cup
	Meat	2	chicken	2 ounces
	Vegetable	1	romaine lettuce	3 cups
Meal 4	Bread	1½	tortilla, flour	1½ items
	Meat	2	chicken	2 ounces
	Vegetable	1	tomato	1 item
Meal 5	Fruit	1	orange	1 item
Meal 6	Bread	1½	potato, baked	½ item
	Meat	6	sirloin	6 ounces
	Vegetable	3	tomato	3 items
Meal 7	Fruit	1	apple	1 item

Week 9

	Category	Exchanges	Sample food	Quantity
Meal 1	Fruit	1	blueberries	1 cup
	Shake	2	whey protein shake	2 scoops
Meal 2	Fruit	1	nectarine	1 item
Meal 3	Bread	1½	lentils	½ cup
	Meat	2	chicken	2 ounces
	Vegetable	2	carrots	1 cup
Meal 4	Bread	1½	potato	¾ cup
	Meat	2	tuna	4 ounces
	Vegetable	1	romaine lettuce	3 cups
Meal 5	Fruit	1	apple	1 item
	Meat (Nut)	1	almond butter	1 tablespoon
Meal 6	Meat	6	turkey	6 ounces
	Vegetable	3	mushrooms	6 cups
Meal 7	Bread	1	popcorn	1 cup
	Fruit	1	orange	1 item

Week 10

	Category	Exchanges	Sample food	Quantity
Meal 1	Fruit	1	mango	½ item
	Shake	2	whey protein shake	2 scoops
Meal 2	Fruit	1	cherries	½ cup
Meal 3	Bread	1½	tortilla, corn	1½ items
	Meat	2	flank steak	2 ounces
	Vegetable	1	peppers	1 cup
Meal 4	Bread	1½	tortilla, flour	1½ items
	Meat	2	chicken	2 ounces
	Vegetable	1	tomato	1 item

Meal 5	Fruit	I	banana	½ item
	Meat (Nut)	I	peanut butter	I tablespoon
Meal 6	Bread	I ½	wild rice	½ cup
	Meat	6	snapper	12 ounces
	Vegetable	2	Brussels sprouts	2 cups

Week 11

	Category	Exchanges	Sample food	Quantity
Meal I	Bread	2	bran flakes	I cup
	Fruit	I	blueberries	I cup
	Meat	I	egg	I item
Meal 2	Fruit	I	grapes	I cup
Meal 3	Bread	I ½	brown rice	½ cup
	Meat	4	salmon	4 ounces
	Vegetable	2	spinach	4 cups
Meal 4	Fruit	I	apple	I item
	Meat (Nut)	I	almonds	⅛ cup
Meal 5	Bread	I ½	corn	¾ cup
	Meat	6	chicken	6 ounces
	Vegetable	3	green beans	3 cups
Meal 6	Bread	I	popcorn	I cup
	Fruit	I	peach	2 small items

Week 12

	Category	Exchanges	Sample food	Quantity
Meal I	Bread	2	oatmeal	I cup
	Fruit	I	grapefruit	I item
	Meat	I	egg	I item
Meal 2	Fruit	I	banana	½ item
	Meat (Nut)	I	almond butter	I tablespoon
Meal 3	Bread	I ½	split peas	½ cup
	Meat	4	salmon	4 ounces
	Vegetable	2	spinach	4 cups
Meal 4	Fruit	I	apple	I item
	Meat (Nut)	I	peanut butter	I tablespoon
Meal 5	Bread	I ½	white rice	½ cup
	Meat	8	halibut	16 ounces
	Vegetable	2	asparagus	2 cups
Meal 6	Bread	I	couscous	½ cup
	Fruit	I	figs	I large item

Level 6

Week 1

Category	Exchanges	Sample food	Quantity
Meal 1			
Bread	3	bagel	1 large item
Fruit	1	cantaloupe	½ item
Meat	2	egg	2 items
Meal 2			
Fruit	1	apple	1 item
Meat (Nut)	1	peanut butter	1 tablespoon
Meal 3			
Bread	3	pita	1½ items
Meat	4	turkey	4 ounces
Vegetable	1	romaine lettuce	3 cups
Meal 4			
Fruit	1	plum	2 items
Meat (Nut)	1	almonds	⅛ cup
Meal 5			
Bread	3	baked potato	1 item
Meat	8	salmon	8 ounces
Vegetable	2	spinach	4 cups
Meal 6			
Bread	1	popcorn	1 cup
Fruit	2	pear	2 items

Week 2

Category	Exchanges	Sample food	Quantity
Meal 1			
Bread	3	oatmeal	1½ cups
Fruit	1	banana	½ item
Meat	2	egg white	6 items
Meal 2			
Fruit	1	peach	2 small items
Meat (Nut)	1	cashews	⅛ cup
Meal 3			
Bread	3	white rice	1 cup
Meat	4	tuna	8 ounces
Vegetable	1	tomato	1 item
Meal 4			
Fruit	1	apple	1 item
Meat (Nut)	1	peanut butter	1 tablespoon
Meal 5			
Bread	3	corn	1½ cups
Meat	8	chicken breast	8 ounces
Vegetable	2	green beans	2 cups
Meal 6			
Bread	1	whole wheat crackers	1 ounce
Fruit	2	strawberries	3 cups

Week 3

Category	Exchanges	Sample food	Quantity
Meal 1			
Bread	3	bran flakes	1½ cups
Fruit	1	raspberries	1 cup
Meat	2	egg	2 items

Meal 2	Fruit	I	watermelon	I cup
	Meat (Nut)	I	cashews	⅛ cup
Meal 3	Bread	I½	white rice	½ cup
	Meat	4	shrimp	8 ounces
	Vegetable	I	zucchini	I cup
Meal 4	Bread	I½	pasta	I½ ounces
	Vegetable	I	broccoli	I cup
Meal 5	Fruit	I	apple	I item
	Meat (Nut)	I	almond butter	I tablespoon
Meal 6	Bread	3	tortilla	3 items
	Meat	8	flank steak	8 ounces
	Vegetable	2	peppers	2 cups
Meal 7	Bread	I	popcorn	I cup
	Fruit	I	orange	I item

Week 4

	Category	Exchanges	Sample food	Quantity
Meal I	Bread	3	cream of wheat	I½ cups
	Fruit	I	grapefruit	I item
	Meat	2	egg white	6 items
Meal 2	Fruit	I	grapes	I cup
	Meat (Nut)	I	walnuts	⅛ cup
Meal 3	Bread	I½	kidney beans	½ cup
	Meat	4	tuna	8 ounces
	Vegetable	I	romaine lettuce	3 cups
Meal 4	Bread	I½	tortilla, flour	I½ items
	Meat	2	chicken	2 ounces
	Vegetable	I	peppers	I cup
Meal 5	Fruit	I	apricot	3 items
	Meat (Nut)	I	Brazil nuts	⅛ cup
Meal 6	Bread	I½	couscous	¾ cup
	Meat	8	chicken	8 ounces
	Vegetable	2	tomato	2 items
Meal 7	Bread	I	popcorn	I cup
	Fruit	I	papaya	½ item

Week 5

	Category	Exchanges	Sample food	Quantity
Meal I	Bread	2	oatmeal	I cup
	Fruit	2	blueberries	2 cups
	Meat	2	egg	2 items

Meal 2	Fruit	1	pear	1 item
	Meat (Nut)	1	almonds	1/8 cup
Meal 3	Bread	1½	corn tortilla	1½ items
	Meat	4	chicken	4 ounces
	Vegetable	2	peppers	2 cups
Meal 4	Bread	1½	corn	¾ cup
	Meat	2	potato	1 cup
	Vegetable	1	romaine lettuce	3 cups
Meal 5	Fruit	1	banana	½ item
	Meat (Nut)	1	peanut butter	1 tablespoon
Meal 6	Bread	1½	wild rice	½ cup
	Meat	8	whitefish	16 ounces
	Vegetable	3	spinach	6 cups
Meal 7	Fruit	1	applesauce	½ cup

Week 6

	Category	Exchanges	Sample food	Quantity
Meal 1	Bread	2	shredded wheat	2 large biscuits
	Fruit	2	strawberries	3 cups
	Meat	2	egg white	6 items
Meal 2	Fruit	1	papaya	½ item
	Meat (Nut)	1	avocado	1/3 item
Meal 3	Bread	1½	artichoke	1½ items
	Meat	4	salmon	4 ounces
	Vegetable	2	asparagus	2 cups
Meal 4	Bread	1½	winter squash	¾ cup
	Meat	2	turkey	2 ounces
	Vegetable	1	tomato	1 item
Meal 5	Fruit	1	kiwi	2 items
	Meat (Nut)	1	Brazil nuts	1/8 cup
Meal 6	Bread	1½	corn	¾ cup
	Meat	8	chicken	8 ounces
	Vegetable	3	broccoli	3 cups

Week 7

	Category	Exchanges	Sample food	Quantity
Meal 1	Fruit	2	banana	1 item
	Shake	2	whey protein shake	2 scoops
Meal 2	Fruit	1	apple	1 item
	Meat (Nut)	1	peanut butter	1 tablespoon

Meal 3	Bread	1½	yams	½ cup
	Meat	4	catfish	4 ounces
	Vegetable	2	collards	4 cups
Meal 4	Bread	1½	garbanzo beans	⅜ cup
	Meat	2	chicken	2 ounces
	Vegetable	1	celery	2 cups
Meal 5	Fruit	1	apricot	3 items
	Meat (Nut)	1	cashews	⅛ cup
Meal 6	Bread	1½	potato, baked	½ item
	Meat	8	chicken	8 ounces
	Vegetable	3	romaine lettuce	9 cups

Week 8

	Category	Exchanges	Sample food	Quantity
Meal 1	Bread	3	corn grits	1½ cups
	Meat	2	egg white	6 items
Meal 2	Fruit	1	banana	½ item
	Meat (Nut)	1	sesame butter	1 tablespoon
Meal 3	Bread	1½	garbanzo beans	⅜ cup
	Meat	4	chicken	4 ounces
	Vegetable	1	romaine lettuce	3 cups
Meal 4	Bread	1½	corn tortilla	1½ items
	Meat	2	pollack	4 ounces
	Vegetable	1	cabbage	2 cups
Meal 5	Fruit	1	apple	1 item
	Meat (Nut)	1	peanut butter	1 tablespoon
Meal 6	Meat	8	sirloin	8 ounces
	Vegetable	3	tomato	3 items
Meal 7	Bread	1	popcorn	1 cup
	Fruit	1	pear	1 item

Week 9

	Category	Exchanges	Sample food	Quantity
Meal 1	Fruit	2	blueberries	2 cups
	Shake	2	whey protein shake	2 scoops
Meal 2	Fruit	1	tangerine	2 items
	Meat (Nut)	1	cashews	⅛ cup
Meal 3	Bread	1½	corn	¾ cup
	Meat	4	chicken	4 ounces
	Vegetable	1	summer squash	1 cup

Meal 4	Bread	1½	lentils	½ cup
	Meat	2	chicken	2 ounces
	Vegetable	1	tomato	1 item
Meal 5	Fruit	1	pear	1 item
	Meat (Nut)	1	walnuts	⅛ cup
Meal 6	Meat	8	turkey	8 ounces
	Vegetable	3	mushrooms	6 cups
Meal 7	Bread	1	cream of wheat	½ cup
	Fruit	1	nectarine	1 item

Week 10

	Category	Exchanges	Sample food	Quantity
Meal 1	Fruit	2	mango	1 item
	Meat	2	egg	2 items
Meal 2	Bread	3	corn	1½ cups
Meal 3	Bread	1½	corn tortilla	1½ items
	Meat	4	flank steak	4 ounces
	Vegetable	1	peppers	1 cup
Meal 4	Bread	1½	wild rice	½ cup
	Meat	2	turkey	2 ounces
	Vegetable	1	spinach	2 cups
Meal 5	Fruit	1	cherries	½ cup
Meal 6	Meat	8	snapper	16 ounces
	Vegetable	3	Brussels sprouts	3 cups

Week 11

	Category	Exchanges	Sample food	Quantity
Meal 1	Fruit	1	banana	½ item
	Shake	2	whey protein shake	2 scoops
Meal 2	Fruit	1	peach	2 small items
	Meat (Nut)	1	cashews	⅛ cup
Meal 3	Bread	1½	lentils	½ cup
	Meat	4	chicken	4 ounces
	Vegetable	1	carrots	½ cup
Meal 4	Bread	1½	pasta	1½ ounces
	Meat	2	chicken	2 ounces
	Vegetable	1	tomato	1 item
Meal 5	Fruit	1	grapes	1 cup

Meal 6	Bread	1½	potato, baked	½ item
	Meat	8	salmon	8 ounces
	Vegetable	3	green beans	3 cups
Meal 7	Fruit	1	pineapple	1 cup

Week 12

	Category	Exchanges	Sample food	Quantity
Meal 1	Bread	3	granola	⅜ cup
	Fruit	2	grapefruit	2 items
	Meat	1	egg	1 item
Meal 2	Fruit	1	apple	1 item
	Meat (Nut)	1	peanut butter	1 tablespoon
Meal 3	Bread	1½	split peas	½ cup
	Meat	4	chicken	4 ounces
	Vegetable	1	spinach	2 cups
Meal 4	Bread	1½	white rice	½ cup
	Meat	2	crab	4 ounces
	Vegetable	1	cucumber	1 cup
Meal 5	Fruit	1	pear	1 item
Meal 6	Bread	1½	sweet potato	½ item
	Meat	8	halibut	16 ounces
	Vegetable	3	asparagus	3 cups
Meal 7	Fruit	1	figs	1 large item

Level 7

Week 1

	Category	Exchanges	Sample food	Quantity
Meal 1	Bread	3	bagel	1 large item
	Fruit	1	cantaloupe	½ item
	Meat	2	egg	2 items
Meal 2	Fruit	1	apple	1 item
	Meat (Nut)	1	peanut butter	1 tablespoon
Meal 3	Bread	3	pita	1½ items
	Meat	4	turkey	4 ounces
	Vegetable	1	romaine lettuce	3 cups
Meal 4	Fruit	1	plum	2 items
	Meat (Nut)	1	almonds	⅛ cup
Meal 5	Fruit	1	watermelon	1 cup
Meal 6	Bread	3	baked potato	1 item
	Meat	8	salmon	8 ounces
	Vegetable	2	spinach	4 cups

| Meal 7 | Bread | 2 | popcorn | 2 cups |
| | Fruit | 2 | pear | 2 items |

Week 2

	Category	Exchanges	Sample food	Quantity
Meal 1	Bread	3	oatmeal	1½ cups
	Fruit	1	banana	½ item
	Meat	2	egg white	6 items
Meal 2	Fruit	1	peach	2 small items
	Meat (Nut)	1	cashews	⅛ cup
Meal 3	Bread	3	white rice	1 cup
	Meat	4	tuna	8 ounces
	Vegetable	1	tomato	1 item
Meal 4	Fruit	1	apple	1 item
	Meat (Nut)	1	peanut butter	1 tablespoon
Meal 5	Fruit	1	nectarine	1 item
Meal 6	Bread	3	corn	1½ cups
	Meat	8	chicken breast	8 ounces
	Vegetable	2	green beans	2 cups
Meal 7	Bread	2	whole wheat crackers	2 ounces
	Fruit	2	strawberries	3 cups

Week 3

	Category	Exchanges	Sample food	Quantity
Meal 1	Bread	3	bran flakes	1½ cups
	Fruit	1	raspberries	1 cup
	Meat	2	egg	2 items
Meal 2	Fruit	1	watermelon	1 cup
	Meat (Nut)	1	cashews	⅛ cup
Meal 3	Bread	3	white rice	1 cup
	Meat	4	shrimp	8 ounces
	Vegetable	1	zucchini	1 cup
Meal 4	Fruit	1	apple	1 item
	Meat (Nut)	1	almond butter	1 tablespoon
Meal 5	Fruit	1	grapes	1 cup
Meal 6	Bread	3	tortilla	3 items
	Meat	8	flank steak	8 ounces
	Vegetable	2	peppers	2 cups
Meal 7	Bread	2	popcorn	2 cups
	Fruit	1	orange	1 item

Week 4

Meal	Category	Exchanges	Sample food	Quantity
Meal 1	Bread	3	cream of wheat	1½ cups
	Fruit	1	grapefruit	1 item
	Meat	2	egg white	6 items
Meal 2	Fruit	1	grapes	1 cup
	Meat (Nut)	1	walnuts	⅛ cup
Meal 3	Bread	3	kidney beans	1 cup
	Meat	4	tuna	8 ounces
	Vegetable	1	romaine lettuce	3 cups
Meal 4	Fruit	1	apricot	3 items
	Meat (Nut)	1	Brazil nuts	⅛ cup
Meal 5	Fruit	1	melon, cantaloupe	½ item
Meal 6	Bread	1½	couscous	¾ cup
	Meat	8	chicken	8 ounces
	Vegetable	2	tomato	2 items
Meal 7	Bread	1	popcorn	1 cup
	Fruit	1	papaya	½ item

Week 5

Meal	Category	Exchanges	Sample food	Quantity
Meal 1	Bread	3	oatmeal	1½ cups
	Fruit	1	blueberries	1 cup
	Meat	2	egg	2 items
Meal 2	Fruit	1	pear	1 item
	Meat (Nut)	1	almonds	⅛ cup
Meal 3	Bread	1½	corn tortilla	1½ items
	Meat	4	chicken	4 ounces
	Vegetable	1	peppers	1 cup
Meal 4	Bread	1½	potato	¾ cup
	Vegetable	1	celery	2 cups
Meal 5	Fruit	1	banana	½ item
	Meat (Nut)	1	peanut butter	1 tablespoon
Meal 6	Bread	1½	wild rice	½ cup
	Meat	8	whitefish	16 ounces
	Vegetable	2	spinach	4 cups
Meal 7	Bread	2	rice cakes	4 items
	Fruit	2	kiwi	4 items

Week 6

	Category	Exchanges	Sample food	Quantity
Meal 1	Bread	3	shredded wheat	3 large biscuits
	Fruit	1	strawberries	1½ cups
	Meat	1	egg white	3 items
Meal 2	Fruit	1	papaya	½ item
	Meat (Nut)	1	avocado	⅓ item
Meal 3	Bread	1½	artichoke	1½ items
	Meat	2	salmon	2 ounces
	Vegetable	1	asparagus	1 cup
Meal 4	Bread	1½	winter squash	¾ cup
	Meat	3	turkey	3 ounces
	Vegetable	1	tomato	1 item
Meal 5	Fruit	1	peach	2 small items
	Meat (Nut)	1	Brazil nuts	⅛ cup
Meal 6	Bread	1½	pasta	1½ ounces
	Meat	8	chicken	8 ounces
	Vegetable	3	broccoli	3 cups
Meal 7	Bread	2	popcorn	2 cups
	Fruit	2	applesauce	1 cup

Week 7

	Category	Exchanges	Sample food	Quantity
Meal 1	Bread	3	cream of rice	1½ cups
	Fruit	1	banana	½ item
	Meat	2	egg	2 items
Meal 2	Fruit	1	plum	2 items
	Meat (Nut)	1	peanut butter	1 tablespoon
Meal 3	Bread	1½	yams	½ cup
	Meat	2	catfish	2 ounces
	Vegetable	2	collards	4 cups
Meal 4	Bread	1½	corn	¾ cup
	Meat	2	turkey	2 ounces
	Vegetable	1	beets	½ cup
Meal 5	Fruit	1	apple	1 item
	Meat (Nut)	1	peanut butter	1 tablespoon
Meal 6	Bread	1½	garbanzo beans	⅜ cup
	Meat	8	chicken	8 ounces
	Vegetable	3	romaine lettuce	9 cups

| Meal 7 | Bread | 1 | granola | ⅛ cup |
| | Fruit | 1 | apricot | 3 items |

Week 8

Meal	Category	Exchanges	Sample food	Quantity
Meal 1	Bread	1	potato	½ cup
	Fruit	2	orange	2 items
	Meat	2	egg white	6 items
Meal 2	Bread	3	corn	1½ cups
Meal 3	Bread	1½	garbanzo beans	⅜ cup
	Meat	2	chicken	2 ounces
	Vegetable	2	romaine lettuce	6 cups
Meal 4	Bread	1½	green peas	¾ cup
	Meat	2	tuna	4 ounces
	Vegetable	2	onions	1 cup
Meal 5	Fruit	1	banana	½ item
Meal 6	Bread	1½	potato, baked	½ item
	Meat	8	sirloin	8 ounces
	Vegetable	3	tomato	3 items
Meal 7	Bread	1	rice cakes	2 items
	Fruit	2	pear	2 items

Week 9

Meal	Category	Exchanges	Sample food	Quantity
Meal 1	Fruit	2	mango	1 item
	Shake	2	whey protein shake	2 scoops
Meal 2	Fruit	1	apple	1 item
	Meat (Nut)	1	cashews	⅛ cup
Meal 3	Bread	3	corn	1½ cups
	Vegetable	3	tomato	3 items
Meal 4	Fruit	1	banana	½ item
	Meat (Nut)	1	peanut butter	1 tablespoon
Meal 5	Meat	2	turkey	2 ounces
	Vegetable	1	tomato	1 item
Meal 6	Bread	1½	artichoke	1½ items
	Meat	8	turkey	8 ounces
	Vegetable	3	mushrooms	6 cups
Meal 7	Bread	1	popcorn	1 cup
	Fruit	1	tangerine	2 items

Week 10

	Category	Exchanges	Sample food	Quantity
Meal 1	Bread	3	oatmeal	1½ cups
	Fruit	1	peach	2 small items
	Meat	2	egg	2 items
Meal 2	Fruit	1	banana	½ item
	Meat (Nut)	1	almond butter	1 tablespoon
Meal 3	Bread	3	white rice	1 cup
	Vegetable	3	carrots	1½ cups
Meal 4	Fruit	1	cherries	½ cup
	Meat (Nut)	1	almonds	⅛ cup
Meal 5	Meat	2	turkey	2 ounces
Meal 6	Bread	1½	black beans	½ cup
	Meat	8	flank steak	8 ounces
	Vegetable	2	peppers	2 cups
Meal 7	Bread	1	cream of wheat	½ cup
	Fruit	1	pear	1 item

Week 11

	Category	Exchanges	Sample food	Quantity
Meal 1	Fruit	2	blueberries	2 cups
	Shake	2	whey protein shake	2 scoops
Meal 2	Meat	2	egg white	6 items
Meal 3	Bread	3	lentils	1 cup
	Meat	2	chicken	2 ounces
	Vegetable	3	carrots	1½ cups
Meal 4	Fruit	1	grapes	1 cup
	Meat (Nut)	1	walnuts	⅛ cup
Meal 5	Meat	2	tuna	4 ounces
Meal 6	Bread	1½	brown rice	½ cup
	Meat	8	salmon	8 ounces
	Vegetable	2	cauliflower	2 cups
Meal 7	Bread	1	popcorn	1 cup
	Fruit	1	peach	2 small items

Week 12

	Category	Exchanges	Sample food	Quantity
Meal 1	Bread	3	bran flakes	1½ cups
	Fruit	1	grapefruit	1 item
	Meat	2	egg	2 items

Meal 2	Fruit	1	apple	1 item
	Meat (Nut)	1	peanut butter	1 tablespoon
Meal 3	Bread	3	split peas	1 cup
	Meat	4	chicken	4 ounces
	Vegetable	2	spinach	4 cups
Meal 4	Bread	1½	pasta	1½ ounces
	Vegetable	1	tomato	1 item
Meal 5	Fruit	1	banana	½ item
	Meat (Nut)	1	soynut butter	1 tablespoon
Meal 6	Bread	1½	potato, baked	½ item
	Meat	8	halibut	16 ounces
	Vegetable	2	asparagus	2 cups
Meal 7	Bread	1	Grapenuts	¼ cup
	Fruit	1	figs	1 large item

Level 8

Week 1

	Category	Exchanges	Sample food	Quantity
Meal 1	Bread	3	bagel	1 large item
	Fruit	1	cantaloupe	½ item
	Meat	2	egg	2 items
Meal 2	Fruit	1	apple	1 item
	Meat (Nut)	1	peanut butter	1 tablespoon
Meal 3	Bread	3	pita	1½ items
	Meat	4	turkey	4 ounces
	Vegetable	1	romaine lettuce	3 cups
Meal 4	Fruit	1	plum	2 items
	Meat (Nut)	1	almonds	⅛ cup
Meal 5	Fruit	1	watermelon	1 cup
	Meat	2	turkey	2 ounces
Meal 6	Bread	3	baked potato	1 item
	Meat	8	salmon	8 ounces
	Vegetable	2	spinach	4 cups
Meal 7	Bread	2	popcorn	2 cups
	Fruit	2	pear	2 items

Week 2

	Category	Exchanges	Sample food	Quantity
Meal 1	Bread	3	oatmeal	1½ cups
	Fruit	1	banana	½ item
	Meat	2	egg white	6 items

Meal 2	Fruit	I	peach	2 small items
	Meat (Nut)	I	cashews	⅛ cup
Meal 3	Bread	3	white rice	I cup
	Meat	4	tuna	8 ounces
	Vegetable	I	tomato	I item
Meal 4	Fruit	I	apple	I item
	Meat (Nut)	I	peanut butter	I tablespoon
Meal 5	Fruit	I	nectarine	I item
	Meat	2	turkey	2 ounces
Meal 6	Bread	3	corn	I ½ cups
	Meat	8	chicken breast	8 ounces
	Vegetable	2	green beans	2 cups
Meal 7	Bread	2	whole wheat crackers	2 ounces
	Fruit	2	strawberries	3 cups

Week 3

	Category	Exchanges	Sample food	Quantity
Meal 1	Bread	3	bran flakes	I ½ cups
	Fruit	I	raspberries	I cup
	Meat	2	egg	2 items
Meal 2	Fruit	I	watermelon	I cup
	Meat (Nut)	I	cashews	⅛ cup
Meal 3	Bread	3	white rice	I cup
	Meat	3	shrimp	6 ounces
	Vegetable	I	zucchini	I cup
Meal 4	Fruit	I	apple	I item
	Meat (Nut)	I	almond butter	I tablespoon
Meal 5	Fruit	I	grapes	I cup
	Meat	2	turkey	2 ounces
Meal 6	Bread	3	tortilla	3 items
	Meat	8	flank steak	8 ounces
	Vegetable	2	peppers	2 cups
Meal 7	Bread	2	popcorn	2 cups
	Fruit	2	orange	2 items

Week 4

	Category	Exchanges	Sample food	Quantity
Meal 1	Bread	3	cream of wheat	I ½ cups
	Fruit	I	grapefruit	I item
	Meat	2	egg white	6 items

	Category	Exchanges	Sample food	Quantity
Meal 2	Fruit	1	grapes	1 cup
	Meat (Nut)	1	walnuts	⅛ cup
Meal 3	Bread	3	kidney beans	1 cup
	Meat	2	tuna	4 ounces
	Vegetable	1	romaine lettuce	3 cups
Meal 4	Fruit	1	papaya	½ item
	Meat	2	turkey	2 ounces
Meal 5	Fruit	1	melon, cantaloupe	½ item
	Meat	2	tuna	4 ounces
Meal 6	Bread	3	couscous	1½ cups
	Meat	8	chicken	8 ounces
	Vegetable	2	tomato	2 items
Meal 7	Fruit	2	apricot	6 items

Week 5

	Category	Exchanges	Sample food	Quantity
Meal 1	Bread	1½	oatmeal	¾ cup
	Fruit	1	blueberries	1 cup
	Meat	2	egg	2 items
Meal 2	Bread	2	popcorn	2 cups
	Fruit	1	pear	1 item
Meal 3	Bread	3	corn tortilla	3 items
	Meat	2	chicken	2 ounces
	Vegetable	2	peppers	2 cups
Meal 4	Fruit	1	apple	1 item
	Meat	2	tuna	4 ounces
Meal 5	Fruit	1	cranberries	1 cup
	Meat	2	turkey	2 ounces
Meal 6	Bread	3	wild rice	1 cup
	Meat	8	whitefish	16 ounces
	Vegetable	2	spinach	4 cups
Meal 7	Fruit	2	strawberries	3 cups

Week 6

	Category	Exchanges	Sample food	Quantity
Meal 1	Bread	1	shredded wheat	1 large biscuit
	Fruit	1	strawberries	1½ cups
	Meat	2	egg white	6 items
Meal 2	Bread	2	granola	¼ cup
	Fruit	1	grapes	1 cup

Meal 3	Bread	1½	artichoke	1½ items
	Meat	4	salmon	4 ounces
	Vegetable	2	asparagus	2 cups
Meal 4	Bread	1½	black beans	½ cup
	Vegetable	1	onions	½ cup
Meal 5	Fruit	1	peach	2 small items
	Meat (Nut)	1	Brazil nuts	⅛ cup
Meal 6	Fruit	1	nectarine	1 item
	Meat	2	turkey	2 ounces
Meal 7	Bread	3	winter squash	1½ cup
	Meat	8	chicken	8 ounces
	Vegetable	2	broccoli	2 cups

Week 7

	Category	Exchanges	Sample food	Quantity
Meal 1	Bread	3	cream of rice	1½ cups
	Fruit	1	raspberries	1 cup
Meal 2	Fruit	1	apple	1 item
	Meat (Nut)	1	peanut butter	1 tablespoon
Meal 3	Bread	1½	yams	½ cup
	Meat	4	catfish	4 ounces
	Vegetable	2	collards	4 cups
Meal 4	Bread	1½	tortilla, flour	1½ items
	Meat	2	egg	2 items
Meal 5	Fruit	1	banana	½ item
	Meat (Nut)	1	almond butter	1 tablespoon
Meal 6	Fruit	1	cantaloupe	½ item
	Meat	2	tuna	4 ounces
Meal 7	Bread	3	garbanzo beans	¾ cup
	Meat	8	chicken	8 ounces
	Vegetable	2	romaine lettuce	6 cups

Week 8

	Category	Exchanges	Sample food	Quantity
Meal 1	Fruit	2	blueberries	2 cups
	Shake	2	whey protein shake	2 scoops
Meal 2	Fruit	1	banana	½ item
	Meat (Nut)	1	sesame butter	1 tablespoon
Meal 3	Bread	1½	garbanzo beans	⅜ cup
	Meat	4	chicken	4 ounces
	Vegetable	1	romaine lettuce	3 cups

Meal 4	Bread	1½	white rice	½ cup
	Meat	2	crab	4 ounces
Meal 5	Fruit	I	pear	I item
	Meat (Nut)	I	walnuts	⅛ cup
Meal 6	Fruit	I	apple	I item
	Meat	2	tuna	4 ounces
Meal 7	Bread	3	potato, baked	I item
	Meat	8	sirloin	8 ounces
	Vegetable	2	spinach	4 cups

Week 9

	Category	Exchanges	Sample food	Quantity
Meal 1	Fruit	2	mango	I item
	Shake	2	whey protein shake	2 scoops
Meal 2	Bread	2	rice cakes	4 items
	Meat (Nut)	I	peanut butter	I tablespoon
Meal 3	Bread	1½	corn	¾ cup
	Meat	4	chicken	4 ounces
	Vegetable	I	summer squash	I cup
Meal 4	Bread	1½	pasta	1½ ounces
	Meat	2	chicken	2 ounces
Meal 5	Fruit	I	orange	I item
	Meat (Nut)	I	almonds	⅛ cup
Meal 6	Fruit	I	grapes	I cup
	Meat	2	egg	2 items
Meal 7	Bread	3	wild rice	I cup
	Meat	8	turkey	8 ounces
	Vegetable	2	mushrooms	4 cups

Week 10

	Category	Exchanges	Sample food	Quantity
Meal 1	Bread	1½	potato	¾ cup
	Fruit	I	orange	I item
	Meat	2	egg white	6 items
Meal 2	Fruit	I	banana	½ item
	Meat (Nut)	I	almond butter	I tablespoon
Meal 3	Bread	1½	tortilla	1½ items
	Meat	4	flank steak	4 ounces
	Vegetable	I	peppers	I cup

Meal 4	Bread	1½	white rice	½ cup
	Meat	2	tuna	4 ounces
Meal 5	Fruit	2	cherries	1 cup
	Meat (Nut)	1	cashews	⅛ cup
Meal 6	Bread	1½	winter squash	¾ cup
	Meat	8	turkey	8 ounces
	Vegetable	2	green beans	2 cups
Meal 7	Bread	1	popcorn	1 cup
	Fruit	1	kiwi	2 items

Week 11

	Category	Exchanges	Sample food	Quantity
Meal 1	Bread	3	bran flakes	1½ cups
	Fruit	1	blueberries	1 cup
	Meat	2	egg white	6 items
Meal 2	Fruit	1	pear	1 item
	Meat (Nut)	1	pecans	⅛ cup
Meal 3	Bread	1½	lentils	½ cup
	Meat	4	chicken	4 ounces
	Vegetable	2	carrots	1 cup
Meal 4	Bread	1½	corn tortilla	1½ items
	Meat	2	halibut	4 ounces
Meal 5	Fruit	2	apple	2 items
	Meat (Nut)	1	peanut butter	1 tablespoon
Meal 6	Bread	1½	brown rice	½ cup
	Meat	8	salmon	8 ounces
	Vegetable	3	asparagus	3 cups
Meal 7	Fruit	1	figs	1 large item

Week 12

	Category	Exchanges	Sample food	Quantity
Meal 1	Bread	3	corn grits	1½ cups
	Fruit	1	grapefruit	1 item
	Meat	2	egg	2 items
Meal 2	Fruit	1	banana	½ item
	Meat (Nut)	1	cashew butter	1 tablespoon
Meal 3	Bread	1½	split peas	½ cup
	Meat	4	chicken	4 ounces
	Vegetable	2	spinach	4 cups

Meal 4	Bread	1½	black beans	½ cup
	Vegetable	1	tomato	1 item
Meal 5	Fruit	2	apple	2 items
	Meat (Nut)	1	soynut butter	1 tablespoon
Meal 6	Bread	1½	sweet potato	½ item
	Meat	8	halibut	16 ounces
	Vegetable	3	broccoli	3 cups
Meal 7	Bread	1	popcorn	1 cup
	Fruit	2	tangerine	4 items

Level 9

Week 1

	Category	Exchanges	Sample food	Quantity
Meal 1	Bread	4	bagel	1⅓ large items
	Fruit	1	cantaloupe	½ item
	Meat	2	egg	2 items
Meal 2	Fruit	1	apple	1 item
	Meat (Nut)	1	peanut butter	1 tablespoon
Meal 3	Bread	3	pita	1½ items
	Meat	8	turkey	8 ounces
	Vegetable	1	romaine lettuce	3 cups
Meal 4	Fruit	1	plum	2 items
	Meat (Nut)	1	almonds	⅛ cup
Meal 5	Fruit	1	watermelon	1 cup
	Meat	2	turkey	2 ounces
Meal 6	Bread	3	baked potato	1 item
	Meat	8	salmon	8 ounces
	Vegetable	2	spinach	4 cups
Meal 7	Bread	2	popcorn	2 cups
	Fruit	2	pear	2 items

Week 2

	Category	Exchanges	Sample food	Quantity
Meal 1	Bread	4	oatmeal	2 cups
	Fruit	1	banana	½ item
	Meat	2	egg white	6 items
Meal 2	Fruit	1	peach	2 small items
	Meat (Nut)	1	cashews	⅛ cup
Meal 3	Bread	3	white rice	1 cup
	Meat	8	tuna	16 ounces
	Vegetable	1	tomato	1 item

Meal 4	Fruit	I	apple	I item
	Meat (Nut)	I	peanut butter	I tablespoon
Meal 5	Fruit	I	nectarine	I item
	Meat	2	turkey	2 ounces
Meal 6	Bread	3	corn	I½ cups
	Meat	8	chicken breast	8 ounces
	Vegetable	2	green beans	2 cups
Meal 7	Bread	2	whole wheat crackers	2 ounces
	Fruit	2	strawberries	3 cups

Week 3

	Category	Exchanges	Sample food	Quantity
Meal 1	Bread	4	bran flakes	2 cups
	Fruit	2	raspberries	2 cups
	Meat	2	egg	2 items
Meal 2	Fruit	I	watermelon	I cup
	Meat (Nut)	I	cashews	⅛ cup
Meal 3	Bread	3	white rice	I cup
	Meat	8	shrimp	16 ounces
	Vegetable	2	zucchini	2 cups
Meal 4	Fruit	I	apple	I item
	Meat (Nut)	I	almond butter	I tablespoon
Meal 5	Fruit	I	melon, honeydew	½ item
	Meat	2	tuna	4 ounces
Meal 6	Bread	3	tortilla	3 items
	Meat	8	flank steak	8 ounces
	Vegetable	2	peppers	2 cups
Meal 7	Bread	2	popcorn	2 cups
	Fruit	2	orange	2 items

Week 4

	Category	Exchanges	Sample food	Quantity
Meal 1	Bread	3	cream of wheat	I½ cups
	Fruit	2	grapefruit	2 items
Meal 2	Fruit	I	grapes	I cup
	Meat (Nut)	I	walnuts	⅛ cup
Meal 3	Bread	3	artichoke	3 items
	Meat	8	shrimp	16 ounces
	Vegetable	2	romaine lettuce	6 cups

Meal 4	Fruit	I	apricot	3 items
	Meat (Nut)	I	Brazil nuts	⅛ cup
Meal 5	Fruit	I	apple	I item
	Meat	2	tuna	4 ounces
Meal 6	Bread	3	couscous	I½ cups
	Meat	I0	chicken	I0 ounces
	Vegetable	2	tomato	2 items
Meal 7	Bread	2	rice cakes	4 items
	Fruit	2	papaya	I item

Week 5

	Category	Exchanges	Sample food	Quantity
Meal I	Bread	4	oatmeal	2 cups
	Fruit	2	blueberries	2 cups
Meal 2	Fruit	I	pear	I item
	Meat (Nut)	I	almonds	⅛ cup
Meal 3	Bread	I½	corn tortilla	I½ items
	Meat	4	chicken	4 ounces
	Vegetable	2	peppers	2 cups
Meal 4	Bread	I½	bulgur wheat	¾ cup
	Meat	4	chicken	4 ounces
	Vegetable	2	eggplant	2 cups
Meal 5	Fruit	2	banana	I item
	Meat (Nut)	I	peanut butter	I tablespoon
Meal 6	Bread	3	wild rice	I cup
	Meat	I0	whitefish	20 ounces
	Vegetable	2	spinach	4 cups
Meal 7	Bread	2	granola	¼ cup
	Fruit	2	grapes	2 cups

Week 6

	Category	Exchanges	Sample food	Quantity
Meal I	Bread	4	shredded wheat	4 large biscuits
	Fruit	2	strawberries	3 cups
Meal 2	Fruit	I	papaya	½ item
	Meat (Nut)	I	avocado	⅓ item
Meal 3	Bread	I½	artichoke	I½ items
	Meat	4	salmon	4 ounces
	Vegetable	2	asparagus	2 cups

Meal 4	Bread	1½	white rice	½ cup
	Meat	4	tuna	8 ounces
	Vegetable	2	cucumber	4 cups
Meal 5	Fruit	2	peach	4 small items
	Meat (Nut)	1	Brazil nuts	⅛ cup
Meal 6	Bread	3	pasta	3 ounces
	Meat	8	chicken	8 ounces
	Vegetable	2	broccoli	2 cups
Meal 7	Bread	1	whole wheat crackers	1 ounce
	Fruit	1	apricot	3 items

Week 7

	Category	Exchanges	Sample food	Quantity
Meal 1	Bread	4	cream of rice	2 cups
	Fruit	1	banana	½ item
Meal 2	Fruit	2	apple	2 items
	Meat (Nut)	1	peanut butter	1 tablespoon
Meal 3	Bread	1½	yams	½ cup
	Meat	4	catfish	4 ounces
	Vegetable	2	collards	4 cups
Meal 4	Bread	1½	corn	¾ cup
	Meat	4	turkey	4 ounces
	Vegetable	2	beets	1 cup
Meal 5	Fruit	2	apricot	6 items
	Meat (Nut)	1	almonds	⅛ cup
Meal 6	Bread	3	potato	1½ cups
	Meat	8	chicken	8 ounces
	Vegetable	2	romaine lettuce	6 cups
Meal 7	Bread	1	popcorn	1 cup
	Fruit	1	plum	2 items

Week 8

	Category	Exchanges	Sample food	Quantity
Meal 1	Bread	4	oatmeal	2 cups
	Fruit	1	orange	1 item
Meal 2	Fruit	2	banana	1 item
	Meat (Nut)	1	sesame butter	1 tablespoon
Meal 3	Bread	1½	garbanzo beans	⅜ cup
	Meat	4	chicken	4 ounces
	Vegetable	2	romaine lettuce	6 cups

Meal 4	Bread	1½	whole wheat crackers	1½ ounces
	Meat	4	tuna	8 ounces
	Vegetable	2	celery	4 cups
Meal 5	Fruit	2	apple	2 items
	Meat (Nut)	1	peanut butter	1 tablespoon
Meal 6	Bread	1½	green peas	¾ cup
	Meat	8	sirloin	8 ounces
	Vegetable	2	tomato	2 items
Meal 7	Bread	1½	couscous	¾ cup
	Fruit	1	mango	½ item

Week 9

	Category	Exchanges	Sample food	Quantity
Meal 1	Bread	1	granola	⅛ cup
	Fruit	2	blueberries	2 cups
	Shake	2	whey protein shake	2 scoops
Meal 2	Fruit	2	cherries	1 cup
	Meat (Nut)	1	cashews	⅛ cup
Meal 3	Bread	1½	brown rice	½ cup
	Meat	4	chicken	4 ounces
	Vegetable	2	summer squash	2 cups
Meal 4	Bread	1½	kidney beans	½ cup
	Meat	4	tuna	8 ounces
	Vegetable	2	romaine lettuce	6 cups
Meal 5	Fruit	2	avocado	⅔ item
	Meat (Nut)	1	papaya	½ item
Meal 6	Bread	1½	wild rice	½ cup
	Meat	8	turkey	8 ounces
	Vegetable	3	mushrooms	6 cups
Meal 7	Bread	1	popcorn	1 cup
	Fruit	1	grapes	1 cup

Week 10

	Category	Exchanges	Sample food	Quantity
Meal 1	Fruit	2	mango	1 item
	Shake	2	whey protein shake	2 scoops
Meal 2	Fruit	2	banana	1 item
	Meat (Nut)	1	almond butter	1 tablespoon
Meal 3	Bread	1½	tortilla	1½ items
	Meat	4	flank steak	4 ounces
	Vegetable	2	peppers	2 cups

Meal 4	Bread	1½	rice cakes	3 items
	Meat	4	tuna	8 ounces
	Vegetable	2	tomato	2 items
Meal 5	Fruit	2	nectarine	2 items
	Meat (Nut)	2	almonds	¼ cup
Meal 6	Bread	1½	yams	½ cup
	Meat	8	turkey	8 ounces
	Vegetable	2	green beans	2 cups
Meal 7	Fruit	1	papaya	½ item

Week 11

	Category	Exchanges	Sample food	Quantity
Meal 1	Bread	3	Grapenuts	¾ cup
	Fruit	1	banana	½ item
	Meat	2	egg	2 items
Meal 2	Fruit	1	apple	1 item
	Meat (Nut)	1	almond butter	1 tablespoon
Meal 3	Bread	1½	lentils	½ cup
	Meat	4	chicken	4 ounces
	Vegetable	2	carrots	1 cup
Meal 4	Bread	1½	potato	¾ cup
	Meat	4	tuna	8 ounces
	Vegetable	2	peppers	2 cups
Meal 5	Fruit	2	melon, honeydew	⅓ item
	Meat (Nut)	2	cashews	¼ cup
Meal 6	Bread	1½	brown rice	½ cup
	Meat	8	salmon	8 ounces
	Vegetable	2	asparagus	2 cups
Meal 7	Fruit	1	pear	1 item

Week 12

	Category	Exchanges	Sample food	Quantity
Meal 1	Bread	3	bran flakes	1½ cups
	Fruit	1	blueberries	1 cup
	Meat	2	egg white	6 items
Meal 2	Fruit	1	apple	1 item
	Meat (Nut)	1	peanut butter	1 tablespoon
Meal 3	Bread	1½	split peas	½ cup
	Meat	4	chicken	4 ounces
	Vegetable	2	spinach	4 cups

Meal 4	Bread	1½	corn	¾ cup
	Meat	4	turkey	4 ounces
	Vegetable	2	Brussels sprouts	2 cups
Meal 5	Fruit	2	pear	2 items
	Meat (Nut)	2	walnuts	¼ cup
Meal 6	Bread	1½	wild rice	½ cup
	Meat	8	halibut	16 ounces
	Vegetable	2	tomato	2 items
Meal 7	Bread	1	rice cakes	2 items
	Fruit	1	figs	1 large item

Level 10

Week 1

	Category	Exchanges	Sample food	Quantity
Meal 1	Bread	4	bagel	1⅓ large items
	Fruit	1	cantaloupe	½ item
	Meat	3	egg	3 items
Meal 2	Fruit	1	apple	1 item
	Meat (Nut)	1	peanut butter	1 tablespoon
Meal 3	Bread	3	pita	1½ items
	Meat	8	turkey	8 ounces
	Vegetable	2	romaine lettuce	6 cups
Meal 4	Fruit	1	plum	2 items
	Meat (Nut)	1	almonds	⅛ cup
Meal 5	Fruit	1	mango	½ item
	Meat	2	turkey	2 ounces
Meal 6	Bread	4	baked potato	1⅓ items
	Meat	8	salmon	8 ounces
	Vegetable	3	spinach	6 cups
Meal 7	Bread	2	popcorn	2 cups
	Fruit	2	pear	2 items

Week 2

	Category	Exchanges	Sample food	Quantity
Meal 1	Bread	4	oatmeal	2 cups
	Fruit	1	banana	½ item
	Meat	3	egg white	9 items
Meal 2	Fruit	1	peach	2 small items
	Meat (Nut)	1	cashews	⅛ cup

Meal 3	Bread	3	white rice	1 cup
	Meat	8	tuna	16 ounces
	Vegetable	2	tomato	2 items
Meal 4	Fruit	1	apple	1 item
	Meat (Nut)	1	peanut butter	1 tablespoon
Meal 5	Fruit	1	nectarine	1 item
	Meat	2	turkey	2 ounces
Meal 6	Bread	4	corn	2 cups
	Meat	8	chicken breast	8 ounces
	Vegetable	3	green beans	3 cups
Meal 7	Bread	2	whole wheat crackers	2 ounces
	Fruit	2	strawberries	3 cups

Week 3

	Category	Exchanges	Sample food	Quantity
Meal 1	Bread	4	bran flakes	2 cups
	Fruit	1	raspberries	1 cup
	Meat	3	egg	3 items
Meal 2	Fruit	1	watermelon	1 cup
	Meat (Nut)	1	Brazil nuts	⅛ cup
Meal 3	Bread	3	white rice	1 cup
	Meat	8	shrimp	16 ounces
	Vegetable	1	zucchini	1 cup
Meal 4	Fruit	1	apple	1 item
	Meat (Nut)	1	almond butter	1 tablespoon
Meal 5	Fruit	1	pear	1 item
	Meat	4	tuna	8 ounces
Meal 6	Bread	3	tortilla	3 items
	Meat	8	flank steak	8 ounces
	Vegetable	3	peppers	3 cups
Meal 7	Bread	2	popcorn	2 cups
	Fruit	2	orange	2 items

Week 4

	Category	Exchanges	Sample food	Quantity
Meal 1	Bread	4	cream of wheat	2 cups
	Fruit	1	grapefruit	1 item
	Meat	4	egg white	12 items

Meal 2	Fruit	I	grapes	I cup
	Meat (Nut)	I	walnuts	⅛ cup
Meal 3	Bread	3	couscous	I ½ cups
	Meat	8	chicken	8 ounces
	Vegetable	2	tomato	2 items
Meal 4	Fruit	I	apricot	3 items
	Meat (Nut)	I	Brazil nuts	⅛ cup
Meal 5	Fruit	I	melon, cantaloupe	½ item
	Meat	2	tuna	4 ounces
Meal 6	Bread	3	potato, baked	I item
	Meat	8	salmon	8 ounces
	Vegetable	3	asparagus	3 cups
Meal 7	Bread	2	popcorn	2 cups
	Fruit	2	papaya	I item

Week 5

	Category	Exchanges	Sample food	Quantity
Meal I	Bread	4	oatmeal	2 cups
	Fruit	2	blueberries	2 cups
	Meat	2	egg	2 items
Meal 2	Fruit	I	pear	I item
	Meat (Nut)	I	almonds	⅛ cup
Meal 3	Bread	3	corn tortilla	3 items
	Meat	8	chicken	8 ounces
	Vegetable	2	peppers	2 cups
Meal 4	Fruit	I	apple	I item
	Meat (Nut)	I	peanut butter	I tablespoon
Meal 5	Fruit	I	cranberries	I cup
	Meat	2	turkey	2 ounces
Meal 6	Bread	3	wild rice	I cup
	Meat	8	whitefish	16 ounces
	Vegetable	3	spinach	6 cups
Meal 7	Bread	I	rice cakes	2 items
	Fruit	2	pear	2 items

Week 6

	Category	Exchanges	Sample food	Quantity
Meal I	Bread	4	shredded wheat	4 large biscuits
	Fruit	2	strawberries	3 cups
	Meat	2	egg white	6 items

Meal 2	Fruit	I	papaya	½ item
	Meat (Nut)	I	avocado	⅓ item
Meal 3	Bread	3	artichoke	3 items
	Meat	4	salmon	4 ounces
	Vegetable	2	spinach	4 cups
Meal 4	Bread	I½	whole wheat crackers	I½ ounces
	Meat	4	tuna	8 ounces
	Vegetable	2	celery	4 cups
Meal 5	Fruit	I	tangerine	2 items
	Meat (Nut)	I	Brazil nuts	⅛ cup
Meal 6	Bread	3	pasta	3 ounces
	Meat	8	chicken	8 ounces
	Vegetable	3	broccoli	3 cups
Meal 7	Bread	I	popcorn	I cup
	Fruit	2	plum	4 items

Week 7

	Category	Exchanges	Sample food	Quantity
Meal I	Bread	4	cream of rice	2 cups
	Meat	2	egg	2 items
Meal 2	Fruit	2	banana	I item
	Meat (Nut)	2	peanut butter	2 tablespoons
Meal 3	Bread	3	yams	I cup
	Meat	4	catfish	4 ounces
	Vegetable	2	collards	4 cups
Meal 4	Bread	I½	green peas	¾ cup
	Meat	4	turkey	4 ounces
	Vegetable	2	tomato	2 items
Meal 5	Fruit	I	tangerine	2 items
	Meat (Nut)	I	almonds	⅛ cup
Meal 6	Bread	3	corn	I½ cups
	Meat	8	chicken	8 ounces
	Vegetable	2	romaine lettuce	6 cups
Meal 7	Bread	I	brown rice	⅓ cup
	Fruit	I	pineapple	I cup

Week 8

	Category	Exchanges	Sample food	Quantity
Meal I	Bread	4	potato	2 cups
	Meat	2	egg white	6 items

Meal 2	Fruit	2	apple	2 items
	Meat (Nut)	2	peanut butter	2 tablespoons
Meal 3	Bread	3	garbanzo beans	¾ cup
	Meat	8	chicken	8 ounces
	Vegetable	2	romaine lettuce	6 cups
Meal 4	Bread	1½	rice	½ cup
	Meat	2	tuna	4 ounces
	Vegetable	1	cucumber	2 cups
Meal 5	Fruit	2	mango	1 item
	Meat (Nut)	1	avocado	⅓ item
Meal 6	Bread	1½	winter squash	¾ cup
	Meat	8	sirloin	8 ounces
	Vegetable	1	tomato	1 item
Meal 7	Bread	1	popcorn	1 cup
	Fruit	1	grapes	1 cup

Week 9

	Category	Exchanges	Sample food	Quantity
Meal 1	Bread	1	granola	⅛ cup
	Fruit	2	mango	1 item
	Shake	2	whey protein shake	2 scoops
Meal 2	Fruit	2	cherries	1 cup
	Meat (Nut)	2	cashews	¼ cup
Meal 3	Bread	1½	pasta	1½ ounces
	Meat	4	chicken	4 ounces
	Vegetable	2	tomato	2 items
Meal 4	Bread	1½	artichoke	1½ items
	Meat	4	tuna	8 ounces
	Vegetable	2	romaine lettuce	6 cups
Meal 5	Fruit	1	banana	½ item
	Meat (Nut)	1	peanut butter	1 tablespoon
Meal 6	Bread	1½	split peas	½ cup
	Meat	8	turkey	8 ounces
	Vegetable	3	mushrooms	6 cups
Meal 7	Bread	1	popcorn	1 cup
	Fruit	1	strawberries	1½ cups

Week 10

	Category	Exchanges	Sample food	Quantity
Meal 1	Fruit	2	banana	1 item
	Shake	2	whey protein shake	2 scoops

Meal 2	Fruit	2	apple	2 items
	Meat (Nut)	2	almond butter	2 tablespoons
Meal 3	Bread	1½	tortilla	1½ items
	Meat	8	flank steak	8 ounces
	Vegetable	2	peppers	2 cups
Meal 4	Bread	1½	garbanzo beans	⅜ cup
	Vegetable	2	cucumbers	4 cups
Meal 5	Fruit	1	pear	1 item
	Meat (Nut)	1	walnuts	⅛ cup
Meal 6	Bread	1½	corn	¾ cup
	Meat	8	snapper	16 ounces
	Vegetable	3	green beans	3 cups
Meal 7	Bread	1	rice cakes	2 items
	Fruit	1	peach	2 small items

Week 11

	Category	Exchanges	Sample food	Quantity
Meal 1	Bread	1	oatmeal	½ cup
	Fruit	2	blueberries	2 cups
	Shake	2	whey protein shake	2 scoops
Meal 2	Fruit	2	cantaloupe	1 item
	Meat (Nut)	2	almonds	¼ cup
Meal 3	Bread	1½	lentils	½ cup
	Meat	6	chicken	6 ounces
	Vegetable	2	carrots	1 cup
Meal 4	Bread	1½	whole wheat crackers	1½ ounces
	Meat	2	tuna	4 ounces
	Vegetable	2	celery	4 cups
Meal 5	Fruit	1	apple	1 item
	Meat (Nut)	1	peanut butter	1 tablespoon
Meal 6	Bread	1½	wild rice	½ cup
	Meat	8	salmon	8 ounces
	Vegetable	3	asparagus	3 cups
Meal 7	Fruit	1	pineapple	1 cup

Week 12

	Category	Exchanges	Sample food	Quantity
Meal 1	Bread	4	bran flakes	2 cups
	Fruit	1	melon, honeydew	⅙ item
	Meat	3	egg white	9 items

Meal 2	Fruit	2	banana	I item
	Meat (Nut)	2	peanut butter	2 tablespoons
Meal 3	Bread	I ½	split peas	½ cup
	Meat	8	chicken	8 ounces
	Vegetable	2	spinach	4 cups
Meal 4	Bread	I ½	potato, baked	½ item
	Meat	2	turkey	2 ounces
	Vegetable	2	tomato	2 items
Meal 5	Fruit	I	apple	I item
	Meat (Nut)	I	soynut butter	I tablespoon
Meal 6	Bread	I ½	couscous	¾ cup
	Meat	8	halibut	16 ounces
	Vegetable	3	Brussels sprouts	3 cups
Meal 7	Bread	I	popcorn	I cup
	Fruit	I	figs	I large item

Level 11

Week I	Category	Exchanges	Sample food	Quantity
Meal I	Bread	4	bagel	I ⅓ large items
	Fruit	2	cantaloupe	I item
	Meat	3	egg	3 items
Meal 2	Fruit	I	apple	I item
	Meat (Nut)	I	peanut butter	I tablespoon
Meal 3	Bread	3	pita	I ½ items
	Meat	8	turkey	8 ounces
	Vegetable	2	romaine lettuce	6 cups
Meal 4	Fruit	I	plum	2 items
	Meat (Nut)	I	almonds	⅛ cup
Meal 5	Fruit	I	watermelon	I cup
	Meat	4	turkey	4 ounces
Meal 6	Bread	4	baked potato	I ⅓ items
	Meat	8	salmon	8 ounces
	Vegetable	3	spinach	6 cups
Meal 7	Bread	2	popcorn	2 cups
	Fruit	2	pear	2 items

Week 2

Category	Exchanges	Sample food	Quantity
Meal 1			
Bread	4	oatmeal	2 cups
Fruit	2	banana	1 item
Meat	3	egg white	9 items
Meal 2			
Fruit	1	peach	2 small items
Meat (Nut)	1	cashews	⅛ cup
Meal 3			
Bread	3	white rice	1 cup
Meat	8	tuna	16 ounces
Vegetable	2	tomato	2 items
Meal 4			
Fruit	1	apple	1 item
Meat (Nut)	1	peanut butter	1 tablespoon
Meal 5			
Fruit	1	nectarine	1 item
Meat	4	turkey	4 ounces
Meal 6			
Bread	4	corn	2 cups
Meat	8	chicken breast	8 ounces
Vegetable	3	green beans	3 cups
Meal 7			
Bread	2	whole wheat crackers	2 ounces
Fruit	2	strawberries	3 cups

Week 3

Category	Exchanges	Sample food	Quantity
Meal 1			
Bread	4	bran flakes	2 cups
Fruit	2	raspberries	2 cups
Meat	3	egg	3 items
Meal 2			
Bread	3	sweet potato	1 item
Meal 3			
Bread	3	white rice	1 cup
Meat	8	shrimp	16 ounces
Vegetable	2	zucchini	2 cups
Meal 4			
Fruit	1	apple	1 item
Meat (Nut)	1	cashews	⅛ cup
Meal 5			
Fruit	1	pear	1 item
Meat	4	tuna	8 ounces
Meal 6			
Bread	3	tortilla	3 items
Meat	8	flank steak	8 ounces
Vegetable	3	peppers	3 cups
Meal 7			
Bread	2	popcorn	2 cups
Fruit	2	orange	2 items

Week 4

Category	Exchanges	Sample food	Quantity
Meal 1			
Bread	4	cream of wheat	2 cups
Fruit	2	grapefruit	2 items
Meat	3	egg white	9 items
Meal 2			
Bread	3	potato, baked	1 item
Meal 3			
Bread	1½	couscous	¾ cup
Meat	8	chicken	8 ounces
Vegetable	2	tomato	2 items
Meal 4			
Bread	1½	garbanzo beans	⅜ cup
Vegetable	1	cucumber	2 cups
Meal 5			
Fruit	2	apricot	6 items
Meat (Nut)	2	Brazil nuts	¼ cup
Meal 6			
Bread	3	wild rice	1 cup
Meat	8	salmon	8 ounces
Vegetable	3	asparagus	3 cups
Meal 7			
Bread	2	papaya	1 item
Fruit	2	rice cakes	4 items

Week 5

Category	Exchanges	Sample food	Quantity
Meal 1			
Bread	4	oatmeal	2 cups
Fruit	2	blueberries	2 cups
Meat	2	egg	2 items
Meal 2			
Fruit	1	pear	1 item
Meat (Nut)	1	almonds	⅛ cup
Meal 3			
Bread	1½	corn tortilla	1½ items
Meat	8	chicken	8 ounces
Vegetable	2	peppers	2 cups
Meal 4			
Bread	1½	winter squash	¾ cup
Meat	4	turkey	4 ounces
Vegetable	1	eggplant	1 cup
Meal 5			
Fruit	2	banana	1 item
Meat (Nut)	2	peanut butter	2 tablespoons
Meal 6			
Bread	3	brown rice	1 cup
Meat	8	whitefish	16 ounces
Vegetable	3	spinach	6 cups
Meal 7			
Bread	1	granola	⅛ cup
Fruit	2	pear	2 items

Week 6

Category	Exchanges	Sample food	Quantity
Meal 1			
Bread	4	shredded wheat	4 large biscuits
Fruit	2	strawberries	3 cups
Meat	1	egg white	3 items
Meal 2			
Fruit	1	papaya	½ item
Meat	2	chicken	2 ounces
Meal 3			
Bread	1½	artichoke	1½ items
Meat	8	salmon	8 ounces
Vegetable	3	spinach	6 cups
Meal 4			
Bread	1½	rice cakes	3 items
Meat	4	tuna	8 ounces
Vegetable	2	celery	4 cups
Meal 5			
Fruit	2	apricot	6 items
Meat (Nut)	2	Brazil nuts	¼ cup
Meal 6			
Bread	1½	pasta	1½ ounces
Meat	8	chicken	8 ounces
Vegetable	3	broccoli	3 cups
Meal 7			
Bread	2	popcorn	2 cups
Fruit	2	plum	4 items

Week 7

Category	Exchanges	Sample food	Quantity
Meal 1			
Bread	4	cream of rice	2 cups
Fruit	2	banana	1 item
Meat	1	egg	1 item
Meal 2			
Fruit	1	apple	1 item
Meat	2	tuna	4 ounces
Meal 3			
Bread	1½	yams	½ cup
Meat	8	catfish	8 ounces
Vegetable	1	collards	2 cups
Meal 4			
Bread	1½	lentils	½ cup
Meat	4	turkey	4 ounces
Vegetable	1	tomato	1 item
Meal 5			
Fruit	2	grapes	2 cups
Meat (Nut)	2	almonds	¼ cup
Meal 6			
Bread	3	black beans	1 cup
Meat	8	chicken	8 ounces
Vegetable	3	romaine lettuce	9 cups
Meal 7			
Fruit	2	applesauce	1 cup

Week 8

Category	Exchanges	Sample food	Quantity
Meal 1			
Bread	4	bran flakes	2 cups
Fruit	2	orange	2 items
Meat	1	egg white	3 items
Meal 2			
Fruit	1	papaya	½ item
Meat	2	chicken	2 ounces
Meal 3			
Bread	1½	garbanzo beans	⅜ cup
Meat	8	chicken	8 ounces
Vegetable	2	romaine lettuce	6 cups
Meal 4			
Bread	1½	corn tortilla	1½ items
Meat	4	pollack	8 ounces
Vegetable	1	cabbage	2 cups
Meal 5			
Bread	1½	black beans	½ cup
Vegetable	1	onions	½ cup
Meal 6			
Bread	3	potato, baked	1 item
Meat	12	sirloin	12 ounces
Vegetable	3	tomato	3 items
Meal 7			
Fruit	1	kiwi	2 items

Week 9

Category	Exchanges	Sample food	Quantity
Meal 1			
Fruit	2	mango	1 item
Shake	2	whey protein shake	2 scoops
Meal 2			
Bread	3	yams	1 cup
Meal 3			
Bread	1½	couscous	¾ cup
Meat	8	chicken	8 ounces
Vegetable	1	tomato	1 item
Meal 4			
Bread	1½	white rice	½ cup
Meat	4	crab	8 ounces
Vegetable	1	cucumber	2 cups
Meal 5			
Fruit	2	apple	2 items
Meat (Nut)	1	peanut butter	1 tablespoon
Meal 6			
Bread	1½	wild rice	½ cup
Meat	12	turkey	12 ounces
Vegetable	2	mushrooms	4 cups
Meal 7			
Bread	1	popcorn	1 cup
Fruit	1	strawberries	1½ cups

Week 10

	Category	Exchanges	Sample food	Quantity
Meal 1	Bread	4	oatmeal	2 cups
	Fruit	2	melon, cantaloupe	1 item
	Meat	2	egg	2 items
Meal 2	Fruit	1	pear	1 item
	Meat (Nut)	1	walnuts	⅛ cup
Meal 3	Bread	1½	tortilla	1½ items
	Meat	8	flank steak	8 ounces
	Vegetable	1	peppers	1 cup
Meal 4	Bread	1½	navy beans	½ cup
	Meat	4	tuna	8 ounces
	Vegetable	1	tomato	1 item
Meal 5	Fruit	2	apple	2 items
	Meat (Nut)	1	peanut butter	1 tablespoon
Meal 6	Bread	1½	corn	¾ cup
	Meat	8	turkey	8 ounces
	Vegetable	2	green beans	2 cups
Meal 7	Fruit	1	peach	2 small items

Week 11

	Category	Exchanges	Sample food	Quantity
Meal 1	Bread	3	corn grits	1½ cups
	Fruit	2	grapefruit	2 items
	Meat	2	egg	2 items
Meal 2	Fruit	1	banana	½ item
	Meat (Nut)	1	sesame butter	1 tablespoon
Meal 3	Bread	3	split peas	1 cup
	Meat	8	sea bass	16 ounces
	Vegetable	2	asparagus	2 cups
Meal 4	Bread	1½	brown rice	½ cup
	Meat	4	chicken	4 ounces
	Vegetable	1	spinach	2 cups
Meal 5	Fruit	2	orange	2 items
	Meat (Nut)	1	almonds	⅛ cup
Meal 6	Bread	1½	potato, baked	½ item
	Meat	12	halibut	24 ounces
	Vegetable	2	Brussels sprouts	2 cups
Meal 7	Bread	1	popcorn	1 cup
	Fruit	1	applesauce	½ cup

Week 12

	Category	Exchanges	Sample food	Quantity
Meal 1	Bread	4	oatmeal	2 cups
	Fruit	2	banana	1 item
	Meat	2	egg white	6 items
Meal 2	Fruit	1	soynut butter	1 tablespoon
	Meat (Nut)	1	apple	1 item
Meal 3	Bread	3	lentils	1 cup
	Meat	8	chicken	8 ounces
	Vegetable	2	carrots	1 cup
Meal 4	Bread	1½	pasta	1½ ounces
	Meat	4	ground beef	4 ounces
	Vegetable	1	tomato	1 item
Meal 5	Fruit	2	grapes	2 cups
	Meat (Nut)	1	pecans	⅛ cup
Meal 6	Bread	1½	wild rice	½ cup
	Meat	8	turkey	8 ounces
	Vegetable	3	cabbage	6 cups
Meal 7	Bread	1	whole wheat crackers	1 ounce
	Fruit	2	figs	2 large item

The Dual-Metabolism Food Program

12-Week Instructions and Meal Plans for Caloric Levels 1–11

Determine your level by choosing the caloric range closest to the caloric number determined by your metabolic scenario:

Level	Caloric Range of Level
1	Under 1,200
2	1,201–1,365
3	1,366–1,480
4	1,481–1,685
5	1,686–1,805
6	1,806–2,180
7	2,181–2,330
8	2,331–2,450
9	2,451–2,765
10	2,766–3,065
11	3,066 and up

Do not forget the option of adding items from the Free Foods List in appendix C to these meal plans. For example, when you are having oatmeal or cereal, you may add ½ cup nonfat milk; when you are having salad, you can add up to 2 tablespoons of low-fat dressing per day; when you have steamed vegetables, you are allowed 1 tablespoon of nondairy butter per day. Also, beverages such as tea, coffee, and diet soda may be added to your meals plans, but they *do not* count toward your daily water intake.

During certain weeks Meal 1 is listed as a Fruit 1 and a two-scoop whey protein shake. The whey shake is not mandatory for the program, but we have chosen to use the shake during some weeks because whey protein offers the highest, most biologically efficient form of protein. To make this shake you need to buy a zero carbohydrate whey shake either at your health food store or from my website, www.pfcnutrition.com. Make sure that one scoop equals between 70 to 85 calories. To make the shake, blend one serving of fruit, two scoops of whey protein powder, some ice, and water according to your desired consistency and drink this as your first meal. If you choose not to do the shake, then the whey portion of Meal 1 becomes a Meat 2, for example, two eggs.

■ Weekly Instructions for the Dual Metabolism (for All Levels)

Below are just a few things to keep in mind as you begin each week of your program, no matter what level you are using.

Week 1. In this first week, also known as your Foundation Food Program, you'll be laying the groundwork for the coming weeks of the program. This week we want you to get used to eating more times during the day, drinking more water, and getting to know your list of foods. If this week seems like a drastic change from your normal eating habits, do the best you can.

Week 2. You'll notice that the meal pattern this week is the same as last week. Your challenge this week, and from now on, is to eliminate from your diet the foods in the Bread subcategory from the larger Bread category. There are lots of great foods in the Bread category that are not what most people think of as "bread," so get to know and love these choices. For optimum results, eliminate, as best you can, all regular rising breads, including bagels, cakes, muffins, and bread. I know this may be a huge challenge, just do the best you can.

Week 3. Congratulations on your success last week! I hope you're getting used to cutting out those breads. This week, you'll be bumping up your percentage of protein and cutting back your carbohydrates just a little, bringing you closer to that even balance of protein, fat, and carb that your dual metabolism needs to function optimally. You'll probably notice only one or two changes in the menu. Keep up the good work and don't forget to drink that water.

Week 4—Reassessment Week. Great job last week! This week, you'll notice that you're moving toward fewer carbohydrates in the evening. Remember, your body needs those carbs during the day when you're active—not at night when you're sleeping. So do your best to stick with this week's plan. The other challenge is to go the whole week without eating *any* red meat. All your Meat category foods should consist of fish, poultry, eggs, and maybe a little soy.

Week 5. Fantastic! You've made it to Week 5, also known as "fish week." Eat fish for dinner every night this week. Any fish you like is fine, but try to enjoy as much fresh fish as you can. Experiment with a type of fish that you've never tried before. Try a new fish recipe you've been meaning to make. If you are allergic to seafood, have skinless chicken breast every night.

Week 6. Congratulations! You've made it to Week 6. You'll notice that we are slowly adding calories and adjusting your balance of carbohydrate and protein in your diet. Don't let yourself get bored—this week, try a new vegetable you've never tried before. You're doing great. How's the water intake?

Week 7. You've made it to lucky Week 7! You must be feeling fantastic by now. You're now at the point where you will be reducing the Bread exchanges in your nighttime meals. You'll be continuing this through Week 12, so you'd better get used to it. Remember, you need protein at night to rebuild your muscle, not carbohydrate. And be sure to keep eating all your meals in order.

Week 8—Reassessment Week. Week 8 is great! You should be getting really good at this by now, keep up the good work. No special instructions for you this week. Just enjoy your success. And we hope you are getting used to avoiding the bread "breads."

Week 9. Week 9! You're really cooking—just don't cook any red meat this week. If you liked Week 4, then you'll love Week 9, because it's another no-red-meat week. Stick with fish, poultry, and eggs in your Meat category. By choosing only low-fat protein sources, you will utilize your own fat stores for energy.

Week 10. Congratulations! You've made it through nine weeks of the Turn Up the Heat program. Right now, be thankful for your dual metabolism. For the other two metabolic types, Week 10 is fondly referred to as "Hell Week." You won't be tortured with nutritional hell because of your highly evolved metabolism. But that means you owe it to yourself to follow your program precisely. You can do it. And here's something to look forward to—a treat day is only six days away.

Week 11. Fantastic job! How do you feel? Since you don't have to go through any real form of nutritional hell, make a point of really following your food program this week and documenting how you feel in your journal. You're getting ready for some big changes, so follow Week 11.

Week 12. Congratulations—you did it! Eleven weeks, wow! Week 12 is the last menu before you start again. Do a good job this week and enjoy your treat day. After this week, you have a choice—you can either reassess your caloric level and continue your weight loss, or you can start your maintenance program. If you choose to continue your weight loss, you will reassess your caloric level and begin again with Week 1 (remember—you were even allowed to have bread back then!), moving down a level, maintaining your current level, or moving up a level, depending on your answers to the reassessment evaluation on page 76. Or, you may be happy with your weight loss and choose to stabilize your current weight and begin your maintenance program, at which point you would maintain the menu pattern for Week 12. Keep up the great work.

Dual-Metabolism Food Program

Level 1

Week 1

Meal	Category	Exchanges	Sample food	Quantity
Meal 1	Bread	2	bagel	⅔ item
	Fruit	1	cantaloupe	½ item
Meal 2	Fruit	1	apple	1 item
Meal 3	Bread	3	pita	1½ items
	Meat	2	turkey	2 ounces
	Vegetable	1	romaine lettuce	3 cups
Meal 4	Fruit	1	plum	2 items
Meal 5	Bread	1½	baked potato	½ item
	Meat	4	salmon	4 ounces
	Vegetable	2	spinach	4 cups
Meal 6	Fruit	1	pear	1 item

Week 2

Meal	Category	Exchanges	Sample food	Quantity
Meal 1	Bread	2	oatmeal	1 cup
	Fruit	1	banana	½ item
Meal 2	Fruit	1	peach	2 small items
Meal 3	Bread	3	white rice	1 cup
	Meat	2	tuna	2 ounces
	Vegetable	1	tomato	1 item
Meal 4	Fruit	1	grapes	1 cup
Meal 5	Bread	1½	corn	¾ cup
	Meat	4	chicken breast	4 ounces
	Vegetable	2	green beans	2 cups
Meal 6	Fruit	1	strawberries	1½ cups

Week 3

Meal	Category	Exchanges	Sample food	Quantity
Meal 1	Bread	2	bran flakes	1 cup
	Meat	1	egg	1 item
Meal 2	Fruit	1	watermelon	1 cup
Meal 3	Bread	3	white rice	1 cup
	Meat	2	shrimp	4 ounces
	Vegetable	1	zucchini	1 cup
Meal 4	Fruit	1	apple	1 item
	Meat (Nut)	1	peanut butter	1 tablespoon

Meal 5	Bread	1½	tortilla, flour	1½ items
	Meat	4	flank steak	4 ounces
	Vegetable	2	asparagus	2 cups
Meal 6	Fruit	1	orange	1 item

Week 4

	Category	Exchanges	Sample food	Quantity
Meal 1	Bread	2	cream of wheat	1 cup
	Meat	1	egg white	3 items
Meal 2	Fruit	1	grapes	1 cup
Meal 3	Bread	3	kidney beans	1 cup
	Meat	2	tuna	4 ounces
	Vegetable	1	romaine lettuce	3 cups
Meal 4	Fruit	1	banana	½ item
	Meat (Nut)	1	almond butter	1 tablespoon
Meal 5	Bread	1½	pasta	1½ ounces
	Meat	4	chicken	4 ounces
	Vegetable	2	peppers	2 cups
Meal 6	Fruit	1	papaya	½ item

Week 5

	Category	Exchanges	Sample food	Quantity
Meal 1	Bread	2	oatmeal	1 cup
	Meat	1	egg	1 item
Meal 2	Fruit	1	apple	1 item
Meal 3	Bread	1½	corn tortilla	1½ items
	Meat	4	chicken	4 ounces
	Vegetable	1	peppers	1 cup
Meal 4	Fruit	1	apricot	3 items
	Meat (Nut)	1	cashews	⅛ cup
Meal 5	Bread	1½	brown rice	½ cup
	Meat	4	whitefish	8 ounces
	Vegetable	2	spinach	4 cups

Week 6

	Category	Exchanges	Sample food	Quantity
Meal 1	Bread	2	shredded wheat	2 large biscuits
	Meat	1	egg white	3 items
Meal 2	Fruit	1	banana	½ item

Meal 3	Bread	1½	artichoke	1½ items
	Meat	2	salmon	2 ounces
	Vegetable	1	asparagus	1 cup
Meal 4	Bread	1½	garbanzo beans	⅜ cup
	Vegetable	1	tomato	1 item
Meal 5	Fruit	1	orange	1 item
Meal 6	Bread	1½	corn	¾ cup
	Meat	4	chicken	4 ounces
	Vegetable	1	broccoli	1 cup

Week 7

	Category	Exchanges	Sample food	Quantity
Meal 1	Bread	2	oatmeal	1 cup
	Meat	1	egg white	3 items
Meal 2	Fruit	1	blueberries	1 cup
Meal 3	Bread	1½	yams	½ cup
	Meat	4	catfish	4 ounces
	Vegetable	1	collards	2 cups
Meal 4	Bread	1½	white rice	½ cup
	Vegetable	1	onions	½ cup
Meal 5	Fruit	1	apple	1 item
	Meat (Nut)	1	cashew butter	1 tablespoon
Meal 6	Meat	4	chicken	4 ounces
	Vegetable	3	romaine lettuce	9 cups

Week 8

	Category	Exchanges	Sample food	Quantity
Meal 1	Bread	1	Grapenuts	¼ cup
	Fruit	1	strawberries	1½ cups
Meal 2	Meat	1	egg	1 item
Meal 3	Bread	1½	garbanzo beans	⅜ cup
	Meat	4	chicken	4 ounces
	Vegetable	1	romaine lettuce	3 cups
Meal 4	Bread	1½	popcorn	1½ cups
	Vegetable	1	jicama	½ cup
Meal 5	Fruit	1	banana	½ item
	Meat (Nut)	1	peanut butter	1 tablespoon
Meal 6	Meat	4	sirloin	4 ounces
	Vegetable	3	tomato	3 items

Week 9

Meal	Category	Exchanges	Sample food	Quantity
Meal 1	Bread	2	bran flakes	1 cup
	Fruit	1	banana	½ item
Meal 2	Meat	1	egg white	3 items
Meal 3	Bread	1½	potato	¾ cup
	Meat	2	tuna	4 ounces
	Vegetable	1	romaine lettuce	3 cups
Meal 4	Bread	1½	lentils	½ cup
	Meat	2	chicken	2 ounces
	Vegetable	1	tomato	1 item
Meal 5	Meat (Nut)	1	soynut butter	1 tablespoon
	Vegetable	1	celery	2 cups
Meal 6	Meat	4	turkey	4 ounces
	Vegetable	3	mushrooms	6 cups

Week 10

Meal	Category	Exchanges	Sample food	Quantity
Meal 1	Fruit	1	mango	½ item
	Shake	2	whey protein shake	2 scoops
Meal 2	Meat	1	egg white	3 items
Meal 3	Bread	1½	tortilla, corn	1½ items
	Meat	2	flank steak	2 ounces
	Vegetable	1	peppers	1 cup
Meal 4	Fruit	1	cherries	½ cup
Meal 5	Meat	2	turkey	2 ounces
	Vegetable	1	cucumber	2 cups
Meal 6	Meat	4	snapper	8 ounces
	Vegetable	3	Brussels sprouts	3 cups

Week 11

Meal	Category	Exchanges	Sample food	Quantity
Meal 1	Fruit	1	blueberries	1 cup
	Shake	2	whey protein shake	2 scoops
Meal 2	Fruit	1	apple	1 item
Meal 3	Bread	1½	tortilla, corn	1½ items
	Meat	4	halibut	8 ounces
	Vegetable	1	cabbage	2 cups
Meal 4	Bread	1½	pasta	1½ ounces
Meal 5	Meat (Nut)	1	peanut butter	1 tablespoon
	Vegetable	1	celery	2 cups
Meal 6	Meat	4	chicken	4 ounces
	Vegetable	2	green beans	2 cups

Week 12

	Category	Exchanges	Sample food	Quantity
Meal 1	Fruit	1	grapefruit	1 item
	Meat	2	egg	2 items
Meal 2	Fruit	1	pear	1 item
Meal 3	Bread	1½	lentil	½ cup
	Meat	2	chicken	2 ounces
	Vegetable	1	spinach	2 cups
Meal 4	Fruit	1	banana	½ item
Meal 5	Meat (Nut)	1	avocado	⅓ item
	Vegetable	1	romaine lettuce	3 cups
Meal 6	Meat	4	salmon	4 ounces
	Vegetable	3	summer squash	3 cups

Level 2

Week 1

	Category	Exchanges	Sample food	Quantity
Meal 1	Bread	2	bagel	⅔ item
	Fruit	1	cantaloupe	½ item
Meal 2	Fruit	1	apple	1 item
Meal 3	Bread	3	pita	1½ items
	Meat	4	turkey	4 ounces
	Vegetable	1	romaine lettuce	3 cups
Meal 4	Fruit	1	plum	2 items
Meal 5	Bread	1½	baked potato	½ item
	Meat	4	salmon	4 ounces
	Vegetable	2	spinach	4 cups
Meal 6	Fruit	1	pear	1 item

Week 2

	Category	Exchanges	Sample food	Quantity
Meal 1	Bread	2	oatmeal	1 cup
	Fruit	1	banana	½ item
Meal 2	Fruit	1	peach	2 small items
Meal 3	Bread	3	white rice	1 cup
	Meat	4	tuna	8 ounces
	Vegetable	1	tomato	1 item
Meal 4	Fruit	1	grapes	1 cup
Meal 5	Bread	1½	corn	¾ cup
	Meat	4	chicken breast	4 ounces
	Vegetable	2	green beans	2 cups
Meal 6	Fruit	1	strawberries	1½ cups

Week 3

Category	Exchanges	Sample food	Quantity
Meal 1			
Bread	2	bran flakes	1 cup
Fruit	1	raspberries	1 cup
Meat	1	egg	1 item
Meal 2			
Fruit	1	watermelon	1 cup
Meal 3			
Bread	3	white rice	1 cup
Meat	4	shrimp	8 ounces
Vegetable	1	zucchini	1 cup
Meal 4			
Fruit	1	apple	1 item
Meal 5			
Bread	1½	tortilla	1½ items
Meat	4	flank steak	4 ounces
Vegetable	2	peppers	2 cups
Meal 6			
Fruit	1	orange	1 item

Week 4

Category	Exchanges	Sample food	Quantity
Meal 1			
Bread	2	cream of wheat	1 cup
Fruit	1	grapefruit	1 item
Meat	1	egg white	3 items
Meal 2			
Fruit	1	grapes	1 cup
Meal 3			
Bread	3	kidney beans	1 cup
Meat	4	tuna	8 ounces
Vegetable	1	romaine lettuce	3 cups
Meal 4			
Fruit	1	apricot	3 items
Meal 5			
Meat	4	chicken	4 ounces
Vegetable	2	tomato	2 items
Meal 6			
Bread	1	popcorn	1 cup
Fruit	1	tangerine	2 items

Week 5

Category	Exchanges	Sample food	Quantity
Meal 1			
Bread	2	oatmeal	1 cup
Fruit	1	blueberries	1 cup
Meat	1	egg	1 item
Meal 2			
Fruit	1	pear	1 item
Meal 3			
Bread	3	corn tortilla	3 items
Meat	4	chicken	4 ounces
Vegetable	1	peppers	1 cup
Meal 4			
Fruit	1	apple	1 item

Meal 5	Meat	6	whitefish	12 ounces
	Vegetable	3	spinach	6 cups
Meal 6	Bread	I	rice cakes	2 items
	Fruit	I	applesauce	½ cup

Week 6

	Category	Exchanges	Sample food	Quantity
Meal I	Bread	2	shredded wheat	2 large biscuits
	Fruit	I	strawberries	I ½ cups
	Meat	I	egg white	3 items
Meal 2	Fruit	I	pineapple	I cup
Meal 3	Bread	I ½	artichoke	I ½ items
	Meat	4	salmon	4 ounces
	Vegetable	I	asparagus	I cup
Meal 4	Fruit	I	apple	I item
	Meat (Nut)	I	peanut butter	I tablespoon
Meal 5	Meat	6	chicken	6 ounces
	Vegetable	3	broccoli	3 cups
Meal 6	Bread	I	popcorn	I cup
	Fruit	I	papaya	½ item

Week 7

	Category	Exchanges	Sample food	Quantity
Meal I	Bread	2	bran flakes	I cup
	Fruit	I	blueberries	I cup
	Meat	I	egg	I item
Meal 2	Fruit	I	mango	½ item
Meal 3	Bread	I ½	yams	½ cup
	Meat	4	catfish	4 ounces
	Vegetable	I	collards	2 cups
Meal 4	Fruit	I	banana	½ item
	Meat (Nut)	I	almond butter	I tablespoon
Meal 5	Bread	I ½	potato, baked	½ item
	Meat	6	chicken	6 ounces
	Vegetable	3	romaine lettuce	9 cups

Week 8

	Category	Exchanges	Sample food	Quantity
Meal I	Bread	2	oatmeal	I cup
	Fruit	I	raspberries	I cup
	Meat	I	egg	I item
Meal 2	Fruit	I	banana	½ item

Meal 3	Bread	1½	garbanzo beans	⅜ cup
	Meat	4	chicken	4 ounces
	Vegetable	1	romaine lettuce	3 cups
Meal 4	Bread	1½	white rice	½ cup
	Meat	2	tuna	4 ounces
Meal 5	Fruit	1	apple	1 item
Meal 6	Meat	6	sirloin	6 ounces
	Vegetable	3	tomato	3 items

Week 9

	Category	Exchanges	Sample food	Quantity
Meal 1	Bread	2	cream of rice	1 cup
	Fruit	1	melon, honeydew	⅛ item
	Meat	1	egg	1 item
Meal 2	Fruit	1	grapes	1 cup
Meal 3	Bread	1½	split peas	½ cup
	Meat	4	tuna	8 ounces
	Vegetable	1	romaine lettuce	3 cups
Meal 4	Fruit	1	pear	1 item
	Meat (Nut)	1	pecans	⅛ cup
Meal 5	Meat	2	turkey	2 ounces
Meal 6	Meat	4	turkey	4 ounces
	Vegetable	3	mushrooms	6 cups

Week 10

	Category	Exchanges	Sample food	Quantity
Meal 1	Fruit	1	banana	½ item
	Shake	2	whey protein shake	2 scoops
Meal 2	Fruit	1	nectarine	1 item
Meal 3	Bread	1½	tortilla, flour	1½ items
	Meat	4	flank steak	4 ounces
	Vegetable	1	peppers	1 cup
Meal 4	Fruit	1	apple	1 item
	Meat (Nut)	1	peanut butter	1 tablespoon
Meal 5	Meat	2	turkey	2 ounces
Meal 6	Meat	4	snapper	8 ounces
	Vegetable	3	Brussels sprouts	3 cups

Week 11

	Category	Exchanges	Sample food	Quantity
Meal 1	Fruit	1	mango	½ item
	Shake	2	whey protein shake	2 scoops
Meal 2	Fruit	1	cherries	½ cup

	Category	Exchanges	Sample food	Quantity
Meal 3	Bread	1½	tortilla, corn	1½ items
	Meat	4	halibut	8 ounces
	Vegetable	1	cabbage	2 cups
Meal 4	Fruit	1	banana	½ item
	Meat (Nut)	1	soynut butter	1 tablespoon
Meal 5	Meat	2	tuna	4 ounces
Meal 6	Bread	1½	wild rice	½ cup
	Meat	4	chicken	4 ounces
	Vegetable	3	green beans	3 cups

Week 12

	Category	Exchanges	Sample food	Quantity
Meal 1	Fruit	1	blueberries	1 cup
	Meat	2	egg	2 items
Meal 2	Fruit	1	pear	1 item
Meal 3	Bread	1½	lentil	½ cup
	Meat	4	chicken	4 ounces
	Vegetable	1	spinach	2 cups
Meal 4	Fruit	1	papaya	½ item
	Meat (Nut)	1	avocado	⅓ item
Meal 5	Meat	2	turkey	2 ounces
Meal 6	Meat	4	salmon	4 ounces
	Vegetable	3	spinach	6 cups
Meal 7	Fruit	1	grapes	1 cup

Level 3

Week 1

	Category	Exchanges	Sample food	Quantity
Meal 1	Bread	2	bagel	⅔ item
	Fruit	1	cantaloupe	½ item
Meal 2	Fruit	1	apple	1 item
Meal 3	Bread	3	pita	1½ items
	Meat	4	turkey	4 ounces
	Vegetable	1	romaine lettuce	3 cups
Meal 4	Fruit	1	plum	2 items
Meal 5	Bread	3	baked potato	1 item
	Meat	4	salmon	4 ounces
	Vegetable	2	spinach	4 cups
Meal 6	Fruit	1	pear	1 item

Week 2

	Category	Exchanges	Sample food	Quantity
Meal 1	Bread	2	oatmeal	1 cup
	Fruit	1	banana	½ item
Meal 2	Fruit	1	peach	2 small items
Meal 3	Bread	3	white rice	1 cup
	Meat	4	tuna	8 ounces
	Vegetable	1	tomato	1 item
Meal 4	Fruit	1	grapes	1 cup
Meal 5	Bread	3	corn	1½ cups
	Meat	4	chicken breast	4 ounces
	Vegetable	2	green beans	2 cups
Meal 6	Fruit	1	strawberries	1½ cups

Week 3

	Category	Exchanges	Sample food	Quantity
Meal 1	Bread	2	bran flakes	1 cup
	Fruit	1	raspberries	1 cup
Meal 2	Fruit	1	watermelon	1 cup
Meal 3	Bread	3	white rice	1 cup
	Meat	4	shrimp	8 ounces
	Vegetable	2	zucchini	2 cups
Meal 4	Fruit	1	apple	1 item
	Meat (Nut)	1	peanut butter	1 tablespoon
Meal 5	Bread	1½	tortilla	1½ items
	Meat	4	flank steak	4 ounces
	Vegetable	2	peppers	2 cups
Meal 6	Fruit	1	orange	1 item

Week 4

	Category	Exchanges	Sample food	Quantity
Meal 1	Bread	2	cream of wheat	1 cup
	Fruit	1	grapefruit	1 item
	Meat	1	egg	1 item
Meal 2	Fruit	1	grapes	1 cup
Meal 3	Bread	3	kidney beans	1 cup
	Meat	4	tuna	8 ounces
	Vegetable	1	romaine lettuce	3 cups
Meal 4	Fruit	1	apricot	3 items
	Meat (Nut)	1	cashews	⅛ cup

Meal 5	Bread	1½	couscous	¾ cup
	Meat	4	chicken	4 ounces
	Vegetable	2	tomato	2 items
Meal 6	Fruit	1	pear	1 item

Week 5

	Category	Exchanges	Sample food	Quantity
Meal 1	Bread	2	oatmeal	1 cup
	Fruit	1	blueberries	1 cup
	Meat	1	egg	1 item
Meal 2	Fruit	1	pear	1 item
	Meat (Nut)	1	walnuts	⅛ cup
Meal 3	Bread	3	corn tortilla	3 items
	Meat	4	chicken	4 ounces
	Vegetable	1	peppers	1 cup
Meal 4	Meat (Nut)	1	peanut butter	1 tablespoon
	Vegetable	1	celery	2 cups
Meal 5	Meat	4	whitefish	8 ounces
	Vegetable	3	spinach	6 cups
Meal 6	Bread	1	popcorn	1 cup
	Fruit	1	peach	2 small items

Week 6

	Category	Exchanges	Sample food	Quantity
Meal 1	Bread	2	shredded wheat	2 large biscuits
	Fruit	1	strawberries	1½ cups
	Meat	1	egg white	3 items
Meal 2	Fruit	1	pineapple	1 cup
	Meat (Nut)	1	almonds	⅛ cup
Meal 3	Bread	1½	artichoke	1½ items
	Meat	4	salmon	4 ounces
	Vegetable	1	asparagus	1 cup
Meal 4	Bread	1½	garbanzo beans	⅜ cup
	Vegetable	1	cucumber	2 cups
Meal 5	Fruit	1	orange	1 item
	Meat (Nut)	1	Brazil nuts	⅛ cup
Meal 6	Bread	1½	potato, baked	½ item
	Meat	4	chicken	4 ounces
	Vegetable	2	broccoli	2 cups
Meal 7	Fruit	1	papaya	½ item

Week 7

	Category	Exchanges	Sample food	Quantity
Meal 1	Bread	2	oatmeal	1 cup
	Fruit	1	blueberries	1 cup
	Meat	1	egg	1 item
Meal 2	Fruit	1	apple	1 item
	Meat (Nut)	1	peanut butter	1 tablespoon
Meal 3	Bread	1½	yams	½ cup
	Meat	4	catfish	4 ounces
	Vegetable	2	collards	4 cups
Meal 4	Bread	1½	brown rice	½ cup
	Vegetable	1	carrot	½ cup
Meal 5	Meat (Nut)	1	almond butter	1 tablespoon
	Vegetable	1	celery	2 cups
Meal 6	Bread	1½	split peas	½ cup
	Meat	4	chicken	4 ounces
	Vegetable	2	romaine lettuce	6 cups
Meal 7	Fruit	1	strawberries	1½ cups

Week 8

	Category	Exchanges	Sample food	Quantity
Meal 1	Bread	2	tortilla, flour	2 items
	Fruit	1	orange	1 item
	Meat	2	egg white	6 items
Meal 2	Fruit	1	banana	½ item
Meal 3	Bread	1½	lentils	½ cup
	Meat	4	salmon	4 ounces
	Vegetable	1	spinach	2 cups
Meal 4	Fruit	1	mango	½ item
	Meat (Nut)	1	avocado	⅓ item
Meal 5	Meat	2	tuna	4 ounces
Meal 6	Bread	1½	potato, baked	½ item
	Meat	4	sirloin	4 ounces
	Vegetable	2	tomato	2 items

Week 9

	Category	Exchanges	Sample food	Quantity
Meal 1	Bread	2	corn grits	1 cup
	Fruit	1	melon, honeydew	⅙ item
	Meat	1	egg	1 item
Meal 2	Fruit	1	cherries	½ cup

Meal 3	Bread	1½	garbanzo beans	⅜ cup
	Meat	4	chicken	4 ounces
	Vegetable	2	romaine lettuce	6 cups
Meal 4	Fruit	1	apple	1 item
	Meat (Nut)	1	peanut butter	1 tablespoon
Meal 5	Meat	2	turkey	2 ounces
	Vegetable	1	tomato	1 item
Meal 6	Meat	4	turkey	4 ounces
	Vegetable	3	mushrooms	6 cups
Meal 7	Fruit	1	applesauce	½ cup

Week 10

	Category	Exchanges	Sample food	Quantity
Meal 1	Fruit	1	banana	½ item
	Shake	2	whey protein shake	2 scoops
Meal 2	Fruit	1	tangerine	2 items
Meal 3	Bread	1½	potato	¾ cup
	Meat	4	tuna	8 ounces
	Vegetable	3	romaine lettuce	9 cups
Meal 4	Fruit	1	apple	1 item
	Meat (Nut)	1	almond butter	1 tablespoon
Meal 5	Meat	2	turkey	2 ounces
Meal 6	Meat	4	snapper	8 ounces
	Vegetable	3	Brussels sprouts	3 cups
Meal 7	Fruit	1	watermelon	1 cup

Week 11

	Category	Exchanges	Sample food	Quantity
Meal 1	Bread	2	bran flakes	1 cup
	Fruit	1	grapefruit	1 item
Meal 2	Meat	2	egg	2 items
Meal 3	Bread	1½	tortilla	1½ items
	Meat	4	flank steak	4 ounces
	Vegetable	2	peppers	2 cups
Meal 4	Fruit	1	nectarine	1 item
	Meat (Nut)	1	almonds	⅛ cup
Meal 5	Meat	2	tuna	4 ounces
Meal 6	Meat	4	chicken	4 ounces
	Vegetable	3	green beans	3 cups

Week 12

	Category	Exchanges	Sample food	Quantity
Meal 1	Bread	2	cream of wheat	1 cup
	Fruit	1	apricot	3 items
	Meat	1	egg white	3 items
Meal 2	Meat	1	egg	1 item
Meal 3	Bread	1½	lentil	½ cup
	Meat	4	chicken	4 ounces
	Vegetable	1	carrots	½ cup
Meal 4	Fruit	1	pear	1 item
	Meat (Nut)	1	pecans	⅛ cup
Meal 5	Meat	2	turkey	2 ounces
Meal 6	Bread	1½	potato, baked	½ item
	Meat	4	halibut	8 ounces
	Vegetable	3	spinach	6 cups

Level 4

Week 1

	Category	Exchanges	Sample food	Quantity
Meal 1	Bread	3	bagel	1 item
	Fruit	1	cantaloupe	½ item
Meal 2	Fruit	1	apple	1 item
Meal 3	Bread	3	pita	1½ items
	Meat	4	turkey	4 ounces
	Vegetable	1	romaine lettuce	3 cups
Meal 4	Fruit	1	plum	2 items
	Meat (Nut)	1	almonds	⅛ cup
Meal 5	Bread	3	baked potato	1 item
	Meat	4	salmon	4 ounces
	Vegetable	2	spinach	4 cups
Meal 6	Bread	1	popcorn	1 cup
	Fruit	1	pear	1 item

Week 2

	Category	Exchanges	Sample food	Quantity
Meal 1	Bread	3	oatmeal	1½ cups
	Fruit	1	banana	½ item
Meal 2	Fruit	1	peach	2 small items
Meal 3	Bread	3	white rice	1 cup
	Meat	4	tuna	8 ounces
	Vegetable	1	tomato	1 item

Meal 4	Fruit	I	apple	I item
	Meat (Nut)	I	peanut butter	I tablespoon
Meal 5	Bread	3	corn	I ½ cups
	Meat	4	chicken breast	4 ounces
	Vegetable	2	green beans	2 cups
Meal 6	Bread	I	whole wheat crackers	I ounce
	Fruit	I	strawberries	I ½ cups

Week 3

	Category	Exchanges	Sample food	Quantity
Meal I	Bread	3	bran flakes	I ½ cups
	Fruit	I	raspberries	I cup
	Meat	I	egg	I item
Meal 2	Fruit	I	banana	½ item
	Meat (Nut)	I	almond butter	I tablespoon
Meal 3	Bread	3	white rice	I cup
	Meat	4	shrimp	8 ounces
	Vegetable	I	zucchini	I cup
Meal 4	Fruit	I	apple	I item
	Meat (Nut)	I	cashew butter	I tablespoon
Meal 5	Bread	3	tortilla	3 items
	Meat	4	flank steak	4 ounces
	Vegetable	2	peppers	2 cups
Meal 6	Fruit	I	orange	I item

Week 4

	Category	Exchanges	Sample food	Quantity
Meal I	Bread	2	cream of wheat	I cup
	Fruit	I	grapefruit	I item
	Meat	2	egg	2 items
Meal 2	Fruit	I	grapes	I cup
	Meat (Nut)	I	pecans	⅛ cup
Meal 3	Bread	I ½	kidney beans	½ cup
	Meat	4	tuna	8 ounces
	Vegetable	I	romaine lettuce	3 cups
Meal 4	Fruit	I	apricot	3 items
	Meat (Nut)	I	Brazil nuts	⅛ cup
Meal 5	Bread	I ½	couscous	¾ cup
	Meat	8	chicken	8 ounces
	Vegetable	3	tomato	3 items
Meal 6	Fruit	I	pear	I item

Week 5

	Category	Exchanges	Sample food	Quantity
Meal 1	Bread	3	oatmeal	1½ cups
	Meat	1	egg	1 item
Meal 2	Fruit	1	pear	1 item
	Meat (Nut)	1	walnuts	⅛ cup
Meal 3	Bread	1½	corn tortilla	1½ items
	Meat	4	chicken	4 ounces
	Vegetable	1	peppers	1 cup
Meal 4	Fruit	1	apple	1 item
	Meat (Nut)	1	peanut butter	1 tablespoon
Meal 5	Bread	1½	wild rice	½ cup
	Meat	8	whitefish	16 ounces
	Vegetable	3	spinach	6 cups
Meal 6	Fruit	1	peach	2 small items

Week 6

	Category	Exchanges	Sample food	Quantity
Meal 1	Bread	3	shredded wheat	3 large biscuits
	Fruit	1	strawberries	1½ cups
Meal 2	Fruit	1	pineapple	1 cup
Meal 3	Bread	1½	artichoke	1½ items
	Meat	4	salmon	4 ounces
	Vegetable	1	asparagus	1 cup
Meal 4	Fruit	1	orange	1 item
	Meat (Nut)	1	Brazil nuts	⅛ cup
Meal 5	Meat	1	egg	1 item
Meal 6	Meat	8	chicken	8 ounces
	Vegetable	3	broccoli	3 cups
Meal 7	Fruit	1	papaya	½ item

Week 7

	Category	Exchanges	Sample food	Quantity
Meal 1	Bread	3	cream of rice	1½ cups
	Fruit	1	blueberries	1 cup
Meal 2	Fruit	1	apple	1 item
Meal 3	Bread	1½	yams	½ cup
	Meat	4	catfish	4 ounces
	Vegetable	1	collards	2 cups
Meal 4	Fruit	1	banana	½ item
	Meat (Nut)	1	almond butter	1 tablespoon

Meal 5	Meat	2	chicken	2 ounces
	Vegetable	1	romaine lettuce	3 cups
Meal 6	Bread	1½	white rice	½ cup
	Meat	8	crab	16 ounces
	Vegetable	2	cucumber	4 cups

Week 8	**Category**	**Exchanges**	**Sample food**	**Quantity**
Meal 1	Fruit	2	orange	2 items
	Meat	2	egg	2 items
Meal 2	Bread	1½	yams	½ cup
Meal 3	Bread	1½	garbanzo beans	⅜ cup
	Meat	4	chicken	4 ounces
	Vegetable	2	romaine lettuce	6 cups
Meal 4	Meat (Nut)	1	avocado	⅓ item
	Vegetable	1	jicama	½ cup
Meal 5	Meat	2	tuna	4 ounces
	Vegetable	1	celery	2 cups
Meal 6	Bread	1½	potato, baked	½ item
	Meat	8	sirloin	8 ounces
	Vegetable	3	tomato	3 items

Week 9	**Category**	**Exchanges**	**Sample food**	**Quantity**
Meal 1	Fruit	1	mango	½ item
	Shake	2	whey protein shake	2 scoops
Meal 2	Fruit	1	nectarine	1 item
	Meat (Nut)	1	cashews	⅛ cup
Meal 3	Bread	1½	lentil	½ cup
	Meat	4	chicken	4 ounces
	Vegetable	1	carrots	½ cup
Meal 4	Meat (Nut)	1	pecans	⅛ cup
	Vegetable	1	spinach	2 cups
Meal 5	Meat	2	turkey	2 ounces
	Vegetable	1	beets	½ cup
Meal 6	Bread	1½	wild rice	½ cup
	Meat	8	turkey	8 ounces
	Vegetable	3	mushrooms	6 cups

Week 10	**Category**	**Exchanges**	**Sample food**	**Quantity**
Meal 1	Fruit	1	banana	½ item
	Shake	2	whey protein shake	2 scoops
Meal 2	Meat	1	egg	1 item

Meal 3	Bread	1½	pasta	1½ ounces
	Meat	4	salmon	4 ounces
	Vegetable	2	spinach	4 cups
Meal 4	Fruit	1	apple	1 item
	Meat (Nut)	1	peanut butter	1 tablespoon
Meal 5	Meat	2	turkey	2 ounces
	Vegetable	1	tomato	1 item
Meal 6	Bread	1½	winter squash	¾ cup
	Meat	8	snapper	16 ounces
	Vegetable	2	Brussels sprouts	2 cups

Week 11

	Category	Exchanges	Sample food	Quantity
Meal 1	Fruit	1	blueberries	1 cup
	Shake	2	whey protein shake	2 scoops
Meal 2	Meat	1	egg	1 item
Meal 3	Bread	1½	tortilla	1½ items
	Meat	4	flank steak	4 ounces
	Vegetable	2	peppers	2 cups
Meal 4	Fruit	1	cherries	½ cup
	Meat (Nut)	1	almonds	⅛ cup
Meal 5	Meat	2	tuna	4 ounces
	Vegetable	1	celery	2 cups
Meal 6	Meat	8	chicken	8 ounces
	Vegetable	3	green beans	3 cups
Meal 7	Fruit	1	fig	1 large item

Week 12

	Category	Exchanges	Sample food	Quantity
Meal 1	Bread	2	oatmeal	1 cup
	Fruit	1	apricot	3 items
	Meat	2	egg white	6 items
Meal 2	Fruit	1	pear	1 item
Meal 3	Bread	1½	split peas	½ cup
	Meat	4	salmon	4 ounces
	Vegetable	1	spinach	2 cups
Meal 4	Fruit	1	papaya	½ item
	Meat (Nut)	1	avocado	⅓ item

Meal 5	Meat	2	turkey	2 ounces
	Vegetable	I	broccoli	I cup
Meal 6	Bread	I½	couscous	¾ cup
	Meat	8	halibut	I6 ounces
	Vegetable	3	asparagus	3 cups

Level 5

Week 1

	Category	Exchanges	Sample food	Quantity
Meal 1	Bread	3	bagel	I item
	Fruit	I	cantaloupe	½ item
	Meat	I	egg	I item
Meal 2	Fruit	I	apple	I item
	Meat (Nut)	I	peanut butter	I tablespoon
Meal 3	Bread	3	pita	I½ items
	Meat	4	turkey	4 ounces
	Vegetable	I	romaine lettuce	3 cups
Meal 4	Fruit	I	plum	2 items
	Meat (Nut)	I	almonds	⅛ cup
Meal 5	Bread	3	baked potato	I item
	Meat	4	salmon	4 ounces
	Vegetable	2	spinach	4 cups
Meal 6	Bread	I	popcorn	I cup
	Fruit	I	pear	I item

Week 2

	Category	Exchanges	Sample food	Quantity
Meal 1	Bread	3	oatmeal	I½ cups
	Fruit	I	banana	½ item
	Meat	I	egg white	3 items
Meal 2	Fruit	I	peach	2 small items
	Meat (Nut)	I	cashews	⅛ cup
Meal 3	Bread	3	white rice	I cup
	Meat	4	tuna	8 ounces
	Vegetable	I	tomato	I item
Meal 4	Fruit	I	apple	I item
	Meat (Nut)	I	peanut butter	I tablespoon

Meal 5	Bread	3	corn	1½ cups
	Meat	4	chicken breast	4 ounces
	Vegetable	2	green beans	2 cups
Meal 6	Bread	1	whole wheat crackers	1 ounce
	Fruit	1	strawberries	1½ cups

Week 3

	Category	Exchanges	Sample food	Quantity
Meal 1	Bread	3	bran flakes	1½ cups
	Fruit	1	raspberries	1 cup
	Meat	2	egg	2 items
Meal 2	Fruit	1	watermelon	1 cup
	Meat (Nut)	1	cashews	⅛ cup
Meal 3	Bread	3	white rice	1 cup
	Meat	4	shrimp	8 ounces
	Vegetable	1	zucchini	1 cup
Meal 4	Fruit	1	apple	1 item
	Meat (Nut)	1	almond butter	1 tablespoon
Meal 5	Bread	3	tortilla	3 items
	Meat	4	flank steak	4 ounces
	Vegetable	2	peppers	2 cups
Meal 6	Bread	1	popcorn	1 cup
	Fruit	1	orange	1 item

Week 4

	Category	Exchanges	Sample food	Quantity
Meal 1	Bread	3	cream of wheat	1½ cups
	Fruit	1	grapefruit	1 item
	Meat	2	egg white	6 items
Meal 2	Fruit	1	grapes	1 cup
	Meat (Nut)	1	walnuts	⅛ cup
Meal 3	Bread	1½	kidney beans	½ cup
	Meat	4	tuna	8 ounces
	Vegetable	1	romaine lettuce	3 cups
Meal 4	Bread	1½	corn tortilla	1½ items
	Vegetable	1	tomato	1 item
Meal 5	Fruit	1	apricot	3 items
Meal 6	Bread	3	couscous	1½ cups
	Meat	8	chicken	8 ounces
	Vegetable	2	summer squash	2 cups
Meal 7	Fruit	1	papaya	½ item

Week 5

Category	Exchanges	Sample food	Quantity
Meal 1			
Bread	3	oatmeal	1½ cups
Fruit	1	blueberries	1 cup
Meat	2	egg	2 items
Meal 2			
Fruit	1	pear	1 item
Meat (Nut)	1	almonds	⅛ cup
Meal 3			
Bread	1½	corn tortilla	1½ items
Meat	4	chicken	4 ounces
Vegetable	1	peppers	1 cup
Meal 4			
Bread	1½	garbanzo beans	⅜ cup
Vegetable	1	tomato	1 item
Meal 5			
Fruit	1	apple	1 item
Meat (Nut)	1	peanut butter	1 tablespoon
Meal 6			
Bread	1½	wild rice	½ cup
Meat	6	whitefish	12 ounces
Vegetable	2	spinach	4 cups
Meal 7			
Fruit	1	plum	2 items

Week 6

Category	Exchanges	Sample food	Quantity
Meal 1			
Bread	3	tortilla, flour	3 items
Meat	2	egg white	6 items
Meal 2			
Fruit	1	papaya	½ item
Meat (Nut)	1	avocado	⅓ item
Meal 3			
Bread	1½	artichoke	1½ items
Meat	4	salmon	4 ounces
Vegetable	2	asparagus	2 cups
Meal 4			
Bread	1½	pasta	1½ ounces
Vegetable	1	broccoli	1 cup
Meal 5			
Meat (Nut)	1	peanut butter	1 tablespoon
Vegetable	1	celery	2 cups
Meal 6			
Bread	1½	black beans	½ cup
Meat	6	chicken	6 ounces
Vegetable	3	peppers	3 cups
Meal 7			
Fruit	1	figs	1 large item

Week 7

Category	Exchanges	Sample food	Quantity
Meal 1			
Bread	3	cream of rice	1½ cups
Fruit	1	banana	½ item
Meat	2	egg	2 items

Meal 2	Fruit	1	apple	1 item
	Meat (Nut)	1	peanut butter	1 tablespoon
Meal 3	Bread	1½	yams	½ cup
	Meat	4	catfish	4 ounces
	Vegetable	2	collards	4 cups
Meal 4	Bread	1½	brown rice	½ cup
	Vegetable	1	onions	½ cup
Meal 5	Meat	2	turkey	2 ounces
Meal 6	Bread	1½	potato, baked	½ item
	Meat	6	chicken	6 ounces
	Vegetable	3	romaine lettuce	9 cups
Meal 7	Fruit	1	kiwi	2 items

Week 8

	Category	Exchanges	Sample food	Quantity
Meal 1	Bread	2	potato	1 cup
	Fruit	1	orange	1 item
	Meat	2	egg white	6 items
Meal 2	Fruit	1	cherries	½ cup
Meal 3	Bread	1½	garbanzo beans	⅜ cup
	Meat	4	chicken	4 ounces
	Vegetable	1	romaine lettuce	3 cups
Meal 4	Fruit	1	banana	½ item
	Meat (Nut)	1	peanut butter	1 tablespoon
Meal 5	Meat	2	tuna	4 ounces
Meal 6	Bread	1½	corn	¾ cup
	Meat	8	sirloin	8 ounces
	Vegetable	3	tomato	3 items

Week 9

	Category	Exchanges	Sample food	Quantity
Meal 1	Fruit	1	blueberries	1 cup
	Shake	2	whey protein shake	2 scoops
Meal 2	Fruit	1	nectarine	1 item
	Meat (Nut)	1	cashews	⅛ cup
Meal 3	Bread	1½	lentil	½ cup
	Meat	4	chicken	4 ounces
	Vegetable	2	carrots	1 cup
Meal 4	Fruit	1	pear	1 item
	Meat (Nut)	1	pecans	⅛ cup

Meal 5	Meat	4	turkey	4 ounces
Meal 6	Bread	1½	peas	¾ cup
	Meat	8	chicken	8 ounces
	Vegetable	2	mushrooms	4 cups

Week 10

	Category	Exchanges	Sample food	Quantity
Meal 1	Fruit	1	mango	½ item
	Shake	2	whey protein shake	2 scoops
Meal 2	Fruit	1	apple	1 item
	Meat (Nut)	1	almond butter	1 tablespoon
Meal 3	Bread	1½	pinto beans	½ cup
	Meat	4	flank steak	4 ounces
	Vegetable	1	peppers	1 cup
Meal 4	Fruit	1	orange	1 item
	Meat (Nut)	1	Brazil nuts	⅛ cup
Meal 5	Meat	2	turkey	2 ounces
Meal 6	Meat	8	snapper	16 ounces
	Vegetable	3	Brussels sprouts	3 cups
Meal 7	Fruit	1	papaya	½ item

Week 11

	Category	Exchanges	Sample food	Quantity
Meal 1	Fruit	1	banana	½ item
	Shake	2	whey protein shake	2 scoops
Meal 2	Fruit	1	melon, honeydew	⅛ item
	Meat (Nut)	1	sunflower seeds	⅛ cup
Meal 3	Bread	1½	potato, baked	½ item
	Meat	4	salmon	4 ounces
	Vegetable	1	spinach	2 cups
Meal 4	Fruit	1	plum	2 items
	Meat (Nut)	1	almonds	⅛ cup
Meal 5	Meat	2	tuna	4 ounces
Meal 6	Bread	1½	yams	½ cup
	Meat	8	chicken	8 ounces
	Vegetable	3	green beans	3 cups

Week 12

	Category	Exchanges	Sample food	Quantity
Meal 1	Bread	2	oatmeal	1 cup
	Fruit	1	grapefruit	1 item
	Meat	2	egg	2 items

Meal 2	Fruit	1	pear	1 item
	Meat (Nut)	1	walnuts	⅛ cup
Meal 3	Bread	1½	split peas	½ cup
	Meat	4	salmon	4 ounces
	Vegetable	1	spinach	2 cups
Meal 4	Fruit	1	apple	1 item
	Meat (Nut)	1	peanut butter	1 tablespoon
Meal 5	Meat	2	turkey	2 ounces
Meal 6	Bread	1½	brown rice	½ cup
	Meat	8	halibut	16 ounces
	Vegetable	3	asparagus	3 cups

Level 6

Week 1

Meal	Category	Exchanges	Sample food	Quantity
Meal 1	Bread	3	bagel	1 item
	Fruit	1	cantaloupe	½ item
	Meat	2	egg	2 items
Meal 2	Fruit	1	apple	1 item
	Meat (Nut)	1	peanut butter	1 tablespoon
Meal 3	Bread	3	pita	1½ items
	Meat	4	turkey	4 ounces
	Vegetable	1	romaine lettuce	3 cups
Meal 4	Fruit	1	plum	2 items
	Meat (Nut)	1	almonds	⅛ cup
Meal 5	Bread	3	baked potato	1 item
	Meat	8	salmon	8 ounces
	Vegetable	2	spinach	4 cups
Meal 6	Bread	1	popcorn	1 cup
	Fruit	2	pear	2 items

Week 2

Meal	Category	Exchanges	Sample food	Quantity
Meal 1	Bread	3	oatmeal	1½ cups
	Fruit	1	banana	½ item
	Meat	2	egg white	6 items
Meal 2	Fruit	1	peach	2 small items
	Meat (Nut)	1	cashews	⅛ cup
Meal 3	Bread	3	white rice	1 cup
	Meat	4	tuna	8 ounces
	Vegetable	1	tomato	1 item

Meal 4	Fruit	1	apple	1 item
	Meat (Nut)	1	peanut butter	1 tablespoon
Meal 5	Bread	3	corn	1½ cups
	Meat	8	chicken breast	8 ounces
	Vegetable	2	green beans	2 cups
Meal 6	Bread	1	whole wheat crackers	1 ounce
	Fruit	2	strawberries	3 cups

Week 3

	Category	Exchanges	Sample food	Quantity
Meal 1	Bread	3	bran flakes	1½ cups
	Fruit	1	raspberries	1 cup
	Meat	2	egg	2 items
Meal 2	Fruit	1	watermelon	1 cup
	Meat (Nut)	1	cashews	⅛ cup
Meal 3	Bread	3	white rice	1 cup
	Meat	4	shrimp	8 ounces
	Vegetable	1	zucchini	1 cup
Meal 4	Fruit	1	apple	1 item
	Meat (Nut)	1	almond butter	1 tablespoon
Meal 5	Meat	2	turkey	2 ounces
	Vegetable	1	tomato	1 item
Meal 6	Bread	1½	tortilla	1½ items
	Meat	8	flank steak	8 ounces
	Vegetable	2	peppers	2 cups
Meal 7	Bread	1	popcorn	1 cup
	Fruit	1	orange	1 item

Week 4

	Category	Exchanges	Sample food	Quantity
Meal 1	Bread	3	cream of wheat	1½ cups
	Fruit	1	grapefruit	1 item
	Meat	2	egg white	6 items
Meal 2	Fruit	1	grapes	1 cup
	Meat (Nut)	1	walnuts	⅛ cup
Meal 3	Bread	3	kidney beans	1 cup
	Meat	4	tuna	8 ounces
	Vegetable	2	romaine lettuce	6 cups
Meal 4	Fruit	1	apricot	3 items
	Meat (Nut)	1	Brazil nuts	⅛ cup
Meal 5	Meat	4	tuna	8 ounces
	Vegetable	1	celery	2 cups

Meal 6	Bread	1½	couscous	¾ cup
	Meat	8	chicken	8 ounces
	Vegetable	2	tomato	2 items
Meal 7	Fruit	1	papaya	½ item

Week 5

Meal	Category	Exchanges	Sample food	Quantity
Meal 1	Bread	2	oatmeal	1 cup
	Fruit	1	blueberries	1 cup
	Meat	3	egg	3 items
Meal 2	Fruit	1	pear	1 item
	Meat (Nut)	1	almonds	⅛ cup
Meal 3	Bread	3	corn tortilla	3 items
	Meat	4	chicken	4 ounces
	Vegetable	2	peppers	2 cups
Meal 4	Fruit	1	apple	1 item
	Meat (Nut)	1	peanut butter	1 tablespoon
Meal 5	Meat	4	chicken	4 ounces
	Vegetable	1	sauerkraut	½ cup
Meal 6	Bread	1½	wild rice	½ cup
	Meat	8	whitefish	16 ounces
	Vegetable	2	spinach	4 cups
Meal 7	Fruit	1	kiwi	2 items

Week 6

Meal	Category	Exchanges	Sample food	Quantity
Meal 1	Bread	3	shredded wheat	3 large biscuits
	Fruit	1	strawberries	1½ cups
	Meat	2	egg white	6 items
Meal 2	Fruit	1	papaya	½ item
	Meat (Nut)	1	avocado	⅓ item
Meal 3	Bread	1½	artichoke	1½ items
	Meat	6	salmon	6 ounces
	Vegetable	2	asparagus	2 cups
Meal 4	Fruit	1	orange	1 item
	Meat (Nut)	1	Brazil nuts	⅛ cup
Meal 5	Meat	4	tuna	8 ounces
	Vegetable	1	jicama	½ cup
Meal 6	Bread	1½	pasta	1½ ounces
	Meat	8	chicken	8 ounces
	Vegetable	2	broccoli	2 cups

Week 7

	Category	Exchanges	Sample food	Quantity
Meal 1	Bread	3	cream of rice	1½ cups
	Fruit	1	banana	½ item
	Meat	2	egg	2 items
Meal 2	Fruit	1	apple	1 item
	Meat (Nut)	1	peanut butter	1 tablespoon
Meal 3	Bread	1½	yams	½ cup
	Meat	6	catfish	6 ounces
	Vegetable	2	collards	4 cups
Meal 4	Bread	1½	whole wheat crackers	1½ ounces
	Meat	2	turkey	2 ounces
Meal 5	Fruit	1	cherries	½ cup
	Meat (Nut)	1	almonds	⅛ cup
Meal 6	Bread	1½	split peas	½ cup
	Meat	8	chicken	8 ounces
	Vegetable	3	romaine lettuce	9 cups
Meal 7	Fruit	1	strawberries	1½ cups

Week 8

	Category	Exchanges	Sample food	Quantity
Meal 1	Bread	3	oatmeal	1½ cups
	Fruit	1	orange	1 item
	Meat	2	egg white	6 items
Meal 2	Fruit	1	banana	½ item
	Meat (Nut)	1	sesame butter	1 tablespoon
Meal 3	Bread	1½	garbanzo beans	⅜ cup
	Meat	6	chicken	6 ounces
	Vegetable	3	romaine lettuce	9 cups
Meal 4	Bread	1½	white rice	½ cup
	Meat	4	tuna	8 ounces
Meal 5	Fruit	1	mango	½ item
	Meat (Nut)	1	avocado	⅓ item
Meal 6	Meat	8	sirloin	8 ounces
	Vegetable	3	tomato	3 items
Meal 7	Fruit	1	pear	1 item

Week 9

	Category	Exchanges	Sample food	Quantity
Meal 1	Fruit	2	blueberries	2 cups
	Shake	2	whey protein shake	2 scoops
Meal 2	Fruit	1	plum	2 items
	Meat (Nut)	1	cashews	⅛ cup

Meal 3	Bread	1½	corn	¾ cup
	Meat	6	chicken	6 ounces
	Vegetable	2	summer squash	2 cups
Meal 4	Bread	1½	corn tortilla	1½ items
	Meat	4	snapper	8 ounces
Meal 5	Fruit	1	apple	1 item
	Meat (Nut)	1	peanut butter	1 tablespoon
Meal 6	Meat	8	turkey	8 ounces
	Vegetable	3	mushrooms	6 cups
Meal 7	Fruit	1	nectarine	1 item

Week 10

	Category	Exchanges	Sample food	Quantity
Meal 1	Bread	2	bran flakes	1 cup
	Fruit	1	raspberries	1 cup
	Meat	3	egg whites	9 items
Meal 2	Fruit	1	apple	1 item
	Meat (Nut)	1	almond butter	1 tablespoon
Meal 3	Bread	1½	corn tortilla	1½ items
	Meat	6	flank steak	6 ounces
	Vegetable	2	peppers	2 cups
Meal 4	Bread	1½	black beans	½ cup
	Meat	4	turkey	4 ounces
Meal 5	Fruit	1	banana	½ item
	Meat (Nut)	1	peanut butter	1 tablespoon
Meal 6	Meat	8	snapper	16 ounces
	Vegetable	3	Brussels sprouts	3 cups

Week 11

	Category	Exchanges	Sample food	Quantity
Meal 1	Fruit	2	mango	1 item
	Shake	2	whey protein shake	2 scoops
Meal 2	Fruit	1	peach	2 small items
	Meat (Nut)	1	pumpkin seeds	⅛ cup
Meal 3	Bread	1½	lentil	½ cup
	Meat	6	chicken	6 ounces
	Vegetable	2	carrots	1 cup
Meal 4	Bread	1½	white rice	½ cup
	Meat	4	tuna	8 ounces

Meal 5	Fruit	1	apple	1 item
	Meat (Nut)	1	almonds	⅛ cup
Meal 6	Bread	1½	potato	¾ cup
	Meat	8	salmon	8 ounces
	Vegetable	3	green beans	3 cups

Week 12

	Category	Exchanges	Sample food	Quantity
Meal 1	Bread	2	oatmeal	1 cup
	Fruit	1	grapefruit	1 item
	Meat	3	egg	3 items
Meal 2	Fruit	1	pear	1 item
	Meat (Nut)	1	walnuts	⅛ cup
Meal 3	Bread	1½	split peas	½ cup
	Meat	6	chicken	6 ounces
	Vegetable	3	spinach	6 cups
Meal 4	Bread	1½	pasta	1½ ounces
	Meat	4	shrimp	8 ounces
Meal 5	Fruit	1	apple	1 item
	Meat (Nut)	1	peanut butter	1 tablespoon
Meal 6	Bread	1½	wild rice	½ cup
	Meat	8	halibut	16 ounces
	Vegetable	3	asparagus	3 cups
Meal 7	Fruit	1	figs	1 large item

Level 7

Week 1

	Category	Exchanges	Sample food	Quantity
Meal 1	Bread	3	bagel	1 item
	Fruit	1	cantaloupe	½ item
	Meat	2	egg	2 items
Meal 2	Fruit	1	apple	1 item
	Meat (Nut)	1	peanut butter	1 tablespoon
Meal 3	Bread	3	pita	1½ items
	Meat	4	turkey	4 ounces
	Vegetable	1	romaine lettuce	3 cups
Meal 4	Fruit	1	plum	2 items
	Meat (Nut)	1	almonds	⅛ cup
Meal 5	Fruit	1	watermelon	1 cup

Meal 6	Bread	3	baked potato	1 item
	Meat	8	salmon	8 ounces
	Vegetable	2	spinach	4 cups
Meal 7	Bread	2	popcorn	2 cups
	Fruit	2	pear	2 items

Week 2

	Category	Exchanges	Sample food	Quantity
Meal 1	Bread	3	oatmeal	1½ cups
	Fruit	1	banana	½ item
	Meat	2	egg white	6 items
Meal 2	Fruit	1	peach	2 small items
	Meat (Nut)	1	cashews	⅛ cup
Meal 3	Bread	3	white rice	1 cup
	Meat	4	tuna	8 ounces
	Vegetable	1	tomato	1 item
Meal 4	Fruit	1	apple	1 item
	Meat (Nut)	1	peanut butter	1 tablespoon
Meal 5	Fruit	1	nectarine	1 item
Meal 6	Bread	3	corn	1½ cups
	Meat	8	chicken	8 ounces
	Vegetable	2	green beans	2 cups
Meal 7	Bread	2	whole wheat crackers	2 ounces
	Fruit	2	strawberries	3 cups

Week 3

	Category	Exchanges	Sample food	Quantity
Meal 1	Bread	3	bran flakes	1½ cups
	Fruit	1	raspberries	1 cup
	Meat	2	egg	2 items
Meal 2	Fruit	1	watermelon	1 cup
	Meat (Nut)	1	cashews	⅛ cup
Meal 3	Bread	3	white rice	1 cup
	Meat	4	shrimp	8 ounces
	Vegetable	1	zucchini	1 cup
Meal 4	Fruit	1	apple	1 item
	Meat (Nut)	1	almond butter	1 tablespoon
Meal 5	Fruit	1	grapes	1 cup
	Meat	2	tuna	4 ounces

Meal 6	Bread	3	corn tortilla	3 items
	Meat	8	flank steak	8 ounces
	Vegetable	2	peppers	2 cups
Meal 7	Bread	2	rice cakes	4 items
	Fruit	2	orange	2 items

Week 4

	Category	Exchanges	Sample food	Quantity
Meal I	Bread	3	cream of wheat	1½ cups
	Fruit	I	grapefruit	I item
	Meat	2	egg whites	6 items
Meal 2	Fruit	I	grapes	I cup
	Meat (Nut)	I	walnuts	⅛ cup
Meal 3	Bread	3	kidney beans	I cup
	Meat	4	tuna	8 ounces
	Vegetable	I	romaine lettuce	3 cups
Meal 4	Fruit	I	apricot	3 items
	Meat (Nut)	I	Brazil nuts	⅛ cup
Meal 5	Fruit	I	melon, cantaloupe	½ item
	Meat	2	tuna	4 ounces
Meal 6	Bread	1½	couscous	¾ cup
	Meat	10	chicken	10 ounces
	Vegetable	2	tomato	2 items
Meal 7	Bread	I	popcorn	I cup
	Fruit	I	papaya	½ item

Week 5

	Category	Exchanges	Sample food	Quantity
Meal I	Bread	3	oatmeal	1½ cups
	Fruit	I	blueberries	I cup
	Meat	2	egg	2 items
Meal 2	Fruit	I	pear	I item
	Meat (Nut)	I	almonds	⅛ cup
Meal 3	Bread	3	corn tortilla	3 items
	Meat	4	chicken	4 ounces
	Vegetable	I	peppers	I cup
Meal 4	Fruit	I	banana	½ item
	Meat (Nut)	I	peanut butter	I tablespoon
Meal 5	Fruit	I	cranberries	I cup
	Meat	2	turkey	2 ounces

Meal 6	Bread	1½	wild rice	½ cup
	Meat	10	whitefish	20 ounces
	Vegetable	2	spinach	4 cups
Meal 7	Fruit	1	pineapple	1 cup

Week 6

	Category	Exchanges	Sample food	Quantity
Meal 1	Bread	3	shredded wheat	3 large biscuits
	Fruit	1	strawberries	1½ cups
	Meat	2	egg white	6 items
Meal 2	Fruit	1	papaya	½ item
	Meat (Nut)	1	avocado	⅓ item
Meal 3	Bread	1½	artichoke	1½ items
	Meat	4	salmon	4 ounces
	Vegetable	1	asparagus	1 cup
Meal 4	Bread	1½	white rice	½ cup
	Meat	4	tuna	8 ounces
Meal 5	Meat (Nut)	1	peanut butter	1 tablespoon
	Vegetable	1	celery	2 cups
Meal 6	Bread	1½	potato, baked	½ item
	Meat	10	chicken	10 ounces
	Vegetable	2	broccoli	2 cups
Meal 7	Fruit	1	nectarine	1 item

Week 7

	Category	Exchanges	Sample food	Quantity
Meal 1	Bread	3	cream of rice	1½ cups
	Fruit	1	banana	½ item
	Meat	2	egg	2 items
Meal 2	Fruit	1	apple	1 item
	Meat (Nut)	1	peanut butter	1 tablespoon
Meal 3	Bread	1½	yams	½ cup
	Meat	4	catfish	4 ounces
	Vegetable	2	collards	4 cups
Meal 4	Bread	1½	whole wheat crackers	1½ ounces
	Meat	4	turkey	4 ounces
Meal 5	Fruit	1	apricot	3 items
	Meat (Nut)	1	almonds	⅛ cup
Meal 6	Meat	10	chicken	10 ounces
	Vegetable	3	romaine lettuce	9 cups
Meal 7	Fruit	1	strawberries	1½ cups

Week 8

Category	Exchanges	Sample food	Quantity
Meal 1			
Bread	2	potato	1 cup
Fruit	1	orange	1 item
Meat	4	egg white	12 items
Meal 2			
Fruit	1	banana	½ item
Meat (Nut)	1	sesame butter	1 tablespoon
Meal 3			
Bread	1½	garbanzo beans	⅜ cup
Meat	4	chicken	4 ounces
Vegetable	1	romaine lettuce	3 cups
Meal 4			
Bread	1½	white rice	½ cup
Meat	4	crab	8 ounces
Meal 5			
Fruit	1	papaya	½ item
Meat (Nut)	1	avocado	⅓ item
Meal 6			
Meat	10	sirloin	10 ounces
Vegetable	3	tomato	3 items

Week 9

Category	Exchanges	Sample food	Quantity
Meal 1			
Bread	2	oatmeal	1 cup
Fruit	1	peach	2 small items
Meat	4	egg	4 items
Meal 2			
Fruit	1	apricot	3 items
Meat (Nut)	1	cashews	⅛ cup
Meal 3			
Bread	1½	corn	¾ cup
Meat	4	chicken	4 ounces
Vegetable	2	summer squash	2 cups
Meal 4			
Bread	1½	artichoke	1½ items
Meat	2	turkey	2 ounces
Meal 5			
Meat (Nut)	1	peanut butter	1 tablespoon
Vegetable	1	celery	2 cups
Meal 6			
Bread	1½	wild rice	½ cup
Meat	10	turkey	10 ounces
Vegetable	3	mushrooms	6 cups

Week 10

Category	Exchanges	Sample food	Quantity
Meal 1			
Fruit	2	mango	1 item
Shake	2	whey protein shake	2 scoops
Meal 2			
Fruit	1	apple	1 item
Meat (Nut)	1	almond butter	1 tablespoon

Meal 3	Bread	1½	tortilla	1½ items
	Meat	4	flank steak	4 ounces
	Vegetable	1	peppers	1 cup
Meal 4	Bread	1½	pasta	1½ ounces
	Meat	4	turkey	4 ounces
Meal 5	Meat (Nut)	1	olives	20 items
	Vegetable	1	cucumbers	2 cups
Meal 6	Bread	1½	potato, baked	½ item
	Meat	10	snapper	20 ounces
	Vegetable	3	Brussels sprouts	3 cups

Week 11

	Category	Exchanges	Sample food	Quantity
Meal 1	Fruit	2	blueberries	2 cups
	Shake	2	whey protein shake	2 scoops
Meal 2	Fruit	1	grapes	1 cup
	Meat (Nut)	1	pumpkin seeds	⅛ cup
Meal 3	Bread	1½	lentil	½ cup
	Meat	4	chicken	4 ounces
	Vegetable	1	carrots	½ cup
Meal 4	Bread	1½	white rice	½ cup
	Meat	2	tuna	4 ounces
Meal 5	Meat (Nut)	1	almonds	⅛ cup
	Vegetable	1	peppers	1 cup
Meal 6	Bread	1½	potato, baked	½ item
	Meat	10	salmon	10 ounces
	Vegetable	3	cauliflower	3 cups

Week 12

	Category	Exchanges	Sample food	Quantity
Meal 1	Bread	1½	Grapenuts	⅜ cup
	Fruit	1	grapefruit	1 item
	Meat	3	egg	3 items
Meal 2	Fruit	1	apple	1 item
	Meat (Nut)	1	peanut butter	1 tablespoon
Meal 3	Bread	1½	split peas	½ cup
	Meat	4	chicken	4 ounces
	Vegetable	1	spinach	2 cups
Meal 4	Bread	1½	popcorn	1½ cups
	Meat	2	turkey	2 ounces

Meal 5	Meat (Nut)	1	soynut butter	1 tablespoon
	Vegetable	1	celery	2 cups
Meal 6	Bread	1½	brown rice	½ cup
	Meat	10	halibut	20 ounces
	Vegetable	3	asparagus	3 cups
Meal 7	Fruit	1	figs	1 large item

Level 8

Week 1

Meal	Category	Exchanges	Sample food	Quantity
Meal 1	Bread	3	bagel	1 item
	Fruit	1	cantaloupe	½ item
	Meat	2	egg	2 items
Meal 2	Fruit	1	apple	1 item
	Meat (Nut)	1	peanut butter	1 tablespoon
Meal 3	Bread	3	pita	1½ items
	Meat	4	turkey	4 ounces
	Vegetable	1	romaine lettuce	3 cups
Meal 4	Fruit	1	plum	2 items
	Meat (Nut)	1	almonds	⅛ cup
Meal 5	Fruit	1	watermelon	1 cup
	Meat	2	turkey	2 ounces
Meal 6	Bread	3	baked potato	1 item
	Meat	8	salmon	8 ounces
	Vegetable	2	spinach	4 cups
Meal 7	Bread	1	popcorn	1 cup
	Fruit	2	pear	2 items

Week 2

Meal	Category	Exchanges	Sample food	Quantity
Meal 1	Bread	3	oatmeal	1½ cups
	Fruit	1	banana	½ item
	Meat	2	egg white	6 items
Meal 2	Fruit	1	peach	2 small items
	Meat (Nut)	1	cashews	⅛ cup
Meal 3	Bread	3	white rice	1 cup
	Meat	4	tuna	8 ounces
	Vegetable	1	tomato	1 item
Meal 4	Fruit	1	apple	1 item
	Meat (Nut)	1	peanut butter	1 tablespoon

Meal 5	Fruit	1	nectarine	1 item
	Meat	2	turkey	2 ounces
Meal 6	Bread	3	corn	1½ cups
	Meat	8	chicken breast	8 ounces
	Vegetable	2	green beans	2 cups
Meal 7	Bread	1	whole wheat crackers	1 ounce
	Fruit	2	strawberries	3 cups

Week 3	Category	Exchanges	Sample food	Quantity
Meal 1	Bread	3	bran flakes	1½ cups
	Fruit	1	raspberries	1 cup
	Meat	2	egg	2 items
Meal 2	Fruit	1	watermelon	1 cup
	Meat (Nut)	1	cashews	⅛ cup
Meal 3	Bread	3	white rice	1 cup
	Meat	4	shrimp	8 ounces
	Vegetable	1	zucchini	1 cup
Meal 4	Fruit	1	apple	1 item
	Meat (Nut)	1	almond butter	1 tablespoon
Meal 5	Fruit	1	grapes	1 cup
	Meat	4	turkey	4 ounces
Meal 6	Bread	1½	tortilla	1½ items
	Meat	8	flank steak	8 ounces
	Vegetable	2	peppers	2 cups
Meal 7	Bread	1	popcorn	1 cup
	Fruit	2	orange	2 items

Week 4	Category	Exchanges	Sample food	Quantity
Meal 1	Bread	3	cream of wheat	1½ cups
	Fruit	1	grapefruit	1 item
	Meat	2	egg white	6 items
Meal 2	Fruit	1	grapes	1 cup
	Meat (Nut)	1	walnuts	⅛ cup
Meal 3	Bread	3	kidney beans	1 cup
	Meat	4	tuna	8 ounces
	Vegetable	1	romaine lettuce	3 cups
Meal 4	Fruit	1	apricot	3 items
	Meat (Nut)	1	Brazil nuts	⅛ cup

Meal 5	Fruit	1	melon, cantaloupe	½ item
	Meat	4	tuna	8 ounces
Meal 6	Bread	1½	couscous	¾ cup
	Meat	10	chicken	10 ounces
	Vegetable	3	tomato	3 items
Meal 7	Bread	1	popcorn	1 cup
	Fruit	2	papaya	1 item

Week 5

	Category	Exchanges	Sample food	Quantity
Meal 1	Bread	3	oatmeal	1½ cups
	Fruit	1	blueberries	1 cup
	Meat	2	egg	2 items
Meal 2	Fruit	1	pear	1 item
	Meat (Nut)	1	almonds	⅛ cup
Meal 3	Bread	1½	corn tortilla	1½ items
	Meat	4	chicken	4 ounces
	Vegetable	2	peppers	2 cups
Meal 4	Fruit	1	banana	½ item
	Meat (Nut)	1	peanut butter	1 tablespoon
Meal 5	Meat	2	turkey	2 ounces
Meal 6	Bread	1½	wild rice	½ cup
	Meat	10	whitefish	20 ounces
	Vegetable	2	spinach	4 cups
Meal 7	Fruit	1	strawberries	1½ cups

Week 6

	Category	Exchanges	Sample food	Quantity
Meal 1	Bread	3	shredded wheat	3 large biscuits
	Fruit	1	strawberries	1½ cups
	Meat	2	egg white	6 items
Meal 2	Fruit	1	papaya	½ item
	Meat (Nut)	1	avocado	⅓ item
Meal 3	Bread	1½	artichoke	1½ items
	Meat	4	salmon	4 ounces
	Vegetable	2	asparagus	2 cups
Meal 4	Meat	4	tuna	8 ounces
Meal 5	Fruit	1	peach	2 small items
	Meat (Nut)	1	Brazil nuts	⅛ cup

Meal 6	Bread	1½	winter squash	¾ cup
	Meat	10	chicken	10 ounces
	Vegetable	2	broccoli	2 cups
Meal 7	Fruit	1	nectarine	1 item

Week 7

	Category	Exchanges	Sample food	Quantity
Meal 1	Bread	4	cream of rice	2 cups
	Fruit	1	banana	½ item
	Meat	2	egg	2 items
Meal 2	Fruit	1	apple	1 item
	Meat (Nut)	1	peanut butter	1 tablespoon
Meal 3	Bread	1½	yams	½ cup
	Meat	4	catfish	4 ounces
	Vegetable	2	collards	4 cups
Meal 4	Meat (Nut)	1	almonds	⅛ cup
	Vegetable	1	cucumber	2 cups
Meal 5	Meat	4	turkey	4 ounces
Meal 6	Meat	12	chicken	12 ounces
	Vegetable	3	romaine lettuce	9 cups
Meal 7	Fruit	1	plum	2 items

Week 8

	Category	Exchanges	Sample food	Quantity
Meal 1	Bread	3	potato	1½ cups
	Fruit	1	orange	1 item
	Meat	2	egg white	6 items
Meal 2	Fruit	1	banana	½ item
	Meat (Nut)	1	sesame butter	1 tablespoon
Meal 3	Bread	1½	garbanzo beans	⅜ cup
	Meat	6	chicken	6 ounces
	Vegetable	2	romaine lettuce	6 cups
Meal 4	Fruit	1	mango	½ item
	Meat (Nut)	1	avocado	⅓ item
Meal 5	Meat	2	tuna	4 ounces
Meal 6	Meat	12	sirloin	12 ounces
	Vegetable	3	spinach	6 cups
Meal 7	Fruit	1	pear	1 item

Week 9

Category	Exchanges	Sample food	Quantity
Meal 1			
Fruit	2	mango	1 item
Shake	2	whey protein shake	2 scoops
Meal 2			
Meat (Nut)	1	cashews	⅛ cup
Vegetable	1	carrots	½ cup
Meal 3			
Bread	1½	corn	¾ cup
Meat	6	chicken	6 ounces
Vegetable	2	summer squash	2 cups
Meal 4			
Fruit	1	apple	1 item
Meat (Nut)	1	peanut butter	1 tablespoon
Meal 5			
Meat	2	turkey	2 ounces
Meal 6			
Meat	12	turkey	12 ounces
Vegetable	3	mushrooms	6 cups

Week 10

Category	Exchanges	Sample food	Quantity
Meal 1			
Bread	3	oatmeal	1½ cups
Fruit	1	blueberries	1 cup
Meat	2	egg	2 items
Meal 2			
Fruit	1	banana	½ item
Meat (Nut)	1	almond butter	1 tablespoon
Meal 3			
Bread	1½	tortilla	1½ items
Meat	4	flank steak	4 ounces
Vegetable	2	peppers	2 cups
Meal 4			
Bread	1½	white rice	½ cup
Meat	4	tuna	8 ounces
Meal 5			
Fruit	1	walnuts	⅛ cup
Meat (Nut)	1	pear	1 item
Meal 6			
Meat	12	turkey	12 ounces
Vegetable	3	green beans	3 cups

Week 11

Category	Exchanges	Sample food	Quantity
Meal 1			
Bread	3	bran flakes	1½ cups
Fruit	1	peach	2 small items
Meat	2	egg white	6 items
Meal 2			
Fruit	1	cherries	½ cup
Meat (Nut)	1	pumpkin seeds	⅛ cup

Meal 3	Bread	1½	lentil	½ cup
	Meat	6	chicken	6 ounces
	Vegetable	2	carrots	1 cup
Meal 4	Bread	1½	whole wheat crackers	1½ ounces
	Meat	2	tuna	4 ounces
Meal 5	Meat (Nut)	1	peanut butter	1 tablespoon
	Vegetable	1	celery	2 cups
Meal 6	Meat	12	salmon	12 ounces
	Vegetable	3	asparagus	3 cups

Week 12

	Category	Exchanges	Sample food	Quantity
Meal 1	Bread	3	corn grits	1½ cups
	Fruit	1	grapefruit	1 item
	Meat	2	egg	2 items
Meal 2	Fruit	1	apple	1 item
	Meat (Nut)	1	peanut butter	1 tablespoon
Meal 3	Bread	1½	split peas	½ cup
	Meat	4	chicken	4 ounces
	Vegetable	2	spinach	4 cups
Meal 4	Bread	1½	tortilla	1½ items
	Meat	2	chicken	2 ounces
Meal 5	Meat (Nut)	1	soynut butter	1 tablespoon
	Vegetable	1	jicama	½ cup
Meal 6	Bread	1½	potato, baked	½ item
	Meat	12	halibut	24 ounces
	Vegetable	3	broccoli	3 cups
Meal 7	Fruit	1	orange	1 item

Level 9

Week 1

	Category	Exchanges	Sample food	Quantity
Meal 1	Bread	4	bagel	1⅓ items
	Fruit	1	cantaloupe	½ item
	Meat	2	egg	2 items
Meal 2	Fruit	1	apple	1 item
	Meat (Nut)	1	peanut butter	1 tablespoon
Meal 3	Bread	3	pita	1½ items
	Meat	8	turkey	8 ounces
	Vegetable	1	romaine lettuce	3 cups

Meal 4	Fruit	I	plum	2 items
	Meat (Nut)	I	almonds	⅛ cup
Meal 5	Fruit	I	watermelon	I cup
	Meat	2	turkey	2 ounces
Meal 6	Bread	3	baked potato	I item
	Meat	8	salmon	8 ounces
	Vegetable	2	spinach	4 cups
Meal 7	Bread	2	popcorn	2 cups
	Fruit	2	pear	2 items

Week 2

	Category	Exchanges	Sample food	Quantity
Meal I	Bread	4	oatmeal	2 cups
	Fruit	I	banana	½ item
	Meat	2	egg white	6 items
Meal 2	Fruit	I	peach	2 small items
	Meat (Nut)	I	cashews	⅛ cup
Meal 3	Bread	3	white rice	I cup
	Meat	8	tuna	16 ounces
	Vegetable	I	tomato	I item
Meal 4	Fruit	I	apple	I item
	Meat (Nut)	I	peanut butter	I tablespoon
Meal 5	Fruit	I	nectarine	I item
	Meat	2	turkey	2 ounces
Meal 6	Bread	3	corn	I½ cups
	Meat	8	chicken breast	8 ounces
	Vegetable	2	green beans	2 cups
Meal 7	Bread	2	whole wheat crackers	2 ounces
	Fruit	2	strawberries	3 cups

Week 3

	Category	Exchanges	Sample food	Quantity
Meal I	Bread	4	bran flakes	2 cups
	Fruit	I	raspberries	I cup
	Meat	2	egg	2 items
Meal 2	Fruit	I	watermelon	I cup
	Meat (Nut)	I	cashews	⅛ cup
Meal 3	Bread	3	white rice	I cup
	Meat	8	shrimp	16 ounces
	Vegetable	I	zucchini	I cup

Meal 4	Fruit	I	apple	I item
	Meat (Nut)	I	almond butter	I tablespoon
Meal 5	Fruit	I	papaya	½ item
	Meat	4	turkey	4 ounces
Meal 6	Bread	I½	tortilla	I½ items
	Meat	8	flank steak	8 ounces
	Vegetable	2	peppers	2 cups
Meal 7	Bread	2	popcorn	2 cups
	Fruit	2	orange	2 items

Week 4

	Category	Exchanges	Sample food	Quantity
Meal I	Bread	3	cream of wheat	I½ cups
	Fruit	I	grapefruit	I item
	Meat	3	egg white	9 items
Meal 2	Fruit	I	grapes	I cup
	Meat (Nut)	I	walnuts	⅛ cup
Meal 3	Bread	3	kidney beans	I cup
	Meat	8	tuna	16 ounces
	Vegetable	I	romaine lettuce	3 cups
Meal 4	Fruit	I	apricot	3 items
	Meat (Nut)	I	Brazil nuts	⅛ cup
Meal 5	Fruit	I	melon, honeydew	⅙ item
	Meat	4	tuna	8 ounces
Meal 6	Bread	I½	couscous	¾ cup
	Meat	8	chicken	8 ounces
	Vegetable	3	tomato	3 items
Meal 7	Bread	2	rice cakes	4 items
	Fruit	2	applesauce	I cup

Week 5

	Category	Exchanges	Sample food	Quantity
Meal I	Bread	3	oatmeal	I½ cups
	Fruit	I	blueberries	I cup
	Meat	3	egg	3 items
Meal 2	Fruit	I	pear	I item
	Meat (Nut)	I	almonds	⅛ cup
Meal 3	Bread	3	corn tortilla	3 items
	Meat	8	chicken	8 ounces
	Vegetable	I	peppers	I cup

Meal 4	Fruit	1	banana	½ item
	Meat (Nut)	1	peanut butter	1 tablespoon
Meal 5	Fruit	1	grapes	1 cup
	Meat	4	turkey	4 ounces
Meal 6	Meat	12	whitefish	24 ounces
	Vegetable	3	spinach	6 cups
Meal 7	Bread	1	whole wheat crackers	1 ounce
	Fruit	1	peach	2 small items

Week 6

	Category	Exchanges	Sample food	Quantity
Meal 1	Bread	3	shredded wheat	3 large biscuits
	Fruit	1	strawberries	1½ cups
	Meat	3	egg white	9 items
Meal 2	Fruit	1	cherries	½ cup
Meal 3	Bread	3	artichoke	3 items
	Meat	8	salmon	8 ounces
	Vegetable	1	asparagus	1 cup
Meal 4	Fruit	1	apricot	3 items
	Meat (Nut)	1	Brazil nuts	⅛ cup
Meal 5	Meat (Nut)	1	peanut butter	1 tablespoon
	Vegetable	1	celery	2 cups
Meal 6	Bread	1½	pasta	1½ ounces
	Meat	12	chicken	12 ounces
	Vegetable	3	broccoli	3 cups
Meal 7	Fruit	1	applesauce	½ cup

Week 7

	Category	Exchanges	Sample food	Quantity
Meal 1	Bread	3	cream of rice	1½ cups
	Fruit	1	banana	½ item
	Meat	3	egg	3 items
Meal 2	Fruit	1	apple	1 item
	Meat (Nut)	1	peanut butter	1 tablespoon
Meal 3	Bread	1½	yams	½ cup
	Meat	4	catfish	4 ounces
	Vegetable	2	collards	4 cups
Meal 4	Bread	1½	potato	¾ cup
	Meat	4	turkey	4 ounces
	Vegetable	1	beets	½ cup

Meal 5	Meat (Nut)	1	almonds	⅛ cup
	Vegetable	1	jicama	½ cup
Meal 6	Bread	1½	black beans	½ cup
	Meat	12	chicken	12 ounces
	Vegetable	3	romaine lettuce	9 cups
Meal 7	Fruit	1	plum	2 items

Week 8

	Category	Exchanges	Sample food	Quantity
Meal 1	Bread	3	bran flakes	1½ cups
	Fruit	1	orange	1 item
	Meat	3	egg white	9 items
Meal 2	Fruit	1	banana	½ item
	Meat (Nut)	1	sesame butter	1 tablespoon
Meal 3	Bread	1½	garbanzo beans	⅜ cup
	Meat	4	chicken	4 ounces
	Vegetable	2	romaine lettuce	6 cups
Meal 4	Bread	1½	rice cakes	3 items
	Meat	4	tuna	8 ounces
	Vegetable	1	celery	2 cups
Meal 5	Fruit	1	papaya	½ item
	Meat (Nut)	1	avocado	⅓ item
Meal 6	Meat	12	sirloin	12 ounces
	Vegetable	3	tomato	3 items
Meal 7	Bread	1	popcorn	1 cup
	Fruit	2	applesauce	1 cup

Week 9

	Category	Exchanges	Sample food	Quantity
Meal 1	Fruit	2	mango	1 item
	Shake	2	whey protein shake	2 scoops
Meal 2	Fruit	1	orange	1 item
	Meat (Nut)	1	cashews	⅛ cup
Meal 3	Bread	1½	brown rice	½ cup
	Meat	4	chicken	4 ounces
	Vegetable	2	summer squash	2 cups
Meal 4	Bread	1½	white rice	½ cup
	Meat	4	crab	8 ounces
	Vegetable	1	cucumber	2 cups

	Category	Exchanges	Sample food	Quantity
Meal 5	Fruit	1	apple	1 item
	Meat (Nut)	1	peanut butter	1 tablespoon
Meal 6	Meat	12	turkey	12 ounces
	Vegetable	3	mushrooms	6 cups
Meal 7	Bread	1	rice cakes	2 items
	Fruit	2	kiwi	4 items

Week 10

	Category	Exchanges	Sample food	Quantity
Meal 1	Fruit	2	banana	1 item
	Shake	2	whey protein shake	2 scoops
Meal 2	Fruit	1	apple	1 item
	Meat (Nut)	1	almond butter	1 tablespoon
Meal 3	Bread	1½	tortilla	1½ items
	Meat	4	flank steak	4 ounces
	Vegetable	1	peppers	1 cup
Meal 4	Bread	1½	corn tortilla	1½ items
	Meat	4	pollack	8 ounces
	Vegetable	1	cabbage	2 cups
Meal 5	Fruit	1	pear	1 item
	Meat (Nut)	1	pecans	⅛ cup
Meal 6	Bread	1½	corn	¾ cup
	Meat	12	turkey	12 ounces
	Vegetable	3	green beans	3 cups
Meal 7	Fruit	2	grapes	2 cups

Week 11

	Category	Exchanges	Sample food	Quantity
Meal 1	Bread	3	bran flakes	1½ cups
	Fruit	1	banana	½ item
	Meat	3	egg	3 items
Meal 2	Fruit	1	cherries	½ cup
	Meat (Nut)	1	pumpkin seeds	⅛ cup
Meal 3	Bread	1½	lentil	½ cup
	Meat	8	chicken	8 ounces
	Vegetable	2	carrots	1 cup
Meal 4	Bread	1½	whole wheat crackers	1½ ounces
	Meat	2	tuna	4 ounces
Meal 5	Meat (Nut)	1	peanut butter	1 tablespoon
	Vegetable	1	jicama	½ cup

Meal 6	Bread	1½	potato, baked	½ item
	Meat	12	salmon	12 ounces
	Vegetable	2	asparagus	2 cups

Week 12

	Category	Exchanges	Sample food	Quantity
Meal 1	Bread	3	bran flakes	1½ cups
	Fruit	1	blueberries	1 cup
	Meat	3	egg white	9 items
Meal 2	Fruit	1	apple	1 item
	Meat (Nut)	1	peanut butter	1 tablespoon
Meal 3	Bread	1½	split peas	½ cup
	Meat	8	chicken	8 ounces
	Vegetable	2	spinach	4 cups
Meal 4	Bread	1½	rice cakes	3 items
	Meat	2	turkey	2 ounces
Meal 5	Fruit	1	banana	½ item
	Meat (Nut)	1	soynut butter	1 tablespoon
Meal 6	Bread	1½	wild rice	½ cup
	Meat	12	halibut	24 ounces
	Vegetable	3	Brussels sprouts	3 cups
Meal 7	Fruit	2	figs	2 large items

Level 10

Week 1

	Category	Exchanges	Sample food	Quantity
Meal 1	Bread	4	bagel	1⅓ items
	Fruit	1	cantaloupe	½ item
	Meat	3	egg	3 items
Meal 2	Fruit	1	apple	1 item
	Meat (Nut)	1	peanut butter	1 tablespoon
Meal 3	Bread	3	pita	1½ items
	Meat	8	turkey	8 ounces
	Vegetable	1	romaine lettuce	3 cups
Meal 4	Fruit	1	plum	2 items
	Meat (Nut)	1	almonds	⅛ cup
Meal 5	Fruit	1	mango	½ item
	Meat	2	turkey	2 ounces

Meal 6	Bread	3	baked potato	1 item
	Meat	12	salmon	12 ounces
	Vegetable	2	spinach	4 cups
Meal 7	Bread	2	popcorn	2 cups
	Fruit	2	pear	2 items

Week 2

	Category	Exchanges	Sample food	Quantity
Meal 1	Bread	4	oatmeal	2 cups
	Fruit	1	banana	½ item
	Meat	3	egg white	9 items
Meal 2	Fruit	1	peach	2 small items
	Meat (Nut)	1	cashews	⅛ cup
Meal 3	Bread	3	white rice	1 cup
	Meat	8	tuna	16 ounces
	Vegetable	1	tomato	1 item
Meal 4	Fruit	1	apple	1 item
	Meat (Nut)	1	peanut butter	1 tablespoon
Meal 5	Fruit	1	nectarine	1 item
	Meat	2	turkey	2 ounces
Meal 6	Bread	3	corn	1½ cups
	Meat	12	chicken	12 ounces
	Vegetable	2	green beans	2 cups
Meal 7	Bread	2	whole wheat crackers	2 ounces
	Fruit	2	strawberries	3 cups

Week 3

	Category	Exchanges	Sample food	Quantity
Meal 1	Bread	4	bran flakes	2 cups
	Fruit	1	raspberries	1 cup
	Meat	3	egg	3 items
Meal 2	Fruit	1	watermelon	1 cup
	Meat (Nut)	1	Brazil nuts	⅛ cup
Meal 3	Bread	3	white rice	1 cup
	Meat	8	shrimp	16 ounces
	Vegetable	1	zucchini	1 cup
Meal 4	Fruit	1	apple	1 item
	Meat (Nut)	1	almond butter	1 tablespoon
Meal 5	Fruit	1	pear	1 item
	Meat	4	tuna	8 ounces

Meal 6	Bread	3	tortilla	3 items
	Meat	12	flank steak	12 ounces
	Vegetable	2	peppers	2 cups
Meal 7	Bread	1	popcorn	1 cup
	Fruit	1	orange	1 item

Week 4

	Category	Exchanges	Sample food	Quantity
Meal 1	Bread	4	cream of wheat	2 cups
	Fruit	1	grapefruit	1 item
	Meat	3	egg white	9 items
Meal 2	Fruit	1	grapes	1 cup
	Meat (Nut)	1	walnuts	⅛ cup
Meal 3	Bread	3	couscous	1½ cups
	Meat	8	chicken	8 ounces
	Vegetable	1	tomato	1 item
Meal 4	Fruit	1	apricot	3 items
	Meat (Nut)	1	Brazil nuts	⅛ cup
Meal 5	Fruit	1	melon, cantaloupe	½ item
	Meat	4	tuna	8 ounces
Meal 6	Bread	1½	wild rice	½ cup
	Meat	12	salmon	12 ounces
	Vegetable	2	asparagus	2 cups
Meal 7	Bread	1	rice cakes	2 items
	Fruit	2	papaya	1 item

Week 5

	Category	Exchanges	Sample food	Quantity
Meal 1	Bread	4	oatmeal	2 cups
	Fruit	1	blueberries	1 cup
	Meat	3	egg	3 items
Meal 2	Fruit	1	pear	1 item
	Meat (Nut)	1	almonds	⅛ cup
Meal 3	Bread	1½	corn tortilla	1½ items
	Meat	8	chicken	8 ounces
	Vegetable	1	peppers	1 cup
Meal 4	Bread	1½	whole wheat crackers	1½ ounces
	Meat (Nut)	1	peanut butter	1 tablespoon
Meal 5	Fruit	1	cranberries	1 cup
	Meat	4	turkey	4 ounces

Meal 6	Bread	1½	lentils	½ cup
	Meat	12	whitefish	24 ounces
	Vegetable	2	spinach	4 cups
Meal 7	Fruit	1	pear	1 item

Week 6

	Category	Exchanges	Sample food	Quantity
Meal 1	Bread	3	shredded wheat	3 large biscuits
	Fruit	1	strawberries	1½ cups
	Meat	4	egg white	12 items
Meal 2	Fruit	1	papaya	½ item
	Meat (Nut)	1	avocado	⅓ item
Meal 3	Bread	1½	artichoke	1½ items
	Meat	8	salmon	8 ounces
	Vegetable	1	spinach	2 cups
Meal 4	Bread	1½	rice cakes	3 items
	Meat (Nut)	1	almond butter	1 tablespoon
Meal 5	Fruit	1	melon, canteloupe	½ item
	Meat	4	tuna	8 ounces
Meal 6	Bread	1½	pasta	1½ ounces
	Meat	12	chicken	12 ounces
	Vegetable	2	broccoli	2 cups
Meal 7	Fruit	1	plum	2 items

Week 7

	Category	Exchanges	Sample food	Quantity
Meal 1	Bread	3	cream of rice	1½ cups
	Fruit	1	raspberries	1 cup
	Meat	4	egg	4 items
Meal 2	Fruit	1	banana	½ item
	Meat (Nut)	1	peanut butter	1 tablespoon
Meal 3	Bread	1½	yams	½ cup
	Meat	8	catfish	8 ounces
	Vegetable	1	collards	2 cups
Meal 4	Bread	1½	white rice	½ cup
	Meat (Nut)	1	almonds	⅛ cup
Meal 5	Fruit	1	mango	½ item
	Meat	4	turkey	4 ounces
Meal 6	Meat	16	chicken	16 ounces
	Vegetable	2	romaine lettuce	6 cups

Week 8

Category	Exchanges	Sample food	Quantity
Meal 1			
Bread	3	potato	1½ cups
Fruit	1	orange	1 item
Meat	4	egg white	12 items
Meal 2			
Meat (Nut)	1	sesame butter	1 tablespoon
Vegetable	1	celery	2 cups
Meal 3			
Bread	1½	garbanzo beans	⅜ cup
Meat	8	chicken	8 ounces
Vegetable	1	romaine lettuce	3 cups
Meal 4			
Bread	1½	white rice	½ cup
Meat	2	tuna	4 ounces
Meal 5			
Fruit	1	papaya	½ item
Meat (Nut)	1	avocado	⅓ item
Meal 6			
Meat	16	sirloin	16 ounces
Vegetable	2	tomato	2 items
Meal 7			
Bread	2	popcorn	2 cups
Fruit	2	applesauce	1 cup

Week 9

Category	Exchanges	Sample food	Quantity
Meal 1			
Fruit	2	blueberries	2 cups
Shake	2	whey protein shake	2 scoops
Meal 2			
Fruit	1	cherries	½ cup
Meat (Nut)	1	cashews	⅛ cup
Meal 3			
Bread	1½	pasta	1½ ounces
Meat	8	chicken	8 ounces
Vegetable	1	tomato	1 item
Meal 4			
Bread	1½	whole wheat crackers	1½ ounces
Meat	2	tuna	4 ounces
Meal 5			
Fruit	1	apple	1 item
Meat (Nut)	1	peanut butter	1 tablespoon
Meal 6			
Meat	16	turkey	16 ounces
Vegetable	2	mushrooms	4 cups
Meal 7			
Bread	2	popcorn	2 cups
Fruit	2	kiwi	4 items

Week 10

Category	Exchanges	Sample food	Quantity
Meal 1			
Bread	3	Grapenuts	¾ cup
Fruit	1	banana	½ item
Meat	4	egg	4 items

Meal 2	Fruit	1	apple	1 item
	Meat (Nut)	1	almond butter	1 tablespoon
Meal 3	Bread	1½	corn tortilla	1½ items
	Meat	8	flank steak	8 ounces
	Vegetable	1	peppers	1 cup
Meal 4	Bread	1½	white rice	½ cup
	Meat	2	crab	4 ounces
Meal 5	Fruit	1	pear	1 item
	Meat (Nut)	1	walnuts	⅛ cup
Meal 6	Bread	1½	wild rice	½ cup
	Meat	16	snapper	32 ounces
	Vegetable	2	green beans	2 cups

Week 11	**Category**	**Exchanges**	**Sample food**	**Quantity**
Meal 1	Fruit	2	mango	1 item
	Shake	2	whey protein shake	2 scoops
Meal 2	Fruit	1	melon, honeydew	⅙ item
	Meat (Nut)	1	pumpkin seeds	⅛ cup
Meal 3	Bread	1½	lentil	½ cup
	Meat	8	chicken	8 ounces
	Vegetable	1	carrots	½ cup
Meal 4	Bread	1½	couscous	¾ cup
	Meat	4	chicken	4 ounces
Meal 5	Meat (Nut)	1	peanut butter	1 tablespoon
	Vegetable	1	celery	2 cups
Meal 6	Bread	1½	corn	¾ cup
	Meat	16	salmon	16 ounces
	Vegetable	2	asparagus	2 cups

Week 12	**Category**	**Exchanges**	**Sample food**	**Quantity**
Meal 1	Bread	3	bran flakes	1½ cups
	Fruit	1	grapes	1 cup
	Meat	4	egg white	12 items
Meal 2	Fruit	1	banana	½ item
	Meat (Nut)	1	peanut butter	1 tablespoon
Meal 3	Bread	1½	split peas	½ cup
	Meat	8	chicken	8 ounces
	Vegetable	1	spinach	2 cups

Meal 4	Bread	1½	whole wheat crackers	1½ ounces
	Meat	4	turkey	4 ounces
Meal 5	Fruit	1	apple	1 item
	Meat (Nut)	1	soynut butter	1 tablespoon
Meal 6	Bread	1½	brown rice	½ cup
	Meat	16	halibut	32 ounces
	Vegetable	2	Brussels sprouts	2 cups
Meal 7	Fruit	1	figs	1 large item

Level 11

Week 1

	Category	Exchanges	Sample food	Quantity
Meal 1	Bread	4	bagel	1⅓ items
	Fruit	2	cantaloupe	1 item
	Meat	3	egg	3 items
Meal 2	Fruit	1	apple	1 item
	Meat (Nut)	1	peanut butter	1 tablespoon
Meal 3	Bread	3	pita	1½ items
	Meat	8	turkey	8 ounces
	Vegetable	1	romaine lettuce	3 cups
Meal 4	Fruit	1	plum	2 items
	Meat (Nut)	1	almonds	⅛ cup
Meal 5	Fruit	1	watermelon	1 cup
	Meat	4	turkey	4 ounces
Meal 6	Bread	3	baked potato	1 item
	Meat	12	salmon	12 ounces
	Vegetable	2	spinach	4 cups
Meal 7	Bread	2	popcorn	2 cups
	Fruit	2	pear	2 items

Week 2

	Category	Exchanges	Sample food	Quantity
Meal 1	Bread	4	oatmeal	2 cups
	Fruit	2	banana	1 item
	Meat	3	egg white	9 items
Meal 2	Fruit	1	peach	2 small items
	Meat (Nut)	1	cashews	⅛ cup
Meal 3	Bread	3	white rice	1 cup
	Meat	8	tuna	16 ounces
	Vegetable	1	tomato	1 item

Meal 4	Fruit	1	apple	1 item
	Meat (Nut)	1	peanut butter	1 tablespoon
Meal 5	Fruit	1	nectarine	1 item
	Meat	4	turkey	4 ounces
Meal 6	Bread	3	corn	1½ cups
	Meat	12	chicken	12 ounces
	Vegetable	2	green beans	2 cups
Meal 7	Bread	2	whole wheat crackers	2 ounces
	Fruit	2	strawberries	3 cups

Week 3

	Category	Exchanges	Sample food	Quantity
Meal 1	Bread	4	bran flakes	2 cups
	Fruit	2	raspberries	2 cups
	Meat	4	egg	4 items
Meal 2	Fruit	1	watermelon	1 cup
	Meat (Nut)	1	cashews	⅛ cup
Meal 3	Bread	3	white rice	1 cup
	Meat	8	shrimp	16 ounces
	Vegetable	1	zucchini	1 cup
Meal 4	Fruit	1	apple	1 item
	Meat (Nut)	1	almond butter	1 tablespoon
Meal 5	Fruit	1	pear	1 item
	Meat	4	tuna	8 ounces
Meal 6	Bread	3	tortilla	3 items
	Meat	16	flank steak	16 ounces
	Vegetable	2	peppers	2 cups
Meal 7	Bread	2	popcorn	2 cups
	Fruit	2	orange	2 items

Week 4

	Category	Exchanges	Sample food	Quantity
Meal 1	Bread	4	cream of wheat	2 cups
	Fruit	2	grapefruit	2 items
	Meat	4	egg white	12 items
Meal 2	Fruit	1	grapes	1 cup
	Meat (Nut)	1	walnuts	⅛ cup
Meal 3	Bread	3	couscous	1½ cups
	Meat	8	chicken	8 ounces
	Vegetable	1	tomato	1 item

Meal 4	Fruit	I	apricot	3 items
	Meat (Nut)	I	Brazil nuts	⅛ cup
Meal 5	Meat	4	tuna	8 ounces
	Vegetable	I	celery	2 cups
Meal 6	Bread	3	wild rice	I cup
	Meat	16	salmon	16 ounces
	Vegetable	2	asparagus	2 cups
Meal 7	Bread	2	papaya	I item
	Fruit	2	rice cakes	4 items

Week 5

	Category	Exchanges	Sample food	Quantity
Meal I	Bread	4	oatmeal	2 cups
	Fruit	2	blueberries	2 cups
	Meat	4	egg	4 items
Meal 2	Fruit	I	pear	I item
	Meat (Nut)	I	almonds	⅛ cup
Meal 3	Bread	3	corn tortilla	3 items
	Meat	8	chicken	8 ounces
	Vegetable	I	peppers	I cup
Meal 4	Fruit	I	banana	½ item
	Meat (Nut)	I	peanut butter	I tablespoon
Meal 5	Meat	4	turkey	4 ounces
	Vegetable	I	eggplant	I cup
Meal 6	Bread	1½	potato	¾ cup
	Meat	16	whitefish	32 ounces
	Vegetable	3	spinach	6 cups
Meal 7	Bread	2	granola	¼ cup
	Fruit	2	pear	2 items

Week 6

	Category	Exchanges	Sample food	Quantity
Meal I	Bread	4	shredded wheat	4 large biscuits
	Fruit	2	strawberries	3 cups
	Meat	4	egg white	12 items
Meal 2	Fruit	I	papaya	½ item
	Meat (Nut)	I	avocado	⅓ item
Meal 3	Bread	1½	artichoke	1½ items
	Meat	8	salmon	8 ounces
	Vegetable	2	spinach	4 cups

Meal 4	Bread	1½	whole wheat crackers	1½ ounces
	Meat	4	turkey	4 ounces
Meal 5	Fruit	1	apple	1 item
	Meat (Nut)	1	almond butter	1 tablespoon
Meal 6	Bread	1½	pasta	1½ ounces
	Meat	16	chicken	16 ounces
	Vegetable	3	broccoli	3 cups
Meal 7	Bread	1	popcorn	1 cup
	Fruit	2	plum	4 items

Week 7

	Category	Exchanges	Sample food	Quantity
Meal 1	Bread	4	cream of rice	2 cups
	Fruit	2	banana	1 item
	Meat	4	egg	4 items
Meal 2	Fruit	1	apple	1 item
	Meat (Nut)	1	peanut butter	1 tablespoon
Meal 3	Bread	1½	yams	½ cup
	Meat	8	catfish	8 ounces
	Vegetable	2	collards	4 cups
Meal 4	Bread	1½	navy beans	½ cup
	Meat	4	tuna	8 ounces
Meal 5	Fruit	2	cherries	1 cup
	Meat (Nut)	2	almonds	¼ cup
Meal 6	Meat	16	chicken	16 ounces
	Vegetable	3	romaine lettuce	9 cups
Meal 7	Fruit	1	applesauce	½ cup

Week 8

	Category	Exchanges	Sample food	Quantity
Meal 1	Bread	4	bran flakes	2 cups
	Fruit	2	strawberries	3 cups
	Meat	4	egg white	12 items
Meal 2	Fruit	1	papaya	½ item
	Meat (Nut)	1	sunflower seeds	⅛ cup
Meal 3	Bread	1½	garbanzo beans	⅜ cup
	Meat	8	chicken	8 ounces
	Vegetable	2	romaine lettuce	6 cups
Meal 4	Bread	1½	white rice	½ cup
	Meat	4	crab	8 ounces

Meal 5	Fruit	1	banana	½ item
	Meat (Nut)	2	cashew butter	2 tablespoons
Meal 6	Bread	1½	potato, baked	½ item
	Meat	16	sirloin	16 ounces
	Vegetable	2	tomato	2 items

Week 9

	Category	Exchanges	Sample food	Quantity
Meal 1	Bread	4	oatmeal	2 cups
	Fruit	2	melon, cantaloupe	1 item
	Meat	4	turkey	4 ounces
Meal 2	Fruit	1	mango	½ item
	Meat (Nut)	1	avocado	⅓ item
Meal 3	Bread	1½	lentils	½ cup
	Meat	8	chicken	8 ounces
	Vegetable	2	tomato	2 items
Meal 4	Bread	1½	rice cakes	3 items
	Meat	4	tuna	8 ounces
Meal 5	Fruit	1	apple	1 item
	Meat (Nut)	2	peanut butter	2 tablespoons
Meal 6	Meat	16	turkey	16 ounces
	Vegetable	3	mushrooms	6 cups
Meal 7	Fruit	1	strawberries	1½ cups

Week 10

	Category	Exchanges	Sample food	Quantity
Meal 1	Fruit	2	mango	1 item
	Shake	2	whey protein shake	2 scoops
Meal 2	Fruit	1	apricot	3 items
	Meat (Nut)	1	almonds	⅛ cup
Meal 3	Bread	1½	tortilla	1½ items
	Meat	8	flank steak	8 ounces
	Vegetable	2	peppers	2 cups
Meal 4	Bread	1½	couscous	¾ cup
	Meat	4	chicken	4 ounces
Meal 5	Meat (Nut)	2	olives	40 items
	Vegetable	1	cucumbers	2 cups
Meal 6	Meat	16	turkey	16 ounces
	Vegetable	2	green beans	2 cups

Week 11

Category	Exchanges	Sample food	Quantity
Meal 1			
Bread	3	corn grits	1½ cups
Fruit	2	grapefruit	2 items
Meat	4	egg	4 items
Meal 2			
Fruit	1	grapes	1 cup
Meat (Nut)	1	pumpkin seeds	⅛ cup
Meal 3			
Bread	1½	winter squash	¾ cup
Meat	8	sea bass	16 ounces
Vegetable	2	asparagus	2 cups
Meal 4			
Bread	1½	corn	¾ cup
Meat	4	chicken	4 ounces
Meal 5			
Meat (Nut)	2	peanut butter	2 tablespoons
Vegetable	1	jicama	½ cup
Meal 6			
Meat	16	halibut	32 ounces
Vegetable	3	Brussels sprouts	3 cups
Meal 7			
Fruit	1	applesauce	½ cup

Week 12

Category	Exchanges	Sample food	Quantity
Meal 1			
Bread	3	bran flakes	1½ cups
Fruit	2	banana	1 item
Meat	4	turkey	4 ounces
Meal 2			
Fruit	1	melon, honeydew	⅙ item
Meat (Nut)	1	sunflower seeds	⅛ cup
Meal 3			
Bread	1½	lentil	½ cup
Meat	8	chicken	8 ounces
Vegetable	2	carrots	1 cup
Meal 4			
Bread	1½	pasta	1½ ounces
Meat	4	ground beef	4 ounces
Meal 5			
Fruit	1	soynut butter	1 tablespoon
Meat (Nut)	1	apple	1 item
Meal 6			
Bread	1½	potato	¾ cup
Meat	16	turkey	16 ounces
Vegetable	3	cabbage	6 cups
Meal 7			
Fruit	1	figs	1 large item

Appendix A

Food List to Determine a 3-Day Caloric Average

This list is to be used before beginning the Turn Up the Heat program. Use this list to calculate your current calories for three days, then determine the average. The list is based on visual references of the foods you eat. It will be accurate within 10 percent of your caloric intake, which is accurate enough for our purposes.

Here are the types of lists you have to work with:

- Restaurant Meals
- Packaged, Canned, and Frozen Foods
- Breakfast Meals
- Lunch Meals
- Fast Foods
- Snacks (including energy bars, protein bars, etc.)
- Desserts
- Itemized source list for many common **single-ingredient foods,** such as chicken breast, fruit, breads, cheese, and many others. This list includes caloric additions for common cooking methods.

Foods in the single-ingredient food list are all based on grill/broil-type cooking methods. There is also a list for caloric adjustments to add calories for frying, sautéing in oil or butter, sauces, and so on.

The serving sizes in the single-ingredient food list are shown.

Serving sizes in the restaurant list are based on normal restaurant portions. If you usually eat half of your meal, modify the calories of that meal accordingly.

Here's how to use the lists:

- First, see if what you're looking for falls under one of the main-category lists. If you cooked the meal yourself, you can still look under the restaurant list. If you think your serving was smaller than typical restaurant servings, just lower the calories by 25 percent.
- If you can't find what you're looking for, use the single-ingredient food list to pick out the ingredients in your meal.

Single-Ingredient Food List

Item	Portion Size	Calories
Fruits		
apples, oranges	whole fruit	75
melons or other cut fruit	1 cup	75
berries	1 cup	75
fruit juice	1 cup	100
dried fruit (raisins, etc.)	¼ cup	125
Vegetables		
any lettuce	2 cups	30
any leafy vegetable	1 cup	30
cut-up vegetables	1 cup	30
Additional calories to add:		
salad dressing or dip	1 tablespoon	100
low-fat or fat-free dressing or dip	1 tablespoon	30
sautéed in oil or butter		150
if deep-fried, add		150
Starchy Vegetables		
corn	½ cup	75
potatoes	½ cup	60
baked potato	1 whole	150
winter squash	½ cup	70
peas	½ cup	60
artichoke hearts	½ cup	40
yams or sweet potato	½ cup	90
Additional calories to add:		
butter or margarine, whipped	1 tablespoon	70
butter or margarine, regular	1 tablespoon	100
sour cream	1 tablespoon	30
salad dressing or mayo, regular	1 tablespoon	100
salad dressing or mayo, low fat	1 tablespoon	40
Beans/Legumes		
whole, cooked beans (pinto, black, lentils, black eyed peas, navy beans, etc.)	½ cup	110
refried beans	½ cup	130
baked beans	½ cup	150

Grains

rice	½ cup	110
couscous	½ cup	100
wild rice	½ cup	80
bulgur	½ cup	75

Breads and Pastries

bagel (any type)	1 large	300
bread (any grain)	1 regular size slice	70
muffin (any type)	1 jumbo	350
muffin (any type)	1 medium	200
muffin (any type)	1 mini	100
croissant, plain	1	250
croissant, sweet or cheese	1	400
English muffin	1	150
pancakes	Two 4-inch pancakes	100
danish	1	400
scone	1	350
doughnut	1 regular size	150
dinner roll	1	100
tortilla, flour	1 large, burrito size	220
tortilla, flour	1 7″	80
tortilla, corn	1	60
Additional calories to add:		
butter	1 pat	40
cream cheese	1 tablespoon	35
jam or jelly	1 teaspoon	15
peanut butter	1 tablespoon	100
syrup	1 tablespoon	55

Pasta

	1 cup	200
Additional calories to add:		
tomato sauce	½ cup	40
olive oil	1 tablespoon	110
parmesan cheese	1 tablespoon	25

Dairy

cheese, soft (like Brie)	1 cubic inch	60
cheese, medium (Cheddar)	1 cubic inch	70
cheese, hard (parmesan)	1 tablespoon, grated	25

cheese, low fat or fat free	I cubic inch	30
cottage cheese	4 ounces	90
cream cheese, regular	I tablespoon	50
cream cheese, whipped	I tablespoon	35
cream cheese, low fat	I tablespoon	30
cream cheese, fat free	I tablespoon	30
whole milk	½ cup	80
low-fat milk (2%)	½ cup	65
low-fat milk (1%)	½ cup	55
nonfat milk	½ cup	50
yogurt (see package for calories)		

Beef

steak, fatty (porterhouse, prime rib, brisket)	4 ounces	400
steak, lean (flank, round, sirloin, tenderloin, T-bone)	4 ounces	250
ribs	4 ounces	350
ground beef	4 ounces (1 patty)	300
beef and/or pork hot dog	I regular	150
chicken or turkey hot dog	I regular	75

Lamb

fatty	4 ounces	325
lean	4 ounces	225

Pork

fatty	4 ounces	275
lean	4 ounces	225
ham	4 ounces	235
salami	I ounce	75
other lunch meats	See package for calories	

Veal

	4 ounces	275

Poultry

skinless, white meat	4 ounces	130
skinless, dark meat	4 ounces	150
white meat, with skin	4 ounces	225
dark meat, with skin	4 ounces	275

Fish

light fish (halibut, snapper, tuna)	4 ounces	150
oily fish (salmon, herring, sardine, catfish, whitefish)	4 ounces	275

canned tuna (in water)	4 ounces	120
shellfish	4 ounces	100
Additional calories to add:		
mayonnaise	1 tablespoon	100
tartar sauce	1 tablespoon	50

Eggs

whole egg	1	75
egg white	1	15
egg substitute	½ cup	50
Additional calories to add:		
cooked in butter or oil		25

Vegetarian Meat

soy burgers, soy or veggie hot dogs, veggie burgers, etc.: see package for calories.

Other Soy Products

tofu, soft	4 ounces	150
tofu, firm	4 ounces	200
soy protein powder	1 scoop	100

Nuts

any nuts	¼ cup	200
peanut butter	1 tablespoon	100

Additional calories to add to any meat, chicken, seafood, etc.:

breaded and fried	250
cream sauce	200
cooked or dipped in oil or butter	100

Restaurant Meals

Item	Calories
Salad	
small green salad	50
add cheese	75
add nuts	75
add croutons	50
add meat	100
add avocado	100
add salad dressing	75
add corn, beans, peas, or artichoke	75
large green salad	75
add cheese	100
add nuts	100
add croutons	75
add meat	150
add avocado	150
add salad dressing	150
add corn, beans, peas, or artichoke	100
coleslaw; potato, macaroni, or carrot salad	150
tuna, chicken, or egg salad	250
Soup	
broth, pureed vegetable or tomato-based soup	75
add chicken, shrimp, or fish	100
add ham, pork, bacon, or other meat	150
bean soup (split pea, lentil, navy, etc.)	200
cream-based soup	250
Appetizers and Side Dishes	
fried appetizers (one serving)	300
seafood appetizers (not fried)	200
mashed potatoes	150
baked potato	150
scalloped potatoes	250
rice pilaf	150
macaroni and cheese	300
onion rings	250
french fries	250
creamed spinach	250

Additional calories to add:

butter, whipped	1 tablespoon	70
butter, regular	1 tablespoon	100
sour cream	1 tablespoon	30
dipping sauce		75

Italian Food

pasta	300
add tomato and/or vegetable sauce	75
add meat sauce	150
add cream sauce	400
add chicken or seafood	150
add butter or oil	200
lasagna, ravioli, or manicotti	500
chicken, veal, or eggplant parmigiana	600
pizza, cheese (per medium slice)	150
add vegetables only	25
add extra cheese	75
add meat	50
bread, per piece	75
garlic bread, per piece	150

Additional calories to add:

butter, whipped	1 tablespoon	70
butter, regular	1 tablespoon	100
parmesean cheese	1 tablespoon	25

Mexican Food

1 taco, crispy	200
1 taco, soft	150
1 chicken enchilada	200
1 cheese enchilada	250
1 tamale	250
1 tostada or taco salad (with any meat)	500
quesadilla	400
fajitas (just the sautéed meat and vegetables)	250
1 large (empty) burrito	150
add beef, pork, chicken, or fish	150

Additional calories to add:

combo plate (rice, beans, sour cream, guacamole)	500
rice	100

refried beans	150
black beans	100
sour cream	100
guacamole	150
cheese	100
1 corn tortilla	60
1 flour tortilla	75
tortilla chips	200

Chinese Food

dumplings (steamed)	200
dumplings (fried)	300
any fried appetizer (egg rolls, shrimp chips, etc.)	300
Chinese chicken salad	600
Kung Pao chicken	700
Moo Sho chicken or pork	500
any "crispy" entrée	700
fried rice	400
steamed rice	200
stir-fried vegetables	200
chow mein or other noodles	250
Add chicken	200
Add beef	300
Add shrimp	200
Add tofu	150

Japanese Food

sushi, 6 pieces	300
edemame	100
sukiyaki	300
tempura	500
teriyaki chicken or fish	400
soup	150

Middle Eastern and Greek Food

pita bread	200
hummus	200
tabouli	200
spanikopita	300
dolmades (rice-and-meat-stuffed grape leaves)	100 each
gyro sandwich	500

Greek salad (with dressing, cheese, olives)	300
lamb	300
chicken	250
Combination platter, without fried items or heavy cheese	450
Combination platter, with fried items or heavy cheese	650

Packaged, Canned, and Frozen Foods

Cereal, crackers, cookies, chips, protein bars, energy bars, canned soups, canned vegetables, frozen foods—See the package for calories. (See the serving size listed on label and multiply calories by the number of servings that you ate!)

"Mall Food"

popcorn	
small	400
medium	600
large	800
add butter	100
soft pretzel	250
chocolate chip cookie (Mrs. Fields)	1/300
frozen yogurt, sorbet, or low-fat ice cream	150
ice cream	250

Breakfast Meals

two eggs	225
three-egg omelet	300
add vegetables	25
add cheese	100
add sausage or other meat	150
bacon, sausage, or ham	150
steak	250
potatoes (hash browns or home fries)	200
fruit	150
pancakes, waffles, or French toast	350
Add butter, per tablespoon	100
Add syrup, per tablespoon	55
oatmeal	200
add sugar, per teaspoon	15
add raisins	100
add milk	50

Lunch Meals

Sandwiches

bread	250
add turkey or roast beef	250
add ham, salami, other meats	300
add tuna, egg, or chicken salad	400
add bacon	100

add cheese	150
add mayo	100
add avocado	100
add oil	100
add vegetables	50

Fast Foods

Burgers

single patty, regular	275
single patty, large	375
double patty	550
add cheese	100
add mayo or special sauce	100
add bacon	100

Chicken or fish sandwich

grilled chicken	350
fried chicken or fish (crispy)	400
add mayo or sauce	100
add cheese	100

Fried chicken

1 serving of nuggets, strips, or other fried chicken	500

French fries

small order	200
medium order	450
large order	550

Shakes

small	350
large	700

Hot dogs

plain w/bun	250
chili dog	300
chili dog with cheese	350

Breakfast

egg and cheese (bagel) sandwich	450
egg and cheese (English muffin) sandwich	225
Add ham	75
Add bacon	75

Snacks

See label for calorie content!

Desserts

ice cream (light or sorbet)	90
ice cream (regular)	150
ice cream (rich)	250
frozen yogurt	90
cake (light)	150
cake (rich)	250
brownie	1/350
cheesecake	350
fruit pie	250
cream pie	300
candy (see label for calorie content)	

Appendix B

Turn Up the Heat Allowable Food Exchange List

Since some foods, such as fruits and vegetables, can vary widely in size, always choose the medium size. This question arises frequently for foods such as tomatoes, potatoes, avocados, peppers, and many others. For the foods listed below, use the guidelines indicated:

Peppers: All types are permitted (green, yellow, red, orange).
Pita: Choose the large size.
Olives: Always use medium green.
Tortillas: Use burrito size.
Cabbage: All types are permitted; for example, Napa, bok choy, green, red, etc.

Vegetable Category

All measurements are based on UNCOOKED vegetables.

Food	One Exchange = Unit	Cals	Pro (g)	Carb (g)	Fat (g)
alfalfa sprouts	3 cups	36	4.0	3.8	0.6
asparagus	1 cup	39	4.1	4.9	0.3
beets	½ cup	32	1	6.8	0.1
beet greens	3 cups	23	2.6	3	0.06
broccoli	1 cup	23	2.6	3	0.06
Brussels sprouts	1 cup	47	3.3	7.8	0.26
cabbage	2 cups	31	1.7	5.5	0.2
carrots	½ cup	25	0.5	5.5	0.1
cauliflower	1 cup	29	1.9	4.9	0.18
celery	2 cups	44	1.6	8.7	0.28
chard, Swiss or red	4 cups	34	2.6	5.3	0.3
collard or mustard greens	1 cup	43	2.9	7	0.4
cucumber	2 cups	31	1.1	6	0.28
eggplant	1 cup	24	0.9	5	0.08
endive	4 cups	40	2.4	6.7	0.4
fennel	1 cup	27	1.1	6.3	0.2
green beans	1 cup	39	2	7.8	0.01
jicama	½ cup	25	0.8	5.3	0.01
kale	1 cup	40	2.2	6.7	0.47

leeks	½ item	40	0.9	8.7	0.18
lettuce, iceberg	3 cups	30	0.2	6.6	0.36
lettuce, romaine	3 cups	30	2.7	3.9	0.36
mung bean sprouts	I cup	38	3	6	0.2
mushrooms	2 cups	39	2.9	6	0.4
okra	I cup	39	2	7.6	0.1
onions, green	I cup	30	1.7	5.5	0.14
onions, mature	½ cup	28	0.6	5.9	0.21
parsley	I cup	33	2.2	5.1	0.4
parsnips	⅓ cup	36	0.8	7.6	0.26
peppers, chili	½ cup	35	1.5	7	0.15
peppers, sweet	I cup	33	2.2	5.1	0.4
pumpkin	½ cup	28	0.9	6	0.08
sauerkraut	½ cup	25	1.2	4.7	0.17
spinach	2 cups	37	3.6	4.8	0.4
squash, summer	I cup	30	1.4	5.5	0.28
tomato	I items	28	1.1	5.3	0.26
tomato juice	½ cup	26	1.1	5.2	0.1
tomato paste	⅛ cup	31	1.1	6	0.25
turnip greens	2 cups	33	1.6	6	0.34
turnips	I cup	41	1.3	8.6	0.13
water chestnuts	¼ cup	35	0.4	8	0
yellow wax beans	I cup	33	1.8	5.8	0.3
Average of Entire Vegetable Category		34	1.9 g	5.9 g	.25 g
			22%	72%	6%

Fruit Category

All measurements are based on UNCOOKED fruits.

Food	One Exchange = Unit	Cals	Pro (g)	Carb (g)	Fat (g)
apple	I medium	89	0.25	21	0.49
applesauce	½ cup	56	0.2	13.75	0.06
apricot	3 items	56	1.48	11.7	0.41
banana	½ item	60	0.9	13.4	0.27
blackberries	I cup	82	1.04	18.3	0.56
blueberries	I cup	91	0.97	20.5	0.55
boysenberries	I cup	91	0.97	20.5	0.55
cherries	½ cup	58	0.87	12	0.69
cranberries	I cup	49	0.37	12	0

currants	1 cup	79	1.57	17.2	0.45
dates	3 items	84	0.54	20.3	0.12
fig	1 item	52	0.48	12.2	0.09
gooseberries	1 cup	74	1.32	15.2	0.87
grapefruit	1 item	86	1.5	19.4	0.24
grapefruit juice	½ cup	49	0.62	11.35	0.13
grapes	1 cup	68	0.58	15.7	0.32
guava	2 items	94	1.43	20.4	0.7
kiwi	2 items	103	1.5	22.6	0.68
loganberries	1 cup	89	2.23	19	0.46
mango	½ item	75	0.53	17.5	0.28
melon, cantaloupe	½ item	103	2.34	22.3	0.54
melon, casaba	⅙ item	79	2.46	16.6	0.27
melon, honeydew	⅙ item	85	0.98	19.7	0.22
mulberries	1 cup	68	2.02	13.7	0.55
nectarine	1 item	74	1.28	16	0.54
orange	1 item	68	1.23	15.4	0.16
papaya	½ item	66	0.93	15	0.21
passion fruit	4 items	78	1.6	16.84	0.52
peach	2 small	84	1.22	19.3	0.16
pear	1 small	91	0.46	20.9	0.51
persimmon	½ item	65	0.4	15.6	0.15
pineapple	1 cup	85	0.6	19.2	0.66
plantain	½ cup	101	0.96	23.6	0.27
plum	2 small	78	1.04	17.18	0.62
prickly pear	2 items	86	1.5	18.7	0.53
prune	3 items	67	0.65	15.81	0.12
raspberries	1 cup	67	1.11	14.2	0.68
rhubarb	3 cups	86	3.27	16.5	0.72
strawberries	1½ cups	73	1.36	15.6	0.62
tangerines	2 items	82	1.06	18.8	0.32
watermelon	1 cup	56	0.99	11.5	0.68
Average for Entire Fruit Category		76	1.14 g	16.99 g	0.4 g
			6%	89%	5%

Bread Category

All measurements are based on COOKED food (unless otherwise specified).

Food	One Unit Exchange =	Cals	Pro (g)	Carb (g)	Fat (g)
Starchy Veggies					
artichoke	1 medium	77	3.4	15.3	0.26
corn	½ cup	76	2.48	14.5	0.9
popcorn	1 cup	56	1.8	10.7	0.7
potato	½ cup	59	1.6	12.85	0.1
potato, baked	⅓ item	75	1.5	16.9	0.08
squash, winter	½ cup	70	1	16	0.19
yams	⅓ cup	72	1.6	16	0.13
Beans/Legumes/Peas					
black beans	⅓ cup	61	4.4	9.9	0.4
chick peas (garbanzo)	¼ cup	69	3.65	11.25	1.05
kidney beans	⅓ cup	75	4.8	13.2	0.3
lentils	⅓ cup	72	5.2	12.8	0
lima beans	⅓ cup	69	3.8	13	0.18
navy beans	⅓ cup	76	4.9	13.4	0.36
peas, green	½ cup	60	3.95	10.5	0.29
peas, split	⅓ cup	77	5.3	13.8	0.1
soybeans (dried/boiled)	¼ cup	75	7.2	4.3	3.8
soybeans (green/immature)	¼ cup	64	5.6	5	2.9
Bread					
bagel	⅓ large	97	3.67	18.7	0.85
bran muffins	1 small	116	3.1	17.2	3.9
corn bread	1 2″ square	94	3.3	13.1	3.2
cracked wheat	1 slice	61	2	12	0.6
English muffin	½ item	61	2.2	12	0.5
graham crackers	1 items	58	1.1	10.4	1.3
mixed grain	1 slice	51	1.9	9.3	0.7
pancakes	1 4″ diameter	52	1.8	6.4	2.15
pita, whole wheat	½ item	69	3	12	1
pumpernickel	1 slice	83	2.9	17	0.4
rolls, dinner	1 item	113	3.1	20.1	2.2
rolls, whole wheat	1 item	96	3.5	18.3	1
rye	1 slice	59	2.1	12	0.3
whole wheat	1 slice	60	2.4	11	0.7
whole wheat muffins	1 small	110	4	20.9	1.1

Cereal

bran flakes	½ cup	89	2.65	18.65	0.4
corn grits	½ cup	72	1.75	15.7	0.25
corn puffs	¾ cup	55	1.25	11.7	0.35
cream of rice	½ cup	61	1	14.2	0
cream of wheat	½ cup	65	1.9	13.85	0.25
granola	⅛ cup	65	1.4	9.4	2.45
Grapenuts	¼ cup	107	3.3	23.2	0.1
oat flakes	½ cup	54	2.65	10.25	0.2
oat puffs	¾ cup	55	1.25	11.7	0.35
oatmeal	½ cup	73	3	12.6	1.2
rice, puffed	1 cup	55	0.9	12.6	0.1
wheat flakes	½ cup	62	3.3	26	0.7
wheat, puffed	1 cup	50	2.0	11	0.1
wheat, shredded	1 lg. biscuit	88	2.6	18.8	0.3
wheat, toasted germ	⅛ cup	58	4.1	7	1.5

Bread Alternatives

macaroni	½ cup	79	2.4	16.1	0.5
pasta	1 ounce (uncooked)	100	5	19.5	0.25
rice cakes	2 items	70	1.4	16	0.1
spaghetti	½ cup	77	2.4	16.1	0.3
tortilla, corn	1 6" diameter	65	1.5	13.5	0.6
tortilla, flour	1 7" diameter	80	2	14	2
tortilla, flour, burrito-size	½ item	110	2.5	13.5	2.5
whole wheat crackers	1 ounce	100	4	17	2

Grains

bulgur wheat	½ cup	76	2.8	16.9	0.2
couscous	½ cup	101	3.4	20.8	0.1
rice, brown	⅓ cup	77	1.64	16.8	0.4
rice, white	⅓ cup	77	1.46	17.4	0.17
rice, wild	⅓ cup	66	2.5	13.4	0.28
Average for Entire Bread Category		74	2.8 g	14 g	0.8 g
			15%	76%	9%

Meat Category

All measurements are based on COOKED meats.

Food	One Unit Exchange =	Cals	Pro (g)	Carb (g)	Fat (g)
Red Meat					
flank steak	I ounce	57	7.7	0	2.9
ground beef	I ounce	71	6.9	0	4.6
round steak	I ounce	47	8.2	0	1.3
sirloin	I ounce	54	8.6	0	1.9
tenderloin	I ounce	58	8	0	2.7
venison	I ounce	34	5.9	0	1.1
Eggs					
dried egg	2 tablespoons	58	4.58	0.48	4.18
egg substitute/replacement	½ cup	50	10	2	0.1
egg white	3 items	45	10.05	1.23	0
whole egg	I item	77	6.07	0.6	5.58
Fish					
bass	2 ounces	45	10	0	0.6
bluefish	2 ounces	66	11.2	0	2.4
catfish	2 ounces	62	10.2	0	2.4
clams	4 large	48	10.2	0	0.76
cod	2 ounces	43	10	0	0.38
crab	2 ounces	45	10.4	0	0.34
flatfish (sole, flounder)	2 ounces	48	10.6	0	0.6
haddock	2 ounces	45	10.8	0	0.2
halibut	2 ounces	80	15.1	0	1.65
lobster	2 ounces	48	10.6	0.28	0.5
mackerel	I ounce	59	5.9	0	3.9
oysters	6 medium	45	5.9	3.2	0.92
orange roughy	2 ounces	65	11.2	0	2.2
perch	2 ounces	50	10.4	0	0.92
pollack	2 ounces	49	11	0	0.54
salmon	I ounce	38	5.6	0	1.7
sardines, in water	I ounce	77	5.7	0	6
scallops	2 ounces	46	9.4	1.2	0.42
sea bass	2 ounces	71	13.4	0	1.45
shark	2 ounces	69	11.8	0	2.4
shrimp	2 ounces	56	11.4	0.5	0.98
snails	2 ounces	72	13.2	4.4	0.22

snapper	2 ounces	53	11.6	0	0.76
swordfish	2 ounces	65	11.2	0	2.2
trout	2 ounces	81	11.8	0	3.7
tuna, canned in water	2 ounces	60	14	0	0.5
tuna, fresh	2 ounces	76	16.7	0	0.7
whitefish	2 ounces	71	10.6	0	3.2
Poultry					
chicken, dark w/out skin	1 ounce	58	7.8	0	2.8
chicken, light w/out skin	1 ounce	49	8.8	0	1.3
quail	1 ounce	53	5.6	0	3.4
turkey, canned, boned	1 ounce	44	6.7	0	1.9
turkey, dark	1 ounce	53	8.1	0	2.1
turkey, light	1 ounce	45	8.5	0	0.9
Vegetarian Meat					
egg substitute/replacement	½ cup	50	10	2	0.1
soy burgers	½ item	40	6.5	4	0
soy deli meal substitute	2 slices	40	7	3	0
soy protein powder	1 scoop	55	11.5	2	0.5
soybean curd (tofu)	3½ ounces	79	7.8	2.4	4.2
soybean milk	1 cup	81	7.7	5	3.4
soybeans (green/immature)	¼ cup	64	5.6	5	2.9
tofu, firm	2 ounces	67	9.3	3.3	2.7
whey protein shake	1 scoop	80	18	2	0
Nuts					
any nuts (almonds, pistachios, cashews, sunflower seeds, walnuts, soy nuts, etc.)	⅛ cup	107	3.6	2.97	8.95
avocado	⅓ item	113	1.3	4.9	10.2
olives	20 large	100	1	4	8.9
peanut butter (or other nut butter)	1 tablespoon	90	3.4	3.6	7.1
Average for Entire Meat Category		60	9 g	1.02 g	2.23 g
			60%	7%	33%

*Nut subcategory is ONLY to be used for Meat/1 snacks (sometimes Meat/2 for higher level meal plans).

Appendix C
Turn Up the Heat Free Foods List

There's no need to eat bland or boring foods. Use any of these free foods or other flavor enhancers that have minimal added sugar and are low fat, low sodium and low calorie.

Condiments: Up to 3 Tablespoons Daily

ketchup

BBQ sauce

yellow or Dijon mustard (avoid honey mustard varieties)

nonfat sour cream

soy sauce or tamari (low sodium)

miso

teriyaki sauce (low sodium)

pickles (one whole or relish)

Worcestershire sauce

Nonfat Mayonnaise: Up to 1 Teaspoon Daily

You can make tartar sauce with mustard and nonfat mayo.

Nonfat Salad Dressings: Up to 3 Tablespoons Daily

Try to find dressings that have fewer than 16 calories per serving.

Butter Substitutes: Up to 1 Tablespoon Daily

cooking sprays included

Sauces, Broths, Juices: 1/3 Cup Daily

salsa

tomato/marinara (any oil-free variety)

fat-free chicken broth

vegetable juice

tomato juice

Dry Seasonings, Spices, and Fresh Herbs: Unlimited Amounts

any low-sodium variety

garlic

chives

Miscellaneous Flavor Enhancers: Unlimited Amounts

lemon juice

lime juice

vinegar

balsamic vinegar

fat-free vegetable broth

horseradish

watercress

radish

vanilla extract

other extracts (orange, almond, etc.)

orange or lemon zest

Jams and Jellies: Up to 2 Tablespoons Daily

choose all fruit or lite varieties

Syrups: Up to 2 Tablespoons Daily

choose lite varieties

Milk: Up to 1 Cup Daily

skim or nonfat milk for coffee, recipes, or cereal

soymilk

Artificial Sweeteners: Use Sparingly

Equal

Twin

Sweet'N Low

Alcohol: Occasionally, in Small Portions

choose vodka, or red or white wine

Glossary

Active Basal Metabolic Rate (ABMR) The number of daily calories your body needs to support its metabolic functions and activities, such as walking, shopping, and exercising.

arteriosclerosis Diseases related to the buildup of plaque in your circulatory system or the degeneration of your arteries.

atherosclerosis One form of arteriosclerosis (see above).

body composition The ratio of fat to lean muscle in the body.

cardiovascular exercise Exercises such as walking, jogging, and bicycling that strengthen your heart and lungs, reduce stress, elevate your HDLs, reduce your LDLs, and promote longevity.

calorie A heat-energy unit.

carbohydrate-efficient metabolism A metabolic type that most efficiently utilizes carbohydrates, requiring a food program composed of 12 percent fat, 20 percent protein, 68 percent carbohydrate.

CHD Risk factors that could cause coronary heart disease such as hypertension, smoking, HDLs ("good" cholesterol) below 35, diabetes, severe obesity, and history of stroke.

cholesterol A type of fat found in animal foods and an essential component of the structural membranes of all cells.

dual metabolism A metabolic type that efficiently utilizes all three nutrients and therefore requires a food program composed of 33.3 percent fat, 33.3 percent protein, 33.3 percent carbohydrate.

fat-and-protein-efficient metabolism A metabolic type that most efficiently utilizes fats and proteins, requiring a food program composed of 25 percent fats, 50 percent protein, 25 percent carbohydrate.

glucose A form of blood sugar used as an energy source, created when the body processes carbohydrates.

HDL (high-density lipid proteins) The "good," or protective, cholesterol that dissolves the plaque laid down in your blood vessels by the LDLs (see low-density lipid proteins).

hyperplasia The process by which fat cells divide to form new ones when they reach their storage capacity.

internal metabolic thermostats Metabolic efficiency is governed by three internal thermostats: (1) the metabolic thermostat, which uses calories as heat-energy units; (2) the hydration thermostat, which uses water to create a consistent temperature pattern internally; and (3) the insulatory thermostat, which stores fat below the skin to maintain temperature.

LDL (low-density lipid proteins) The "bad" type of cholesterol that collects in your blood vessels as plaque and clogs them if too much of it is present in your bloodstream, or if there is not a sufficient amount of HDL to counteract it.

metabolism The sum total of all the physical and chemical changes that take place within the body, including the transformation of food into energy, the formation of hormones and enzymes, the growth of bone and muscle tissue, and the destruction of body tissue.

metabolic temperature On a scale of 0 to 150, the efficiency of your metabolism, as determined by the ratio between daily caloric intake and ABMR. Unless you are someone like a bodybuilder, who carries an unusually large amount of lean muscle on your frame, your ideal metabolic temperature would be 100 degrees (representing 100 percent efficiency).

Resting Basal Metabolic Rate (RBMR) The number of calories your body needs to complete all of its complex functions, such as digestion, breathing, and the circulation of your blood each day.

target heart rate The heart rate zone at which you are maintaining an aerobic intensity appropriate for consistently using fat as an energy source during exercise.

total cholesterol Found only in animal-derived foods, cholesterol is an essential component of the structural membranes of all cells. Mathematically, it is your HDL plus your LDL plus your triglycerides divided by five.

triglyceride A type of fat that is the major storage form of energy in the body. The liver synthesizes carbohydrates and stores them as triglyeride fat. Elevated triglyceride levels can be a precursor to diabetes and/or sugar sensitivities.

Index